T0233254

50 Big Debates
in Gynecologic Oncology

50 Big Debates in Gynecologic Oncology

Edited by

Dennis S. Chi
Memorial Sloan-Kettering Cancer Center, New York, NY

Nisha Lakhi
Richmond University Medical Center, Staten Island, NY

Nicoletta Colombo
University of Milan-Bicocca

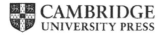
CAMBRIDGE
UNIVERSITY PRESS

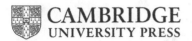

Shaftesbury Road, Cambridge CB2 8EA, United Kingdom

One Liberty Plaza, 20th Floor, New York, NY 10006, USA

477 Williamstown Road, Port Melbourne, VIC 3207, Australia

314–321, 3rd Floor, Plot 3, Splendor Forum, Jasola District Centre, New Delhi – 110025, India

103 Penang Road, #05–06/07, Visioncrest Commercial, Singapore 238467

Cambridge University Press is part of Cambridge University Press & Assessment,
a department of the University of Cambridge.

We share the University's mission to contribute to society through the pursuit of
education, learning and research at the highest international levels of excellence.

www.cambridge.org
Information on this title: www.cambridge.org/9781108940801

DOI: 10.1017/9781108935579

First published 2023

A catalogue record for this publication is available from the British Library.

A Cataloging-in-Publication data record for this book is available from the Library of Congress

ISBN 978-1-108-94080-1 Paperback

Cambridge University Press & Assessment has no responsibility for the persistence
or accuracy of URLs for external or third-party internet websites referred to in this
publication and does not guarantee that any content on such websites is, or will
remain, accurate or appropriate.

....

Every effort has been made in preparing this book to provide accurate and up-to-date information
that is in accord with accepted standards and practice at the time of publication. Although case
histories are drawn from actual cases, every effort has been made to disguise the identities of the
individuals involved. Nevertheless, the authors, editors, and publishers can make no warranties that
the information contained herein is totally free from error, not least because clinical standards are
constantly changing through research and regulation. The authors, editors, and publishers therefore
disclaim all liability for direct or consequential damages resulting from the use of material contained
in this book. Readers are strongly advised to pay careful attention to information provided by the
manufacturer of any drugs or equipment that they plan to use.

Contents

Section IV: Endometrial Cancer

Section V: Cervical Cancer

Section VI: Vaginal and Vulvar Cancer

Contributors

Giovanni Damiano Aletti
Division of Gynecologic Oncology, IEO, European Institute of Oncology IRCCS, Milan, Italy – Department of Oncology and Hemato-Oncology, University of Milan, Milan, Italy

Alessia Aloisi
Division of Gynecologic Oncology, IEO, European Institute of Oncology IRCCS, Milan, Italy

Duaa H. Al-Rawi
Department of Medicine, MemorialSloan Kettering Cancer Center, New York, NY, USA

Shannon D. Armbruster
Division of Gynecologic Oncology, Department of Obstetrics and Gynecology Virginia Tech Carilion School of Medicine, VA, USA

S. Lot Aronson
Department of Gynecologic Oncology., Netherlands Cancer Institute, Amsterdam

Daniele Xavier Assad
Hospital Sírio-Libanês, Brasília-DF, Brazil

Ibraheem O. Awowole
Department of Obstetrics, Gynaecology and Perinatology, Obafemi Awolowo University, Osun State, Nigeria.

Chris Awtrey
Intermountain Health Peaks Region Medical Group, Denver, CO, USA

Olusegun O. Badejoko
Department of Obstetrics, Gynaecology and Perinatology, Obafemi Awolowo University, Osun State, Nigeria

Jamie N. Bakkum-Gamez
Division of Gynecologic Oncology Surgery, Mayo Clinic, Rochester, MN, USA

Janos Balega
Pan-Birmingham Gynaecological Cancer Centre, Birmingham, UK

Susana Banerjee
The Royal Marsden NHS Foundation Trust and Institute of Cancer Research, London, UK

Joyce N. Barlin
Women's Cancer Care Associates, Albany, NY and Albany Medical Center, Albany, NY, USA

Sabrina Marie Bedell
Department of Obstetrics and Gynecology, Cleveland Clinic, Cleveland, OH, USA

Alice Bergamini
Department of Obstetrics and Gynecology, IRCCS San Raffaele and Vita-Salute San Raffaele University, Milan, Italy

Ilaria Betella
Division of Gynecologic Oncology, IEO, European Institute of Oncology IRCCS, Milan, Italy

Félix Blanc-Durand
Medical Department, Gustave-Roussy Cancer Center, Villejuif, France

Luca Bocciolone
Department of Obstetrics and Gynecology, IRCCS San Raffaele and Vita-Salute San Raffaele University, Milan, Italy

Thomas Boerner
Gynecology Service, Department of

Surgery, Memorial Sloan Kettering Cancer Center, New York, NY, USA

Stefano Bogliolo
Department of Gynecology Oncology, European Institute of Oncology-Milan, Italy

Stephanie M. de Boer
Department of Radiation Oncology, Leiden University Medical Center, Leiden, Netherlands

Mareike Bommert
Department of Gynecology and Gynecologic Oncology; Evangelische Kliniken Essen-Mitte, Evangelische Huyssens-Stiftung Essen-Huttrop, Germany

Sara Bouberhan
Department of Hematology/Medical Oncology, Massachusetts General Hospital, Boston, MA, USA

Donal J. Brennan
UCD Gynaecological Oncology Group, UCD School of Medicine, Catherine McAuley Research Centre, Mater Misericordiae University Hospital, Dublin, Ireland

Robert E Bristow
Department of Obstetrics & Gynecology, University of California, Irvine, CA, USA

Kristina Butler
Department of Medical and Surgical Gynecology, Mayo Clinic, Phoenix, Arizona, USA

Karen Cadoo
St James's Hospital, Trinity College Dublin, Trinity St. James's Cancer Institute Dublin, Ireland

David F. Cantú de León
Ginecología Oncológica, Dirección de Investigación, Instituto Nacional de Cancerología, Mexico

Laura M. Chambers
Division of Gynecologic Oncology; Obstetrics, Gynecology and Women's Health Institute, Cleveland Clinic, Cleveland, OH, USA

John K. Chan
Director of Gynecologic Oncology, California Pacific; Palo Alto Medical Foundation; and Sutter Research Institute, San Francisco, CA, USA

Cyrus Chargari
Unit INSERM 10–30, and Department of Radiation Therapy, Gustave Roussy Cancer Campus, Villejuif, France

Anca Chelariu-Raicu
Department of Obstetrics and Gynecology, University Hospital, LMU Munich, Germany

Dennis Chi
Gynecology Service, Department of Surgery, Memorial Sloan Kettering Cancer Center, New York, NY, USA and Weill Cornell Medical College, New York, NY, USA

Luis Chiva
Director of Department of Obstetrics and Gynecology, Clinica Universidad de Navarra. Spain

Supriya Chopra
Advanced Centre for Treatment, Research and Education in Cancer, Tata Memorial Centre and Homi Bhabha National Institute, Mumbai, India

William A. Cliby
Professor Obstetrics and Gynecology, *Virgil S. Counseller M.D. Professor of Surgery*, Mayo Clinic, Rochester, MN, USA

Robert L. Coleman
Sarah Cannon Research Institute (SCRI), Nashville, TN, USA

Nicoletta Colombo
IRCCS European Institute of Oncology
(IEO), University of Milan-Bicocca, 20126
Milan, Italy.

Fernando Cotait Maluf
Hospital Israelita Albert Einstein, São
Paulo, Brazil and Beneficência Portuguesa
de São Paulo, Brazil

Allan Covens
Division of Gynecologic Oncology, Odette
Cancer Centre, Sunnybrook, Health
Sciences Centre, Toronto, Ontario,
Canada

Michelle Davis
Dana Farber Cancer Institute and Brigham
and Women's Hospital, Division of
Gynecologic Oncology, Boston, MA,
USA

Robert Debernardo
Division of Gynecologic Oncology;
Obstetrics, Gynecology and Women's
Health Institute, Cleveland Clinic,
Cleveland, OH, USA

Marcela G. del Carmen
Division of Gynecologic Oncology,
Massachusetts General Hospital, Harvard
Medical School, Boston, MA, USA

Alexandra Diggs
Department of Obstetrics and Gynecology,
College of Physicians and Surgeons,
Columbia University, NY, USA

Nasuh Utku Dogan
Akdeniz University Faculty of Medicine,
Department of Gynecology, Antalya, Turkey

Selen Dogan
Akdeniz University Faculty of Medicine,
Department of Gynecology, Antalya, Turkey

Sean C. Dowdy
Division of Gynecologic Oncology, Mayo
Clinic, Rochester, MN, USA

Paul Downey
Department of Pathology, National
Maternity Hospital, Dublin

Willemien J. van Driel
Department of Gynecologic Oncology.,
Netherlands Cancer Institute, Amsterdam

Andreas du Bois
Department of Gynecology and Gynecologic
Oncology, Evangelische Kliniken
Essen-Mitte, Evangelische Huyssens-
Stiftung Essen-Huttrop, Germany

Eseohi Ehimiaghe
Northwestern University, Evanston, IL,
USA

Sarah Ehmann
Department of Gynecology and
Gynecologic Oncology; Evangelische
Kliniken Essen-Mitte, Evangelische
Huyssens-Stiftung Essen-Huttrop,
Germany and Gynecology Service,
Department of Surgery, Memorial
Sloan-Kettering Cancer Center,
NY, USA

Britt K Erickson
Division of Gynecologic Oncology,
Department of Obstetrics, Gynecology and
Women's Health, University of Minnesota,
Minneapolis, MN USA

Kevin Espino
New York University Langone Health,
Department of Obstetrics and Gynecology,
Division of Gynecologic Oncology, New
York, NY, United States

Amanda N. Fader
The Kelly Gynecologic Oncology Service,
Department of Gynecology and Obstetrics,
Johns Hopkins University School of
Medicine, Baltimore, MD, USA

Lorena Fariñas-Madrid
Gynaecologic Cancer Programme. Vall
d'Hebron Institute of Oncology (VHIO),

Hospital Universitari Vall d'Hebron, Vall d'Hebron Barcelona Hospital Campus, Barcelona, Spain

Olga T. Filippova
Gynecology Service, Department of Surgery, Memorial Sloan Kettering Cancer Center, NY, USA

Gini F. Fleming
University of Chicago Medical Center, Chicago, IL, USA

Daniel Flores Alatriste
Servicio de Oncología Ginecológica. Hospital Militar de Especialidades de la Mujer y Neonatología. Ciudad de México.

Jean Sebastien Frenel
ICO Saint-Herblain, Boulevard Jacques Monod, 44805 Saint-Herblain, France

Michael L. Friedlander
School of Clinical Medicine, University of New South Wales and Gynaecologic Cancer Centre, Royal Hospital for Women, Sydney, Australia

Claire Friedman
Memorial Sloan Kettering Cancer Center and Weill Cornell Medical College, New York, NY, USA

Melissa K. Frey
Division of Gynecologic Oncology, Department of Obstetrics and Gynecology, Weill Cornell Medicine, NY NY USA

Michael Frumovitz
Department of Gynecologic Oncology and Reproductive Medicine, MD Anderson Cancer Center, Houston, TX, USA

Annalisa Garbi
Division of Gynecologic Oncology, IEO, European Institute of Oncology IRCCS, Milan, Italy

Ginger J. Gardner
Memorial Sloan Kettering Cancer Center, NY, USA

John P. Geisler
Specialty Cancer Care, MG Wellness, Columbus, GA, USA

Melissa A. Geller
University of Minnesota, Division of Gynecologic Oncology, Department of Obstetrics Gynecology and Women's Health, Minneapolis, MN. USA

David M. Gershenson
Department of Gynecologic Oncology and Reproductive Medicine, The University of Texas MD Anderson Cancer Center, Houston, TX, USA

Lilian T. Gien
Division of Gynecologic Oncology, Odette Cancer Centre, Sunnybrook Health Sciences Centre, Toronto, Ontario, Canada

Antonio González-Martín
Department of Medical Oncology and Program in Solid Tumors (Cima), Cancer Center Clínica Universidad de Navarra (CCUN), Madrid and Pamplona, Spain.

Sebastien Gouy
Department of Gynecologic Surgery, Gustave Roussy Cancer Campus, Villejuif, France

Francisco Grau
Gynaecologic Cancer Programme.Vall d'Hebron Institute of Oncology (VHIO), Hospital Universitari Vall d'Hebron, Vall d'Hebron Barcelona Hospital Campus, Barcelona, Spain

Rachel N. Grisham
Department of Medicine, Memorial Sloan Kettering Cancer Center and Weill Cornell Medical College, New York, NY, USA

Whitfield B. Growdon
Massachusetts General Hospital, Boston, MA, USA

Dr. Sudeep Gupta
Advanced Centre for Treatment, Research
and Education in Cancer; Tata Memorial
Centre and Homi Bhabha National
Institute, Mumbai, India

Philipp Harter
Department of Gynecology & Gynecologic
Oncology, Ev. Kliniken Essen-Mitte, Essen,
Germany

Laura J. Havrilesky
Division of Gynecology Oncology,
Department of Obstetrics and Gynecology,
Duke Cancer Institute, Duke University
Medical Center, Durham, NC, USA

Thomas J. Herzog
University of Cincinnati Division of
Gynecology Oncology and University of
Cincinnati Cancer Center, Cincinnati,
OH, USA

Claire V. Hoppenot
Department of Obstetrics and Gynecology,
Section of Gynecologic Oncology, Baylor
College of Medicine, Houston, TX, USA

Frederick M. Howard
University of Chicago Medical Center,
Chicago, IL, USA

Haesen Jolien
Division of Gynecologic Oncology,
Department of Gynaecology and
Obstetrics, Leuven Cancer Institute,
University Hospitals Leuven, Leuven,
Belgium

Ryan M. Kahn
Memorial Sloan Kettering Cancer Center,
Department of Surgery, New York,
USA

Daniel S. Kapp
Department of Radiation Oncology,
Stanford University School of Medicine,
Stanford, CA, USA

Payam Katebi Kashi
The Kelly Gynecologic Oncology
Service, Department of Gynecology and
Obstetrics, Johns Hopkins University
School of Medicine, Baltimore,
MD, USA

Sean Kehoe
Oxford Gynaecological Cancer Centre,
Churchill Hospital, Oxford, UK

Wui-Jin Koh
National Comprehensive Cancer Network,
Plymouth Meeting, PA, USA

Amanika Kumar
Department of Obstetrics and Gynecology,
Division of Gynecologic Surgery, Mayo
Clinic, Rochester, MN, USA.

Chrisann Kyi
Department of Medicine, Memorial Sloan
Kettering Cancer Center, New York, NY and
Department of Medicine, Weill-Cornell
Medical College, New York, NY,
USA

Nisha Lakhi
Department of Obstetrics and Gynecology,
New York Medical College School of
Medicine, Valhalla, NY, USA and
Department of Gynecologic Oncology,
Richmond Univesrity Medical Center,
Staten Island, NY, USA

Brooke M. Lamparello
Albany Medical Center, Albany,
NY, USA

Olivia Lara
Division of Gynecologic Oncology,
University of North Carolina, Chapel Hill,
NC, USA

Olivia Le Saux
Medical Oncology Department, Centre
Léon Bérard, University Claude Bernard,
Lyon, France

Jonathan A. Ledermann
Department of Oncology, UCL Cancer
Institute, University College
London, UK

Alvin Jun Xing Lee
Department of Oncology, UCL Cancer
Institute, University College London, UK

Mario M. Leitao, Jr
Gynecology Service, Department of
Surgery, Memorial Sloan Kettering Cancer
Center and Department of Obstetrics and
Gynecology, Weill Cornell Medical College,
New York, NY, USA

Ernst Lengyel
Department of Obstetrics and Gynecology/
Section of Gynecologic Oncology, The
University of Chicago, Chicago, IL, USA

Julianne Lima
The Royal Marsden NHS Foundation
Trust, London, UK

Chrissy Liu
SUNY Downstate Health Sciences
University, NY, US

Beverly Long
Division of Gynecologic Oncology,
Sarasota Memorial Healthcare System,
Sarasota, FL

Kara Long Roche
Gynecology Service, Department of
Surgery, Memorial Sloan Kettering Cancer
Center and Department of Obstetrics &
Gynecology, Weill Cornell Medical Center,
NY, USA

Domenica Lorusso
Catholic University of Sacred Heart and
Fondazione Policlinico Gemelli IRCCS,
Rome, Italy

Paul Magtibay
The Department of Medical and Surgical

Gynecology, Mayo Clinic, Phoenix,
AZ, USA

Javier F. Magrina
The Department of Medical and Surgical
Gynecology, Mayo Clinic, Phoenix,
AZ, USA

Amita Maheshwari
Tata Memorial Centre and Homi Bhabha
National Institute, Mumbai, India

Sven Mahner
Department of Obstetrics and Gynecology,
University Hospital, LMU Munich,
Munich, Germany

Vicky Makker
Gynecologic Medical Oncology Service,
Memorial Sloan Kettering Cancer Center,
New York, NY, USA and Department of
Medicine, Weill Cornell Medical College,
New York, NY, USA

Kelly J. Manahan
Specialty Cancer Care, MG Wellness,
Columbus, GA, USA

Gioriga Mangili
Department of Obstetrics and Gynecology,
IRCCS San Raffaele and Vita-Salute San
Raffaele University, Milan, Italy

Zibi Marchocki
Department of Obstetrics and
Gynaecology, Division of Gynaecologic
Oncology, University College Cork, Cork,
Ireland

Daniel Margul
University of Cincinnati Department of
Obstetrics and Gynecology and University
of Cincinnati Cancer Center˙ Cincinnati,
OH, USA

Andrea Mariani
Division of Gynecologic Surgery, Mayo
Clinic, Rochester, MN, USA

Daniela Matei
Diana Princess of Wales Professor in
Cancer Research, Division of Gynecology
Oncology, Department of Obstetrics and
Gynecology, Northwestern University
Feinberg School of Medicine, Chicago, Il

Ursula Matulonis
Dana Farber Cancer Institute, Boston,
MA, USA

Amandine Maulard
Surgical Department, Gustave-Roussy
Cancer Center, Villejuif, France

Joanie Mayer Hope
Founding Partner, Alaska Women's Cancer
Care and Director of Gynecologic
Oncology, Alaska Native Medical Center &
Providence Alaska Cancer Center, AK,
USA

David S. Miller
Division of Gynecologic Oncology,
Department of Obstetrics & Gynecology,
University of Texas Southwestern
Medical Center, Dallas, Texas,
U.S.A.

Kathryn Miller
Gynecology Service, Department of
Surgery, Memorial Sloan Kettering Cancer
Center, NY, USA

Arwa Mohammad
Division of Gynecologic Oncology, Mayo
Clinic, Rochester, MN,
USA

Philippe Morice
Department of Gynecologic Surgery,
Gustave Roussy Cancer Campus, Villejuif,
France; University Paris Sud, Bures-sur-
Yvette, France

Molly Morton
Obstetrics, Gynecology and Women's
Health Institute, Cleveland Clinic,
Cleveland, OH, USA

Lea A. Moukarzel
Gynecology Service, Department of
Surgery, Memorial Sloan Kettering Cancer
Center, New York, New York, USA.

Francesco Multinu
Department of Gynecology Oncology,
European Institute of Oncology, Milan, Italy

Joo-Hyun Nam
Department of Obstetrics and Gynecology,
University of Ulsan College of Medicine,
Asan Medical Center, Seoul, Republic of
Korea

Deepa Maheswari Narasimhulu
Department of Obstetrics and Gynecology,
Division of Gynecologic Oncology, Mayo
Clinic, Rochester, MN, USA

Steven A. Narod
Women's College Research Institute,
Women's College Hospital and Dalla
Lana School of Public Health,
University of Toronto, Toronto,
ON, Canada

Roni Nitecki
Gynecologic Oncology and Reproductive
Medicine, MD Anderson Cancer Center,
Houston, TX, US

Angelica Nogueira-Rodrigues
Federal University of Minas Gerais, Belo
Horizonte, Brazil

Roisin O'Cearbhaill
Gynecologic Medical Oncology Service,
Department of Medicine, Memorial Sloan
Kettering Cancer Center and Department
of Medicine, Weill Cornell Medical College,
NY, USA

Ana Oaknin
Gynaecologic Cancer Programme, Vall
d'Hebron Institute of Oncology (VHIO),
Hospital Universitari Vall d'Hebron, Vall
d'Hebron Barcelona Hospital Campus,
Barcelona, Spain

Kutluk Oktay
Department of Obstetrics, Gynecology and
Reproductive Sciences, Yale University
School of Medicine, New Haven, CT, USA
and Innovation Institute for Fertility
Preservation and IVF, New York, NY, USA

Jeong-Yeol Park
Department of Obstetrics and Gynecology,
University of Ulsan College of Medicine,
Asan Medical Center, Seoul, Republic of
Korea

Jessica E. Parker
Division of Gynecologic
Oncology, Department of Obstetrics and
Gynecology, Indiana University,
Indianapolis, IN, USA

Patricia Pautier
Medical Department, Gustave-Roussy
Cancer Center, Villejuif, France

Richard T. Penson
Massachusetts General Hospital, Boston,
MA, USA

Milagros Pérez Quintanilla
Ginecología Oncológica, Instituto Nacional
de Cancerología, Mexico

Marie Plante
Division of Gynecologic Oncology,
Department of Obstetrics and
Gynaecology, Laval University, Quebec
City, Canada

Bhavana Pothuri
Department of Obstetrics and Gynecology,
Perlmutter Cancer Center, NYU Langone
Health, NY, USA

Aaron M. Praiss
Gynecology Service, Department of
Surgery, Memorial Sloan Kettering Cancer
Center, NY, USA

Eric Pujade-Lauraine
Medical Director, ARCAGY Paris, France

Pedro T. Ramirez
Department of Obstetrics & Gynecology,
The Houston Methodist Hospital,
Houston, TX, USA

Salihi Rawand
Division of Gynecologic Oncology,
Department of Gynaecology and Obstetrics,
Leuven Cancer Institute, University
Hospitals Leuven, Leuven, Belgium

Isabelle Ray-Coquard
Medical Oncology Department, Centre Léon
Bérard, University Claude Bernard, Lyon,
France

Patricia Rivera
Department of Obstetrics and Gynecology,
Ascension Health, Racine, WI, USA

Matteo Repetto
Division of Early Drug Development for
Innovative Therapies, IEO, European
Institute of Oncology IRCCS, Milan,
Italy

Gordon J. S. Rustin
Mount Vernon Cancer Centre, Northwood,
Middlesex, UK

Dib Sassine
Gynecology Service, Department of
Surgery, Memorial Sloan Kettering Cancer
Center, NY, USA

Brooke A. Schlappe
Department of Gynecologic Oncology,
Advocate Aurora Health, Milwaukee,
WI, USA

Michael J. Seckl
Department of Medical Oncology, Charing
Cross Hospital Campus of Imperial College
London, London, UK

Angeles Alvarez Secord
Division of Gynecology Oncology,
Department of Obstetrics and
Gynecology, Duke Cancer Institute, Duke

University Medical Center, Durham, NC, USA

Karin K. Shih
Division of Gynecologic Oncology, Department of Obstetrics and Gynecology, Zucker School of Medicine at Hofstra University/Northwell Health, New Hyde Park, NY

Rachel C. Sisodia
Harvard Medical School, Massachusetts General Hospital, MA, USA

Gabe S. Sonke
Department of Medical Oncology, Netherlands Cancer Institute, Amsterdam

Yukio Sonoda
Gynecology Service, Department of Surgery, Memorial Sloan Kettering Cancer Center and Department of Obstetrics & Gynecology, Weill Cornell Medical Center, NY, USA

Richard Schwameis
Department of Gynecology & Gynecologic Oncology, Ev. Kliniken Essen-Mitte, Essen, Germany and Department of General Gynecology and Gynecologic Oncology, Gynecologic Cancer Unit, Comprehensive Cancer Center, Medical University of Vienna, 1080 Vienna, Austria.

Edward Tanner
Department of Obstetrics and Gynecology, Northwestern University, Chicago, IL, USA

Enes Taylan
Department of Obstetrics and Gynecology, Wayne State University School of Medicine, Detroit, MI, USA and Department of Obstetrics, Gynecology and Reproductive Sciences, Yale University School of Medicine, New Haven, CT, USA

Beatrice Seddon
Department of Oncology, University College

Hospital NHS Foundation Trust, London, UK

Kavita Singh
Pan-Birmingham Gynaecological Cancer Centre, Birmingham, UK

Pamela T. Soliman
Department of Gynecologic Oncology and Reproductive Medicine, MD Anderson Cancer Center, Houston, TX, USA

Krishnansu S. Tewari
Department of Obstetrics & Gynecology, University of California, Irvine, CA, USA

Lauren Thomaier Bollinger
Division of Gynecologic Oncology, University of Minnesota, Minneapolis, MN, USA

Federica Tomao
IEO, European Institute of Oncology IRCCS, Milan, Italy

Tiffany Y. Sia
Gynecology Service, Department of Surgery, Memorial Sloan Kettering Cancer Center, USA

Federica Tomao
Department of Gynecology Oncology, European Institute of Oncology-Milan, Italy

Yien Ning Sophia Wong
Department of Oncology, UCL Cancer Institute, University College London, UK

William P. Tew
Gynecologic Medical Oncology Service, Department of Medicine, Memorial Sloan Kettering Cancer Center, NY, USA

Anastasios Tranoulis
Pan-Birmingham Gynaecological Cancer Centre, Birmingham, UK

Fabian Trillsch
Department of Obstetrics and Gynecology,

University Hospital, LMU Munich,
Munich, Germany

Hélène Vanacker
Medical Oncology Department, Centre
Léon Bérard, University Claude Bernard,
Lyon, France

Fidel A. Valea
Department of Obstetrics and
Gynecology Virginia Tech Carilion School
of Medicine, VA, USA

Ignace B. Vergote
Division of Gynecologic Oncology,
Department of Gynaecology and Obstetrics,
Leuven Cancer Institute, University
Hospitals Leuven, Leuven, Belgium

Roberto Vargas
Division of Gynecologic Oncology;
Obstetrics, Gynecology and Women's
Health Institute, Cleveland Clinic,
Cleveland, OH, USA

Simrit Warring
Department of Obstetrics and
Gynecology, Division of Gynecologic
Surgery, Mayo Clinic, Rochester,
MN, USA

Jill S. Whyte
Division of Gynecologic Oncology,
Department of Obstetrics and Gynecology,
Zucker School of Medicine at Hofstra
University/Northwell Health, New Hyde
Park, NY

Michael Wilkinson
UCD Gynaecological Oncology Group,
UCD School of Medicine, Catherine
McAuley Research Centre, Mater
Misericordiae University Hospital, Dublin,
Ireland

Jason D. Wright
Columbia University College of
Physicians and Surgeons;
Herbert Irving Comprehensive Cancer

Center; and New York
Presbyterian Hospital, NY, USA

Thomas C. Wright
Columbia University, NY,
USA

Sumer K. Wallace
Division of Gynecologic Oncology,
University of Wisconsin School of
Medicine and Public Health, Madison,
WI, USA

Juliet E. Wolford
University of Cincinnati Department of
Obstetrics and Gynecology and University
of Cincinnati Cancer Center' Cincinnati,
OH, USA

S. Diane Yamada
Department of Obstetrics and
Gynecology/Section of Gynecologic
Oncology, The University of Chicago,
Chicago, IL, USA

Jason Yap
University of Birmingham and
Pan-Birmingham Gynaecological Cancer
Center, Birmingham, UK

Catheryn M. Yashar
Department of Radiation Oncology,
University of California San Diego, San
Diego, CA, USA

Benoit You
Université Lyon, Université Claude
Bernard Lyon 1, Faculté de Médecine Lyon-
Sud, EA3738 CICLY; Medical Oncology,
Institut de Cancérologie des Hospices
Civils de Lyon (IC-HCL), CITOHL,
EPSILYON, Lyon, France and GINECO,
Paris France

Camilla Yu
The Kelly Gynecologic Oncology
Service, Department of Gynecology and
Obstetrics, Johns Hopkins University
School of Medicine, Baltimore,
MD, USA

Eleonora Zaccarelli
Department of Gynecology Oncology,
European Institute of Oncology, Milan, Italy

Dmitriy Zamarin
Department of Medicine, Memorial Sloan
Kettering Cancer Center, New York, NY
and Department of Medicine, Weill-
Cornell Medical College, NY, USA

William A. Zammarrelli III
Gynecology Service, Department of Surgery,
Memorial Sloan Kettering Cancer Center,
New York, NY, USA and Weill Cornell
Medical College, New York, NY, USA

Vanna Zanagnolo
Department of Gynecology Oncology,
European Institute of Oncology, Milan,
Italy

Oliver Zivanovic
Gynecology Service, Department of
Surgery, Memorial Sloan Kettering Cancer
Center, New York, NY, USA and Weill
Cornell Medical College, New York,
NY, USA

Chrissy Liu
SUNY Downstate Health Sciences
University

1A

Should Routine Mechanical Bowel Preparation be Performed before Primary Debulking Surgery?

Yes

Lea A. Moukarzel and Oliver Zivanovic

Debate

Maximal reduction of postoperative residual disease is a well-established prognostic factor in advanced or recurrent ovarian and uterine cancer. Intestinal surgery is often required in order to achieve complete gross resection of malignant disease. Given the anatomical location of these primary tumors in the pelvis, a significant portion of these intestinal surgeries encompass rectosigmoid and ileocecal resections. One key perioperative intervention that has been employed for many years to optimize these procedures is mechanical bowel preparations (MBPs).

There are several reasons as to why mechanical bowel preparations have been used in surgeries requiring colonic or rectal resections. A clean colon can facilitate bowel manipulation, passage and firing of surgical staplers, and significantly improves visualization during intraoperative proctoscopy or colonoscopy. Additionally, MBP has also shown potential reduction in postoperative complications including surgical site infections (SSIs) and anastomotic leaks. This effect is most pronounced when used in combination with oral antibiotic bowel preparations (OABPs).

Mechanical Bowel Preparation is a Commonly Used and Safe Intervention

Regarding the safety of MBP, studies have repeatedly shown it to be a safe and feasible intervention. Some might speculate that the rate of *clostridium difficile* colitis might increase among patients undergoing bowel preparation. However, in line with multiple other studies, Kim et al. found that *C. difficile colitis* was actually less likely among those with who received bowel preparation with combination oral antibiotics and MBP as compared to those who received no bowel preparation (0.5% vs. 1.8%; p=0.01) [1].

Mechanical Bowel Preparation Decreases Postoperative Complications, Specifically Surgical Site Infection

The impact of MBP on reducing surgical morbidity, primarily surgical site infections, remains the most debated aspect of bowel preparation. Colon and rectal surgery are among the most significant surgeries associated with SSIs and therefore any intervention that could decrease this morbidity rate is of critical value. Based on a recent review of the literature, the American Society of Colon and Rectal Surgeons recently released recommendations supporting the use of combined MBP with OABP in elective colorectal resections [2]. This recommendation was assigned a level 1B grade as a strong recommendation that can apply to most patients in most circumstances without reservation based on moderate-quality evidence.

Two randomized control trials formed the foundation for this recommendation where the use of combined MBP and oral antibiotics was associated with a significant decrease in SSI rates [3,4]. This includes the study by Nichols et al., which reported a marked reduction in SSI with the combination of MBP with OABP as compared to MBP alone. Clark et al. performed a similar study where the combination therapy demonstrated a reduction in postoperative complications including not only SSI, but also anastomotic leaks. Multiple studies have subsequently reproduced these findings.

More recently, Morris et al. performed propensity matching on 8,415 patients having undergone colorectal surgery through the National Surgical Quality Improvement Program (NSQIP) database [5]. They found on multivariate analysis that the use of OABP was protective against SSI (OR=0.46, 95% CI: 0.63–0.58) as compared to no bowel preparation. Importantly, among these patients, 92% had also received a MBP. A protective effect against SSI was also present with the use of MBP alone (OR=0.85, 95% CI: 0.72–0.99). In addition to the reduction in SSI, both OABP and MBP alone were associated with a decrease in readmission as compared to no preparation. Importantly, there was also a significant reduction in frequency of anastomotic leaks, postoperative ileus, return to the operating room, acute renal injury, and sepsis among patients that received MBP with or without OABP as compared to those that did not receive any form of bowel preparation.

These findings led to several studies in the colorectal literature that have demonstrated a reduction in SSIs after introduction of SSI bundles that included MBP along with OABP. More recently, there has been similar studies performed in the gynecologic oncology literature with comparable results. This includes a study by Schiavone et al. which reported a significant decrease in the incidence of SSI from 37% to 12% (p<0.001) after the implementation of a SSI reduction bundle that included the use of preoperative OABP with almost routine use of MBP [6].

Mechanical Bowel Preparation Improves Visualization during Intraoperative Proctoscopy or Colonoscopy

Surgical interventions are continuously advancing in order to improve postoperative morbidity and mortality from debulking surgery. One such morbidity is anastomotic leaks after colorectal resection. Proctoscopy is increasingly being used to visualize the anastomosis and aid in assessing its integrity. More recently data has suggested that the addition of near-infrared (NIR) angiography via proctoscopy might reduce anatomic leak rates and is associated with fewer postoperative abscesses and diverting ostomies after rectosigmoid resection performed during surgeries for gynecologic malignancies [7]. In order to use proctoscopy with or without NIR angiography, optimization of visual assessment is paramount. The use of MBPs would assist in insuring adequate visualization of the anastomosis via proctoscopy.

Conclusions

Based on the emergence of data supporting the use of combination bowel prep, four large societies currently recommend the use of combination bowel preparation. These include the American Society of Colon and Rectal Surgeons, the Society of American Gastrointestinal and Endoscopic Surgeons, the American Society for Enhanced Recovery, and the Perioperative Quality Initiative. In addition, the American Society of Colon and Rectal Surgeons specifically states that OABP alone, without mechanical preparation, is generally not recommended. This is largely based on the lack of any randomized trials evaluating the use of oral antibiotics without concurrent MBP. These recommendations in combination with the literature support the standard use of OABP with MBP among patients at risk of requiring colonic resection, such as in the setting of primary debulking surgery for gynecologic malignancy. The benefit of MBP appears to be synergistic with the use of OABP and therefore we recommend it always be used in combination, while the use of MBP alone should fall out of practice.

References

1. Kim EK, et al. A statewide colectomy experience: the role of full bowel preparation in preventing surgical site infection. *Ann Surg* 2014;259(2):310–314.

2. Migaly J, et al. The American Society of Colon and Rectal Surgeons Clinical Practice Guidelines for the Use of Bowel Preparation in Elective Colon and Rectal Surgery. *DC&R* 2019;62(1):3–8.

3. Clarke JS, et al. Preoperative oral antibiotics reduce septic complications of colon operations: results of prospective, randomized, double-blind clinical study. *Ann Surg* 1977;186(3):251–259.

4. Nichols RL, et al. Effect of preoperative neomycin-erythromycin intestinal preparation on the incidence of infectious complications following colon surgery. *Ann Surg* 1973;178(4):453–462.

5. Morris MS, et al. Oral antibiotic bowel preparation significantly reduces surgical site infection rates and readmission rates in elective colorectal surgery. *Ann Surg* 2015;261(6):1034–1040.

6. Schiavone MB, et al. Surgical site infection reduction bundle in patients with gynecologic cancer undergoing colon surgery. *Gynecol Oncol* 2017;147(1):115–119.

7. Moukarzel LA, et al. The impact of near-infrared angiography and proctoscopy after rectosigmoid resection and anastomosis performed during surgeries for gynecologic malignancies. *Gynecol Oncol* 2020;158(2):397–401.

Should Routine Mechanical Bowel Preparation be Performed before Primary Debulking Surgery?

No

Shannon D. Armbruster and Fidel A. Valea

Debate

Since the early 1970s, surgeons have debated the value of preoperative mechanical bowel preparation (MBP) for patients undergoing bowel surgery. Proponents claim that MBP decreases rates of surgical site infections and anastomotic leaks; however, current literature does not support these assertions. In fact, negative impacts of MBP including patient discomfort, dehydration, and electrolyte abnormalities have been reported. For gynecologic oncologists, this debate rages on, as gynecologic oncology-based evidence is limited. Nevertheless, the debate can be settled upon review of the colorectal literature, as suggested by the Enhanced Recovery After Surgery (ERAS) Society Gynecologic Oncology guidelines published in 2019 [1].

The most recent Cochrane Review, published in 2011, included 4595 patients who underwent elective colorectal surgery with (n=2305) and without (n=2290) preoperative MBP. When comparing those patients receiving MBP to those who did not, no differences were observed in rates of anastomotic leak for low anterior resections (8.8% vs. 10.3%, OR=0.88, 95% CI: 0.55, 1.4), anastomotic leak for colon surgery (3.0% vs. 3.5%, OR=0.85, 95%CI: 0.58, 1.26), and overall anastomotic leakage (4.4% vs. 4.5%, OR=0.99, 95% CI: 0.74, 1.31). Furthermore, no differences were seen in the secondary outcomes of mortality (1.6% vs. 1.8%, OR=0.93, 95% CI: 0.58, 1.47), peritonitis (2.2% vs. 3.0%, OR=0.74, 95% CI: 0.5, 1.08), wound infection (9.6% vs. 8.5%, OR=1.16, 95% CI: 0.95, 1.42), reoperation (6.1% vs. 5.8%, OR=1.06, 95% CI: 0.83, 1.37), infectious extra-abdominal complication (11.4% vs. 11.1%, OR=1.05, 95% CI: 0.85, 1.3), or non-infectious extra-abdominal complications (6.4% vs. 6.6%, OR=0.98, 95% CI: 0.71, 1.36) [2]. These data were confirmed in a National Surgery Quality Improvement Program (NSQIP) database review including patients undergoing elective colorectal surgery with (n=11,836) and without (n=8640) MBP. No differences were observed in rates of any surgical site infection (OR= 0.92, 95% CI: 0.84, 1.02), anastomotic leak (OR=0.91, 95% CI 0.77, 1.08), return to the operating room (OR=1.03, 95% CI: 0.88, 1.21), readmission (OR=0.98, 95% CI: 0.89, 1.08), or death (OR=0.77, 95% CI: 0.57, 1.05). Furthermore, patient organ-related outcomes were similar, including cardiac complications (OR=0.83, 95% CI: 0.59, 1.18), renal complications (OR=0.92; 95% CI: 0.65, 1.31), or postoperative ileus (OR=1.04, 95% CI: 0.95, 1.18) [3]. Given these findings, the American Society of Colon and Rectal Surgery does not recommend MBP alone for patients undergoing elective colorectal surgery, a recommendation supported by strong evidence [4].

Colorectal surgery results and national guidelines influence gynecology and gynecologic oncology-specific MBP recommendations. In 2018, a surgical technical evidence review by the Agency for Healthcare Research and Quality Safety Program for Improving Surgical Care and Recovery noted a paucity of gynecology-driven data, and thus the need to examine data from the colorectal surgery population. In this review, Kalogera et al. included results from four meta-analyses demonstrating that patients receiving MBPs derived no benefit in overall mortality, surgical site infection, incidence of anastomotic leak, or reoperation compared to those not undergoing MBP. They concluded with the moderate-strength recommendation that MBP alone is discouraged, unless combined with oral antibiotics [5]. In accord, the Enhanced Recovery After Surgery (ERAS) Society guidelines for gynecologic oncology were updated in 2019 and recommended that MBP alone should not be used to decrease postoperative morbidity in laparotomy cases, and should not be used at all for minimally invasive gynecologic surgery cases [1].

Conclusion

In conclusion, the 50-year debate can be laid to rest. Strong data from the colorectal literature has led to national and international recommendations to avoid MBP alone for patients undergoing bowel surgery. The value of oral antibiotic bowel preparation versus no MBP was observed in a retrospective study, while the addition of an MBP did not add further benefit [5]. Therefore, MBP should only be considered when combined with oral antibiotic preparations.

References

1. Nelson G, et al. Guidelines for perioperative care in gynecologic/oncology: Enhanced Recovery After Surgery (ERAS) Society recommendations – 2019 update. *Int J Gynecol Cancer* 2019;29(4):651–668. https://doi.org/10.1136/ijgc-2019-000356

2. Güenaga KF, et al. Mechanical bowel preparation for elective colorectal surgery. *Cochrane Database Syst Rev* 2011;9: CD001544. https://doi.org/10.1002/14651858.CD001544.pub4

3. Koller SE, et al. Comparative effectiveness and risks of bowel preparation before elective colorectal surgery. *Ann Surg* 2018;267(4):734–742. https://doi.org/10.1097/SLA.0000000000002159

4. Migaly J, et al. The American Society of Colon and Rectal Surgeons Clinical Practice Guidelines for the Use of Bowel Preparation in Elective Colon and Rectal Surgery. *Dis Colon Rectum* 2019;62(1):3–8. https://doi.org/10.1097/dcr.0000000000001238

5. Kalogera E, et al. Surgical technical evidence review for gynecologic surgery conducted for the Agency for Healthcare Research and Quality Safety Program for Improving Surgical Care and Recovery. *Am J Obstet Gynecol* 2018;219(6):563.e561–563.e519. https://doi.org/10.1016/j.ajog.2018.07.014

Should Preoperative Carbohydrate Loading be Routine prior to Debulking Surgery?

Yes

Arwa Mohammad, Deepa Maheswari Narasimhulu, and Sean C. Dowdy

Debate

Preoperative fasting was the surgical dogma for over 100 years, but has been challenged and modified within the last few decades. An abundance of evidence supports the safety of reducing preoperative fasting to six hours for solids and two hours for clear liquids. This practice does not increase the risk of pulmonary aspiration and is supported by the American Society of Anesthesiology [1]. In fact, rather than withholding nutrition, preoperative carbohydrate loading (typically a beverage containing 50 grams of carbohydrates) has been shown to mitigate metabolic derangements related to surgical stress by converting the fasted catabolic state to a fed, anabolic state [1]. The concept of carbohydrate loading was first studied in performance athletes and was found to increase muscle glycogen stores and improve performance during endurance exercise.

The endocrine and immunologic systems demonstrate the most pronounced response to surgical stress. The magnitude of this response is proportional to surgical complexity, and is mediated by the release of catecholamines, cortisol, glucagon, growth hormone and cytokines, causing immunosuppression and insulin resistance [2]. The result is a catabolic state characterized by hyperglycemia, impaired protein metabolism, and lipolysis which may lead to muscle weakness and delayed wound healing. This catabolic state is exacerbated by preoperative fasting [1].

Carbohydrate loading improves insulin resistance and patient comfort measures such as hunger, thirst, anxiety, and nausea, with no delay in gastric emptying or change in gastric pH [1,2]. While a direct cause-and-effect relationship between carbohydrate loading and improvements in clinically significant endpoints has not been proven, reduced insulin resistance has been associated with improved bowel function and decreases in infectious morbidity [1,3]. A National Institute for Health and Care Excellence (NICE) guideline evidence review showed that compared to fasting, preoperative carbohydrate loading decreased length of stay for major abdominal surgery and orthopedic surgery, but not for minor and intermediate abdominal surgery. No differences were found for other types of surgery compared to placebo [2].

Although the quality of evidence supporting carbohydrate loading is low to moderate, there are no clear risks. Some have raised theoretical concerns about the risk of pulmonary aspiration and hyperglycemia. Gastric emptying time for a preoperative carbohydrate solution is only 90 to 120 minutes. No significant increase in preoperative gastric volumes or risk of pulmonary aspiration has been shown with carbohydrate loading [1]. However, beverages containing fat or those with high osmolality may slow gastric emptying and should not be used. Although hyperglycemia is a common event after major abdominal surgery even in nondiabetic patients, carbohydrate loading minimizes the risk of perioperative hyperglycemia by improving insulin resistance.

Most trials investigating carbohydrate loading have excluded diabetics due to concerns of delayed gastric emptying and hyperglycemia. One small trial with 35 patients demonstrated no difference in gastric emptying times [4]. The improvement in perioperative insulin sensitivity seen with carbohydrate loading should theoretically benefit noninsulin-dependent diabetic patients, but not those who are insulin dependent. A study of type 2 diabetics undergoing colorectal surgery found no relationship between preoperative carbohydrate loading and postoperative glycemic control, however, preoperative glucose levels were higher [4]. More studies are awaited to guide optimal care in diabetics, but together with concerns about delays in gastric emptying, water may be substituted for a carbohydrate drink in diabetic patients. Patients with known delayed gastric emptying may be at higher risk of aspiration with oral preoperative carbohydrate loading. Intravenous preoperative carbohydrate loading has been studied and may be an option for nondiabetics.

Apart from calories, protein is crucial for postoperative recovery as it promotes anabolism, slows muscle catabolism, and shortens the postsurgical inflammatory phase. Many practices have added nutritional supplements containing protein in the postoperative period as an element of their Enhanced Recovery After Surgery (ERAS) protocol. There has been recent interest in studying the value of adding whey protein to the preoperative carbohydrate drink. Yi et al. randomized 118 patients undergoing elective surgery for gynecological cancer to preoperative carbohydrate-only loading versus whey protein-infused carbohydrate loading. The whey protein-infused carbohydrate loading group had shorter hospital stay, lower readmission rates, less weight loss, lower C-reactive protein–albumin ratio, preserved muscle mass, and better handgrip strength when compared to the preoperative carbohydrate-only loading group. No significant differences were noted in mid-upper arm circumference and serum albumin level upon discharge [5].

Conclusion

Proven reductions in insulin resistance provide the physiologic rationale for the use of oral carbohydrate loading before surgery to attenuate surgical stress and improve healing. While evidence of clinical benefit is of low to moderate quality, preoperative carbohydrate loading is neither costly nor labor intensive, improves patient satisfaction and well-being, and should be incorporated into Enhanced Recovery After Surgery protocols given the very low risk of harm. Recognizing the high surgical complexity of cytoreductive surgery in patients with ovarian cancer and the high incidence of mild to moderate nutritional compromise, these patients may have comparatively more to gain from carbohydrate loading. ERAS® Society guidelines for gynecologic surgery provide a strong recommendation grade for ingesting a 50-gram preoperative carbohydrate drink up until two hours prior to induction of anesthesia, with the exception of patients with risk factors for delayed gastric emptying [3].

References

1. Pillinger NL, et al. Nutritional prehabilitation: physiological basis and clinical evidence. *Anaesth Intensive Care* 2018;46(5):453–462.

2. National Institute for Health and Care Excellence. Perioperative care in adults. [H] Evidence review for pre-operative fasting. NICE guideline NG180 Perioperative care. Available at: www.nice.org.uk/guidance/n g180/documents/evidence-review-7 [last accessed October 17, 2022].

3. Nelson G, et al. Guidelines for perioperative care in gynecologic/oncology: Enhanced Recovery After Surgery (ERAS) Society recommendations – 2019 update. *Int J Gynecol Cancer* 2019;29(4):651–668.

4. Cua S, et al. The effect of an enhanced recovery protocol on colorectal surgery patients with diabetes. *J Surg Res* 2021;257:153–160.

5. Yi HC, et al. Impact of enhanced recovery after surgery with preoperative whey protein-infused carbohydrate loading and postoperative early oral feeding among surgical gynecologic cancer patients: an open-labelled randomized controlled trial. *Nutrients* 2020;12(1):264.

Should Preoperative Carbohydrate Loading be Routine prior to Debulking Surgery?
No

Kathryn Miller, Dib Sassine, and Yukio Sonoda

Debate

In patients undergoing surgery, nutritional status is a key component in the body's ability to mount an appropriate metabolic response to postoperative inflammation and stress. The negative effects of long-term protein and caloric deficits on outcomes for surgical patients have been well-established in the literature and are associated with higher risk of poor wound healing, sepsis, and mortality. Frequently, the patients at highest risk of poor preoperative nutritional status are those for whom surgery cannot be avoided: oncology, geriatrics, or critical care patients.

To correct nutritional deficits for patients at high metabolic risk, studies have shown that 10–14 days of enteral or parenteral nutritional support confers some benefit. Even with these interventions, measurable change may not be induced in body composition or serum albumin concentration. Prehabilitation, a comprehensive program which combines preoperative nutritional support and exercise has been shown to decrease rates of complications in patients undergoing abdominal surgery and those with cancer, but meaningful changes may take up to four to six weeks to occur.

Of course, delaying surgery in the cancer patient to fully optimize preoperative nutritional status may not be feasible, for numerous reasons. To address nutritional status in the short term, preoperative nutritional support has been added as an element of fast-track recovery or Enhanced Recovery After Surgery (ERAS) programs now in widespread use across surgical disciplines. ERAS preoperative nutrition guidelines generally advise against prolonged periods of fasting and include recommendations for carbohydrate-rich beverages prior to surgery [1]. Typical guidelines are to consume a beverage containing roughly 100 grams of carbohydrates the night before surgery and 50 grams on the day of surgery.

The goal of preoperative carbohydrate-loading is prevention and mitigation of insulin resistance, which has been associated with immune suppression, poor wound healing, and longer hospital stays. However, the impact of its use on outcomes has not been clearly supported throughout various surgical subspecialties, and many studies have demonstrated no benefit. In cohorts of colorectal patients, carbohydrate loading decreased rates of insulin resistance but did not affect complication rates. A large randomized trial of 142 patients undergoing open colorectal or liver surgery did not demonstrate differences in early plasma glucose sensitivity or insulin resistance compared with the control group, and showed no differences in outcomes. Trials in cardiothoracic surgery similarly did not demonstrate

9

differences in insulin resistance, with one study demonstrating increased postoperative nausea and vomiting in the carbohydrate-loading group.

Several recent meta-analyses and a Cochrane Database systematic review have been performed to summarize these studies and determine the benefit of carbohydrate treatment in the preoperative setting [2–5]. One meta-analysis found that carbohydrate loading conferred a slightly shorter length of stay (LOS) compared with fasting, but showed no benefit over water or placebo [2]. The systematic review demonstrated a small reduction in LOS (between 0.04 to 0.56 days) in the carbohydrate treatment group compared with the fasting or placebo groups, but showed no effect on complication rates [4]. All meta-analyses and the systematic review concluded that the evidence from published trials is of low quality and fraught with inconsistencies, and that very few studies have demonstrated meaningful differences in clinical outcomes based on carbohydrate loading alone.

Conclusion

While it is obvious that improvement in nutritional status prior to surgery is ideal, it has been shown that weeks of nutritional support and prehabilitation are needed to truly make a difference in a patient's nutritional profile. Unfortunately, many cancer patients do not have the luxury of delaying necessary surgical interventions. For these patients, one night of carbohydrate loading is insufficient to induce meaningful metabolic change, and may be considered "too little, too late." While many components of ERAS have proven beneficial in improving patient outcomes, preoperative carbohydrate loading is unsupported by the evidence. Its use does not appear to improve outcomes in patients undergoing debulking surgery.

References

1. Nelson G, et al. Guidelines for perioperative care in gynecologic/oncology: Enhanced Recovery After Surgery (ERAS) Society recommendations – 2019 update. *Int J Gynecol Cancer* 2019;29(4):651–668.

2. Amer MA, et al. Network meta-analysis of the effect of preoperative carbohydrate loading on recovery after elective surgery. *Br J Surg* 2017;104(3):187–197.

3. Li L, et al. Preoperative carbohydrate loading for elective surgery: a systematic review and meta-analysis. *Surg Today* 2012;42(7):613–624.

4. Smith MD, et al. Preoperative carbohydrate treatment for enhancing recovery after elective surgery. *Cochrane Database Syst Rev* 2014;8:CD009161. https://doi.org/10.1002/14651858.CD009161.pub2

5. Bilku DK, et al. Role of preoperative carbohydrate loading: a systematic review. *Ann R Coll Surg Engl* 2014;96(1):15–22.

3A Should Women with BRCA Mutations be Offered Bilateral Salpingectomy with Delayed Oophorectomy for Ovarian Cancer Risk Reduction?

Yes

Thomas Boerner and Kara Long Roche

Debate

Hereditary ovarian cancer syndromes are associated with increased risk of developing pelvic high grade serous carcinomas (HGSC), with lifetime risks ranging from 10% to 58% depending on the identified mutation [1]. As the genetic landscape of ovarian cancer broadens beyond *BRCA1* and *BRCA2* with the discovery and inclusion of additional moderate penetrance genetic mutations (for example: *RAD51C*, *RAD51D*, *BRIP1*, *PALB2*), patients are significantly more likely to be identified as carrying a pathologic variant than in decades past. Patients are appropriately seeking, and being referred, for genetic assessment at earlier ages, and thus there is an increasing need for improved, patient center risk-reduction strategies.

There is no effective screening test for ovarian cancer. Risk-reducing bilateral salpingectomy (RRSO) is the current gold standard procedure for decreasing the risk of HGSC in patients at elevated genetic risk [1]. RRSO results in robust protection with a decrease in the risk of developing HGSC of up to 96% [2]. However, infertility and abrupt surgical menopause are inevitable sequelae of this procedure, resulting in significant and detrimental impacts on overall health and quality of life. Cardiovascular disease, osteoporosis, dyslipidemia, sexual dysfunction, and cognitive decline have all been shown to be associated with premature menopause. Additionally, quality of life is impacted with the onset of hot flashes, insomnia, and dyspareunia. Some of these toxicities, notably the decline in sexual function, persist despite the use of hormone replacement therapy. Recently published prospective data from GOG-199 support the validity of these concerns, as seen in the significant decline in sexual function in women who underwent RRSO [3]. These side effects are unacceptable to many and undoubtedly, there is a need to improve options for high-risk patients.

There is overwhelming evidence that the fimbriated end of the fallopian tube plays an important role in the pathogenesis of pelvic HGSC. The identification of serous tubal intraepithelial carcinomas (STIC lesions), believed to be the precursor to HGSC, as well as molecular markers and gene expression profiles support a tubal origin for the majority of HGSC. As the data continues to amass implicating the fallopian tube in this process, the concept of salpingectomy as a risk-reducing strategy has emerged. Similar to RRSO, salpingectomy can be performed via an outpatient, minimally invasive procedure and should incorporate a comprehensive evaluation of the peritoneal cavity (e.g., inspection and peritoneal washings for cytology) and a pathological assessment of the fallopian tube via Sectioning and Extensively Examining the Fimbriated End (SEE-FIM protocol). Salpingectomy performed early, with oophorectomy delayed until the guideline-based recommended age (or possibly beyond) has been proposed as an additional option for patients seeking risk-reduction and is currently under investigation. This approach allows for the preservation of endogenous hormone production and fertility potential, the opportunity for identification of early precursor lesions such as STIC lesions, and has been hypothesized to result in an increased degree of risk-reduction.

The majority of high-risk patients welcome a salpingectomy option. In a study by Gaba et al., RRESDO in a trial setting was acceptable to approximately 70% of premenopausal patients. Currently, there are four major ongoing prospective trials looking at RRESDO as compared to standard RRSO in the high-risk population. Enrolment in these trials has been steady, however the oncologic data regarding salpingectomy alone as a risk-reduction strategy is unlikely to be available for many years. Therefore, the most appropriate use of salpingectomy remains within the context of a RRESDO strategy. Patients motivated to pursue risk-reduction earlier than guideline age, who have completed childbearing or who have elected to utilize assisted reproductive techniques to allow for preimplantation genetic diagnosis, may be ideal candidates for RRESDO. Additionally, many patients who are not eligible for hormone replacement therapy due to a personal history of breast cancer, may opt for RRESDO as a way to delay oophorectomy to the latter end of guideline-based recommendations, or possibly beyond. RRESDO may also provide a more palatable option for patients who would otherwise decline RRSO due to concerns about health and quality of life. While concerns have been raised about the feasibility of this approach, and specifically the need for patients to undergo two separate surgical procedures, overall data supports its safety. Ovarian function does not appear to be compromised and moreover, the approach is cost effective when quality of life is considered [4].

Conclusion

In summary, the incorporation of RRESDO represents a valuable and compelling option for patients with an elevated risk of ovarian cancer. Shared decision making incorporating specific genetic mutation profiles, family history, desires for childbearing, eligibility for hormone replacement therapy, surgical risk, and individual preferences should guide planning for high-risk patients.

References

1. National Comprehensive Care Network. Genetic/familial high-risk assessment: breast, ovarian, and pancreatic. Version 2. 2021. Available from: www.nccn.org

2. Rebbeck TR, et al. Prophylactic oophorectomy in carriers of BRCA1 or BRCA2 mutations. *N Engl J Med* 2002;346 (21):1616–1622

3. Mai PL, et al. Prospective follow-up of quality of life for participants undergoing risk-reducing salpingo-oophorectomy or ovarian cancer screening in GOG-0199: and NRG Oncology/GOG Study. *Gynecol Oncol* 2020;156(1):131–139.

4. Long Roche KC, et al. Risk-reducing salpingectomy: let us be opportunistic. *Cancer* 2017;123(10):1714–1720.

Chapter 3B

Should Women with BRCA Mutations be Offered Bilateral Salpingectomy with Delayed Oophorectomy for Ovarian Cancer Risk Reduction?

No

Steven A. Narod

Debate

The hope that we can prevent ovarian cancer in women at high risk by removing their fallopian tubes while leaving their ovaries intact is based on the belief that many, if not most, high-grade serous ovarian cancers originate in the tubes. The current recommendation for surgical prevention is bilateral salpingo-oophorectomy (BSO). Salpingectomy alone is not yet the standard of care for women with a *BRCA1* of *BRCA2* mutation, but is being proposed widely and is offered in many centers.

Ovarian tumors have long been thought to arise from the ovarian surface epithelium or from ovarian surface inclusion cysts. Emerging data support an alternate model whereby the fallopian tubes are the site of origin for a large proportion of high-grade serous cancers [1]. Studies of occult cancers diagnosed at oophorectomy in asymptomatic mutation carriers often report finding lesions in both the tubes and the ovaries – and sometimes in the tubes alone – but rarely on one ovary alone. If the tumour is symptomatic, it is usually widespread in the pelvis. It may be that the fallopian tube is the origin and nascent cancer cells migrate outwards and are manifest later in the ovary or on the peritoneum. Pathologists have described a tubal lesion Serous Tubal Intraepithelial Carcinoma (STIC) and have proposed this to be a precursor to high-grade serous ovarian cancer. Sequencing studies of p53 and other genes have shown genetic identity between STICs and accompanying high-grade serous tumors, consistent with a shared lineage.

The lifetime risk of ovarian cancer is estimated at 45% for *BRCA1* mutation carriers and 20% for *BRCA2* mutation carriers. The majority of ovarian cancers which arise in BRCA mutation carriers are of the serous histology and are diagnosed at an advanced stage. The best preventive strategy is surgery. At present, we cannot offer chemoprevention, lifestyle change, or screening as a rational alternative. Both oral contraceptives and breastfeeding have been associated with a reduced risk of ovarian cancer in *BRCA1* and *BRCA2* carriers. We recently reported that, compared to women who never breastfed, breastfeeding for seven or more months was associated with a 32% reduction in risk [2]. The combination of breastfeeding and oral contraceptive use was strongly protective (OR=0.47). A good recommendation, but not strong enough to forego surgery.

With regards to screening, the evidence from large clinical trials does not support a reduction in mortality associated with annual cancer antigen 125 (CA-125) or ultrasound imaging among women in the general population. In Poland, we screened *BRCA1* mutation carriers with annual ultrasound [3]. Among the 1,196 women who had one or more ultrasound examinations and no oophorectomy, there were 73 incident cancers detected and 27 deaths from ovarian/fallopian cancer. The ten-year cumulative risk of death was 2.0%. Among the 659 women who had a preventive oophorectomy there were 12 incident cancers and two deaths from ovarian cancer. The ten-year cumulative risk of death was 0.5%.

Based on the age distribution of occult cancers identified at surgery, salpingo-oophorectomy is recommended at age 35 to 40 for *BRCA1* mutation carriers and at age 45 for *BRCA2* mutation carriers. However, potential negative consequences associated with early surgical menopause are manifold and include infertility, vasomotor symptoms, a decline in sexual functioning and a diminishment in quality of life. If salpingectomy alone were equally effective as salpingo-oophorectomy, both fertility and quality of life could be maintained.

Oophorectomy (or salpingo-oophorectomy) has been shown to be effective in preventing cancer incidence and cancer mortality in *BRCA1* and *BRCA2* carriers. In an early study, we estimated the hazard ratio for incident ovarian, fallopian, or peritoneal cancer associated with bilateral oophorectomy to be 0.20 (95% CI: 0.13–0.30; P<.001) [4]. Among women who had no history of cancer at baseline, the hazard ratio for all-cause mortality to age 70 years associated with an oophorectomy was 0.23 (95% CI: 0.13–0.39; P<.001). The benefit of salpingo-oophorectomy extends beyond preventing ovarian and fallopian cancer. Surprisingly, several studies have also shown that oophorectomy prevents death from breast cancer [4–6]. This includes deaths from breast cancer in women who had the oophorectomy before getting breast cancer as well as in women who had the oophorectomy after getting breast cancer. For example, Metcalfe and colleagues reported that oophorectomy confers a significant reduction in breast cancer mortality among *BRCA* mutation carriers with a personal history of breast cancer (HR=0.46; 95% CI: 0.27–0.79) [5]. Recently we describe a 55% decline in breast cancer mortality among women with breast cancer and a *BRCA2* mutation who had an oophorectomy after diagnosis [6]. The ten-year breast cancer survival for women who had a bilateral oophorectomy was 89% and for women who did not have an oophorectomy was 59% (adjusted HR=0.45; 95% CI: 0.28–0.72; p=0.001)

It is not clear why oophorectomy prevents death from breast cancer. Surprisingly, it was effective for both ER-positive pre- and post-menopausal women, and in *BRCA1* and *BRCA2* carriers [5,6]. It worked for oophorectomies done before a diagnosis of breast cancer and for oophorectomies done after diagnosis [4]. It is not clear why the effect is not restricted to premenopausal oophorectomies in women with ER-positive breast cancers and the possibility of bias in study design cannot be excluded. Based on these results, the author is reluctant to recommend an unproven alternative (salpingectomy) when the gold standard (salpingo-oophorectomy) has been shown to have a profound impact on cancer incidence and mortality. In any case, the author would be more comfortable if offering salpingectomy to women who had a bilateral preventive mastectomy.

There is little empirical evidence that salpingectomy is effective and the recommendation is based on theoretical grounds and surveys of patient satisfaction. It is less contentious to offer salpingectomy to women without a *BRCA* mutation because for these women, the risk of ovarian cancer is not high enough to warrant preventive oophorectomy.

There are no long-term research studies comparing cancer incidence and mortality according to the two surgical approaches. Chi and colleagues reported a woman with a *BRCA1* mutation who underwent prophylactic mastectomy and bilateral salpingectomy with ovarian retention before the age of 40 years. She later developed stage IV high-grade serous ovarian cancer – four years after her initial surgery [7]. But to be fair, there are also many cases of women developing primary peritoneal cancer after undergoing oophorectomy.

Large-scale prospective studies that describe the impact of salpingectomy on cancer incidence and mortality, as well as menopausal symptoms or quality of life, are warranted. Trials currently recruiting *BRCA* mutation carriers have the more limited goal of evaluating the impact of salpingectomy (with delayed oophorectomy) on non-cancer endpoints, including safety, acceptability, menopausal symptoms, and quality of life. It remains to be seen whether women who are at a substantially elevated risk of developing serous cancer return for ovarian removal.

Conclusion

Salpingectomy alone should not be offered to high-risk women as a prevention strategy outside of research studies until prospective data on risk and mortality are available. To reach this goal it is important that gynecologists who perform the operation enrol the patients in appropriate research studies with this goal in mind.

References

1. Bowtell DD, et al. Rethinking ovarian cancer II: reducing mortality from high-grade serous ovarian cancer. *Nat Rev Cancer* 2015;15(11):668–679.

2. Kotsopoulos J, et al. Hereditary Ovarian Cancer Clinical Study Group. Breastfeeding and the risk of epithelial ovarian cancer among women with a BRCA1 or BRCA2 mutation. *Gynecol Oncol* 2020;2020:S0090–8258.

3. Gronwald J, et al. A comparison of ovarian cancer mortality in women with BRCA1 mutations undergoing annual ultrasound screening or preventive oophorectomy. *Gynecol Oncol* 2019;155 (2):270–274. https://doi.org/10.1016/j.ygyno.2019.08.034

4. Finch AP, et al. Impact of oophorectomy on cancer incidence and mortality in women with a BRCA1 or BRCA2 mutation. *J Clin Oncol* 2014;32(15):1547–1553.

5. Metcalfe K, et al. Effect of oophorectomy on survival after breast cancer in BRCA1 and BRCA2 mutation carriers. *JAMA Oncol* 2015;1(3):306–313.

6. Evans DG, et al. Survival from breast cancer in women with a BRCA2 mutation by treatment. *Br J Cancer* 2021;124 (9):1524–1532.

7. Lugo Santiago N, et al. Ovarian cancer after prophylactic salpingectomy in a patient with germline BRCA1 mutation. *Obstet Gynecol* 2020;135(6):1270–1274. https://doi.org/10.1097/AOG.0000000000003864

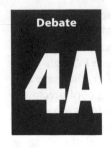

Can High-risk HPV Testing be Used Alone as the Primary Screening Modality for Cervical Cancer?
Yes

Thomas C. Wright

Debate

Cervical cytology reduced cervical cancer incidence by approximately 70% in countries with widespread screening. Despite cytology's success, there is interest in improving screening by incorporating sensitive molecular testing for high-risk HPV genotypes that cause most cervical cancer. This is because cytology is now recognized to have a sensitivity of only 50–75% for high-grade cervical neoplasia (CIN3+). Low sensitivity means cytology needs to be repeated frequently to obtain high levels of protection.

HPV testing can be incorporated into screening in two ways. One is to replace cytology with HPV testing (i.e., primary HPV screening). The other is to combine HPV testing with cytology (i.e., co-testing). Nonrandomized studies and seven randomized screening trials have evaluated the safety and effectiveness of these two approaches [1]. These studies clearly demonstrate that HPV testing increases the detection of CIN3+ at the initial round of screening compared to cytology alone and reduces CIN3+ found at subsequent screening rounds. A meta-analysis of long-term follow-up data from several randomized trials found a 40% lower incidence of invasive cervical cancer in women screened with HPV compared to cytology. Therefore, some countries have adopted HPV primary screening for their national screening programs. These include Australia, United Kingdom, Netherlands, Denmark, Sweden, Turkey, and regions of Italy. In contrast, United States policy makers initially adopted co-testing, which was cleared by the United States Food and Drug Administration (US FDA) for use in women ≥30 years in 2003 and classified as the preferred screening approach for women ≥30 years by the American Cancer Society in 2012.

The reasons why co-testing was initially preferred in the United States include that clinicians want to reduce cervical cancer risk to a minimum and believed two tests would provide the greatest protection. This is not the case. The National Cancer Institute (NCI) analyzed over one million women co-tested at Kaiser Permanente and found that risk of CIN3+ was similar among HPV-negative and co-test-negative women [2]. After three years, the cumulative risk of CIN3+ was 0.07% in HPV-negative women compared to 0.05% for co-test-negative women. The risk in women with a negative cytology was 0.19%.

Three US FDA registration trials of HPV primary screening with up to three years of follow-up have been completed (Table 4A.1). The first is the ATHENA study that evaluated the Roche cobas 4800 HPV test. In ATHENA, all women received HPV testing and cytology and HPV-positive and/or cytology-positive women received colposcopy, as did a random subset of women negative on both tests. This allowed verification bias adjustment. In ATHENA, women without CIN2+ who underwent colposcopy were followed for three

16

Table 4A.1 Verification bias adjusted comparative performance of HPV primary screening and co-testing algorithms for detection of CIN3+ in women >25 years

	ATHENA[1]	BD Onclarity[2]	IMPACT[3]
Number of subjects	40,901	29,633	34,807
HPV (+) rate	10.5%	12.7%	15.1%
>ASCUS	6.4%	8.4%	9.8%
HPV primary screening			
Sensitivity (%)	76.1	64.2	79.9
Specificity (%)	93.5	94.4	92.9
Positive predictive value (%)	12.9	9.0	9.0
Negative predictive value (%)	99.7	99.7	99.8
Colposcopy referral (%)	9.2	6.1	7.7
Co-testing			
Sensitivity (%)	61.7	57.7	77.6
Specificity (%)	94.6	94.2	92.5
Positive predictive value (%)	12.6	7.9	8.4
Negative predictive value (%)	99.5	99.6	99.8
Colposcopy referral (%)	7.6	6.2	8.1
Cytology alone			
Sensitivity (%)	47.8	49.2	66.1
Specificity (%)	97.1	92.0	90.7
Positive predictive value (%)	17.0	5.0	5.9
Negative predictive value (%)	99.3	99.5	99.7
Colposcopy referral (%)	4.7	8.4	9.8

[1] Algorithm performance was assessed after three years of follow-up and is verification bias adjusted. Co-testing algorithm performance does not include HPV testing (i.e., uses cytology only) for women 25–29 years of age.
[2] Algorithm performance was assessed at baseline and is verification bias adjusted.
[3] Algorithm performance was assessed at baseline and is verification bias adjusted. Co-testing algorithm performance does not include HPV testing (i.e., uses cytology only) for women 25–29 years of age.

years. This allowed evaluation of the performance of different screening algorithms over a three-year screening cycle [3]. The HPV primary screening algorithm that was evaluated is shown in Figure 4A.1, as is the co-testing algorithm. The HPV primary screening algorithm incorporates HPV 16/18 genotyping and HPV 16-/18-positive women receive colposcopy. The performance characteristics of the HPV primary screening and co-testing algorithms for CIN3+ in women >30 years are shown in Table 4A.1. HPV primary screening detected more cases of CIN3+ over the three-year period than did co-testing. It is important to recognize that the sensitivity and specificities shown in Table 4A.1 are those of the screening algorithms, not simply the screening test, and have been adjusted for verification bias. The sensitivity of HPV testing, as opposed to the algorithm, for CIN3+ without verification bias adjustment is typically higher, about 90%.

The two other US FDA registration trials are the Onclarity HPV study and the IMPACT study [4,5]. Both trials had similar study designs to that of ATHENA and evaluated HPV primary screening and co-testing algorithms that were similar to ATHENA's. Table 4A.1

HPV Primary Screening

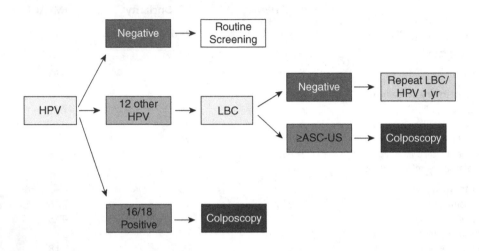

Cotesting *(Used only for women >30 yrs. Women 25–29 yrs received cytology only)*

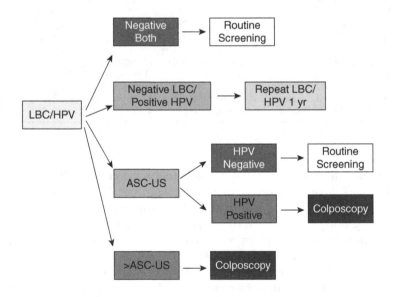

LBC, liquid-based cytology

Figure 4A.1 Screening algorithms evaluated in ATHENA.

shows the comparative performance characteristics of HPV primary screening and co-testing. Both the BD Onclarity HPV assay (Becton, Dickinson, and Company) and the Roche cobas 6800 HPV assay are now FDA cleared for HPV primary screening in women ≥25 years using the algorithm incorporating HPV 16/18 genotyping and cytology triage of women with 12 "other" HPV genotypes.

Conclusion

Data from the European randomized clinical trials, the large NCI-Kaiser Permanente real-world follow-up study, and the three US FDA registration trials clearly demonstrate that HPV primary screening is safe and effective. Moreover, co-testing which combines both HPV testing and cytology offers minimal, if any, benefit compared to HPV primary testing. Co-testing increases costs, requires follow-up of HPV-negative women with ASCUS and LSIL that can lead to unnecessary colposcopies/biopsies, and retains the medico-legal risk of false-negative cytology results. It is also expected that as HPV vaccination reduces the prevalence of CIN3+, the performance of cytology will decrease more than the performance of HPV testing. HPV primary screening is now classified as the preferred screening approach for women ≥25 years by the 2020 American Cancer Society guidelines.

References

1. US Preventive Services Task Force, et al. Screening for cervical cancer: US Preventive Services Task Force Recommendation Statement. *JAMA* 2018;320:674–686.

2. Gage JC, et al. Reassurance against future risk of precancer and cancer conferred by a negative human papillomavirus test. *J Natl Cancer Inst* 2014;56(5):106.

3. Wright TC, et al. Primary cervical cancer screening with human papillomavirus: end of study results from the ATHENA study using HPV as the first-line screening test. *Gynecol Oncol* 2015;136:189–197.

4. Food and Drug Administration. FDA Summary of Safety and Effectiveness Data; cobas HPV for use on the cobas 6800/8800 System. 2020.

5. Food and Drug Administration. FDA Summary of Safety and Effectiveness Data; BD Onclarity HPV Assay. 2018.

Debate

Can High-risk HPV Testing be Used Alone as the Primary Screening Modality for Cervical Cancer?
No

Ibraheem O. Awowole and Olusegun O. Badejoko

Debate: High-risk HPV is Insufficient as a Stand-alone Primary Screening Modality for Cervical Cancer

Cervical cancer, with its global incidence of 570,000, and annual mortality of 311,000 (which represents 7.5% of all female cancer deaths), is the second most common cancer in women living in developing countries [1]. In the United States, cervical cancer used to be the leading cause of cancer death among women, but this narrative has changed significantly over the last four decades. The statistics are similar in other developed countries, due to the impact of the established screening program, which is estimated to prevent up to 80% of cervical cancers [1].

The reduction in the incidence of cervical cancer and associated mortality in developed countries was hinged on conventional and liquid-based cytology screening. The discourse however continues to evolve, concerning what the best modality of screening should be, with some countries gradually transitioning towards high-risk HPV-based primary screening. HPV is a group of about 200 related viruses, 14 of which have been identified as high-risk HPV (Hr-HPV). These 14 Hr-HPV are reportedly found in 99% of cervical cancer specimens, with HPV 16 and 18 alone accounting for at least 70% of all cervical cancers. This knowledge has been utilized extensively in the primary (vaccination) and secondary (screening) prevention of cervical cancer [1]. A meta-analysis involving 140,000 women concluded that primary screening with Hr-HPV was more sensitive than liquid-based cytology (LBC) for CIN2+, with a pooled sensitivity estimate of 89.9% vs. 72.9% (Relative Sensitivity=1.18). Pooled specificity estimate of Hr-HPV is however slightly lower, with a Relative Specificity Estimate of 0.96 (95% CI: 0.95–0.97). Hr-HPV-based screening may also lead to the detection of more CIN2+ lesions [2].

Despite these benefits however, Hr-HPV alone is insufficient as a screening test for cervical cancer. Almost all sexually active women below the age of 30 years will screen positive for HPV at some point, with about 50% being the Hr-HPV serotypes [1,3]. These infections are however transient and more than 90% are cleared by the host immunity within two years, thereby preventing progression to CIN or invasive cancers, which is only seen in persistent cases. Cervical cancer is therefore a low-probability event compared with the total number of HPV-infected women in this age group, making screening with Hr-HPV less effective. This was confirmed by Koliopoulos et al. [2] in their systematic review, which concluded that screening with Hr-HPV may be less likely to miss cases of CIN2+, but will lead to more unnecessary referrals. WHO also recommended that screening with Hr-HPV should not start until the age of 30 years [1], while the U.S. Preventative Task Force (USPTF) and the American College of Obstetricians and Gynecologists (ACOG) currently recommend that LBC, not Hr-HPV should be used for screening women aged 21–29 years [3].

NHS England and the American Cancer Society [4,5] adopted a middle ground, recommending transitioning to Hr-HPV-based screening from 25 years as the preferred option, with LBC or LBC/Hr-HPV co-testing as alternatives. This option may reduce the unnecessary follow-up testing for women <25 years, but it is not without its limitation. Between 2011 and 2015, some 108 new cervical cancers were reported annually among women <25 years in the American Cancer Registry [3]. This was despite over a decade of HPV vaccination, with many of those that were vaccinated now in the 20–24 years group. Suspending screening in that group may leave them vulnerable, especially in settings where vaccination is yet to be established. Screening women <29 years with LBC, and not Hr-HPV therefore appears to be the pragmatic option.

Women that are aged 30–65 years with negative Hr-HPV can be reasonably assured of being at very low risk for cervical cancer. The utility of Hr-HPV is however limited to the negative predictive value. The test is inadequate among women with positive Hr-HPV, as a substantial proportion of these infections will only be transient as well. Cytological triage is therefore essential to design a plan of care, for evaluation of the cytopathic effects of HPV which are only seen in persistent infections. Screening with Hr-HPV alone, without recourse to cytology for women with positive Hr-HPV will therefore be associated with unnecessary referrals to colposcopy and treatment. Furthermore, there is a subset of high grade squamous intraepithelial lesion (HGSIL) cytology and cervical carcinomas that are Hr-HPV negative. The American Society for Clinical Pathology (ASCP) expressed concerns that 9–10% of invasive cancers and that 8.3–14% of HGSIL cases may test negative with commercially available Hr-HPV kits, leading to delayed diagnosis that may result in higher stage tumors, especially in the setting of a longer screening interval of five years. To avoid this, the ASCP advised that Hr-HPV alone may be insufficient, and women should have cytological examination at some point during their screening.

Lastly, concerns have been expressed that some women may test positive to Hr-HPV due to a reactivation of an old, supposedly cleared infection, akin to the phenomenon in chickenpox. LBC co-testing remains the best plan of care for such patients, while research continues on the subject.

Conclusion

Hr-HPV is insufficient as a stand-alone primary screening test for cervical cancer. As countries transition to Hr-HPV for cervical cancer screening, it is important to acknowledge the limitations of the test and refine its utilization across different populations.

References

1. World Health Organization. Human papillomavirus (HPV) and cervical cancer. Geneva: WHO, 2018. Available at: www.who.int/en/news-room/fact-sheets/detail/human-papillomavirus-(hpv)-and-cervical-cancer [last accessed October 18, 2022].

2. Koliopoulos G, et al. Cytology versus HPV testing for cervical cancer screening in the general population. *Cochrane Database Syst Rev* 2017;8(8):CD008587.

3. United States Preventive Service Task Force. Cervical Cancer: Screening. 2018. Available at: www.uspreventiveservices taskforce.org/uspstf/recommendation/cervical-cancer-screening [last accessed October 18, 2022].

4. Public Health England with NHS England and NHS Improvement Public Health Commissioning. NHS public health functions agreement 2019–2020 Service specification No.25; Cervical Screening Programme. PHE England, 2020.

5. Fontham ETH, et al. Cervical cancer screening for individuals at average risk: 2020 Guideline Update from the American Cancer Society. *CA Cancer J Clin* 2020;70 (5):321–346.

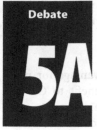

Debate

Should CA-125 Surveillance be Performed after Completion of Primary Treatment for Ovarian Cancer Patients in Remission?

Yes

Eseohi Ehimiaghe and Edward Tanner

Debate

Serum CA-125 levels have been widely used to assess disease status in patients with advanced epithelial ovarian cancer. Although CA-125 is only elevated in half of patients with early-stage disease, the majority of patients with advanced stage disease will have an elevation at diagnosis. The rate of CA-125 decline following cytoreductive surgery and chemotherapy predicts treatment response and recurrence risk [1,2]. Increases in serum CA-125 levels generally herald disease recurrence, with CA-125 levels rising at recurrence in at least 70% of patients with an elevated level at baseline [3]. Even small increases in CA-125 levels have a strong association with recurrence risk. For example, Piatek et al. found a seven-fold increased risk of recurrence when serum CA-125 levels increased by as little as 5 U/ml from baseline [4].

Conventional wisdom suggests that early detection of recurrent disease would lead to superior post-recurrence survival – much like the diagnosis of early-stage disease results in superior survival versus advanced stage disease [5]. Surprisingly, this correlation is not as strong as one may assume. A large European Organisation for Research and Treatment of Cancer (EORTC) trial, which randomized patients with advanced ovarian cancer in first remission to CA-125 surveillance as a mechanism to detect disease recurrence versus identification based on symptoms [6], showed early initiation of salvage chemotherapy based on increased CA-125 levels led to earlier initiation of chemotherapy but did not improve survival. While it is difficult to disagree with the results of a well conducted randomized trial, the results were limited by the fact that only 19% of patients underwent secondary surgery. Two recently completed randomized trials demonstrate a mixed benefit of secondary surgery [7,8], so we must consider the value CA-125 has in subsets of patients. Most surgeons agree that healthy women with a long progression-free interval and high likelihood of complete secondary cytoreduction benefit from surgery and multiple retrospective studies have found that women who have a recurrence identified by CA-125 elevation without symptoms have a higher chance of complete secondary cytoreduction [3,9]. Given these findings, and the small proportion of patients who underwent secondary surgery in the EORTC trial, as oncologists, we could consider CA-125 surveillance as part of the follow-up plan for patients who are good candidates for secondary cytoreduction.

Conclusion

Even if CA-125 surveillance does not provide an objective survival advantage for most patients with ovarian cancer, there may still be a patient-centered benefit to CA-125 surveillance. Many patients recognize loss of control as a leading cause of anxiety after a cancer diagnosis. While some patients feel that earlier identification of recurrence without survival advantage would lead to unnecessary anxiety during a time when they are otherwise well, others feel that knowing their disease status adds a level of control and life planning that is beneficial to their health and well-being [10]. While our focus as gynecology oncologists is often on quantifiable improvement in clinical outcomes and mortality, patients might consider the heralding impact of CA-125 changes as important information to guide life decisions [11,12]. We must be willing to discuss the benefits and harms of CA-125 surveillance with our patients, so that we provide them with options that empower decision making.

References

1. Rodriguez N, et al. Changes in serum CA-125 can predict optimal cytoreduction to no gross residual disease in patients with advanced stage ovarian cancer treated with neoadjuvant chemotherapy. *Gynecol Oncol* 2012;125:362–366. https://doi.org/10.1016/j.ygyno.2012.02.006

2. Rustin GJS, et al. Definitions for response and progression in ovarian cancer clinical trials incorporating Response Evaluation Criteria In Solid Tumors (RECIST) 1.1 and CA-125 agreed by the gynecological cancer intergroup (GCIG). *Int J Gynecol Cancer* 2011;21:419–423. https://doi.org/10.1097/IGC.0b013e3182070f17

3. Fleming ND, et al. CA-125 surveillance increases optimal resectability at secondary cytoreductive surgery for recurrent epithelial ovarian cancer. *Gynecol Oncol* 2011;121:249–252. https://doi.org/10.1016/j.ygyno.2011.01.014

4. Piatek S, et al. Rising serum CA-125 levels within the normal range is strongly associated recurrence risk and survival of ovarian cancer. *J Ovarian Res* 2020;13:102. https://doi.org/10.1186/s13048-020-00681-0

5. Pignata S, et al. Follow-up with CA-125 after primary therapy of advanced ovarian cancer: in favor of continuing to prescribe CA-125 during follow-up. *Ann Oncol Off J Eur Soc Med Oncol* 2011;22(Suppl. 8): viii40–viii44. https://doi.org/10.1093/annonc/mdr470

6. Rustin GJS, et al. Early versus delayed treatment of relapsed ovarian cancer (MRC OV05/EORTC 55955): a randomised trial., *Lancet* 2010;376:1155–1163. https://doi.org/10.1016/S0140-6736(10)61268-8

7. Coleman RL, et al. Secondary surgical cytoreduction for recurrent ovarian cancer. *N Engl J Med* 2019;381:1929–1939. https://doi.org/10.1056/NEJMoa1902626

8. Du Bois A, et al. Randomized phase III study to evaluate the impact of secondary cytoreductive surgery in recurrent ovarian cancer: final analysis of AGO DESKTOP III/ENGOT-ov20. *J Clin Oncol* 2020;38:6000. https://doi.org/10.1200/JCO.2020.38.15_suppl.6000

9. Tanner EJ, et al. Surveillance for the detection of recurrent ovarian cancer: survival impact or lead-time bias? *Gynecol Oncol* 2010;2010:117. https://doi.org/10.1016/j.ygyno.2010.01.014

10. Jordens CFC, et al. Cancergazing? CA-125 and post-treatment surveillance in advanced ovarian cancer. *Soc Sci Med* 2010;71:1548–1556. https://doi.org/10.1016/j.socscimed.2010.07.033

11. Tsai L-Y, et al. Life experiences and disease trajectories in women coexisting with ovarian cancer. *Taiwan J Obstet Gynecol* 2020;59:115–119. https://doi.org/10.1016/j.tjog.2019.11.032

12. Jolicoeur LJA, et al. Women's decision-making needs related to treatment for recurrent ovarian cancer: a pilot study. *Can Oncol Nurs J* 2009;19:117–121. https://doi.org/10.5737/1181912x193117121

Debate

5B

Should CA-125 Surveillance be Performed after Completion of Primary Treatment for Ovarian Cancer Patients in Remission?

No

Gordon J. S. Rustin

Debate

Relapse diagnosed by CA-125 is detected about six months earlier than relapse diagnosed through development of symptoms. If earlier treatment of relapse improves survival and/or quality of life, patients should be advised to have CA-125 surveillance. However, if earlier diagnosis of relapse and earlier treatment do not improve survival and lead to a worse quality of life, patients should be advised against having CA-125 surveillance.

The only randomized trial that investigated the role of CA-125 surveillance found that routine CA-125 measurements did not benefit patients. The MRC OV05/ EORTC 55955 trial enrolled 1442 patients with a CA-125 level within the normal range following platinum-based chemotherapy for epithelial ovarian cancer [1]. If CA-125 levels rose to more than twice the upper limit of normal, patients were randomized to immediate or delayed chemotherapy. Those randomized in the early arm started chemotherapy a median of 4.8 months earlier than those on the delayed arm. There was no difference in survival between the early and delayed arms, with worse quality of life of patients in the early arm.

This led to a change in practice in some centers with 80% of patients in a retrospective audit choosing not to have routine CA-125 follow-up [2]. However, an audit of six United States cancer centres showed that routine use of CA-125 did not change and there was no lengthening of time from CA-125 doubling to re-treatment [3]. Why do some patients opt for CA-125 surveillance and some do not?

A major reason why patients want CA-125 surveillance is the belief that earlier detection of relapsed disease will lead to longer survival. The OVO5 trial clearly showed that earlier starting of chemotherapy does not help, but too few patients had second surgery in that trial to determine whether surgery improves survival. Retrospective studies have suggested that asymptomatic patients whose relapse was detected by surveillance are more likely to receive optimal surgery and have longer survival following surgery than those who relapsed with symptoms. Lead time bias could explain some of this difference as could selection of patients for surgery.

The results of two trials randomizing patients to secondary surgery followed by chemotherapy or chemotherapy alone, have unfortunately not resolved this dilemma. The GOG213 trial failed to show any survival benefit from surgery, but the DESKTOP 3 trial showed a significantly longer survival in the surgery arm [4,5]. The GOG trial was performed in a country where most patients had frequent CA-125 measurements during follow-up. The DESKTOP 3 trial was performed in countries where patients were recommended not to have routine CA-125 surveillance. One can envisage that asymptomatic relapse just detected by CA-125 is more likely to be associated with peritoneal thickening or just ascites, that is not helped by surgery, whilst those with symptomatic relapse might be more likely to have resectable disease. As most surgeons would not consider secondary surgery before patients are treatment-free for at least 12 months, there is no point in measuring CA-125 during the first year of follow-up.

Patient decision making as to what surveillance policy to adopt is likely to be influenced by the local culture and the opinions of their oncologist. If the culture supports maximal intervention regardless of cost (both financial and impact on quality of life) patients will expect intense surveillance and the oncologist might go along with it to appear to be fighting hard for their patient. Those doctors who are happy that their patients erroneously believe that cure of relapsed ovarian cancer is still possible, are likely to be in favor of routine CA-125 measurements. If the culture is to be guided by experts who accurately inform patients of the scientific evidence, patients entering remission should be offered the following options:

1. Not to have routine CA-125 measurements if they are well and have no symptoms suggesting relapse.
2. To continue having CA-125 measurements but not be told the results. This option is particularly useful if they are in a clinical trial.
3. To have routine CA-125 measurements so that they have more warning as to when they might require relapse chemotherapy.

Further requirements to enable safe follow-up of ovarian cancer patients who opt for no routine CA-125 measurements are: (1) A leaflet about follow-up which includes a list of likely symptoms that should prompt an early clinic appointment (see http://links.lww.com /IGC/A456); (2) Facilities for patients to make urgent appointments; (3) Availability of a support nurse for telephone advice.

Conclusion

After completion of primary treatment for ovarian cancer, some patients are started on maintenance therapy with bevacizumab or a PARP inhibitor. These patients need monitoring by CA-125 and scans. Most patients are not on maintenance therapy and risk having their remission shortened and hope of cure destroyed by being told their CA-125 is rising. Worrying about CA-125 results increases anxiety before clinic appointments. Once patients are aware of a rising CA-125 level it becomes difficult to delay starting relapse therapy. Patients need to be told before embarking on CA-125 surveillance that it could lead to a worse quality of life with more chemotherapy than needed, for no survival benefit.

References

1. Rustin GJ, et al. Early versus delayed treatment of relapsed ovarian cancer (MRCOV05/EORTC 55955): a randomised trial. *Lancet* 2010;376:1155–1163.

2. Krell D, et al. Audit of CA-125 follow-up after first-line therapy for ovarian cancer. *Int J Gynecol Cancer* 2017;27:1118–1122.

3. Esselen KM, et al. Use of CA-125 tests and CT scans for surveillance in ovarian cancer. *JAMA Oncol* 2016;2(11):1427–1433.

4. Coleman RL, et al. Secondary surgical cytoreduction for recurrent ovarian cancer. *N Engl J Med* 2019;381(20):1929–1939.

5. Du Bois A, et al. Randomized phase III study to evaluate the impact of secondary cytoreductive surgery in recurrent ovarian cancer: final analysis of AGO DESKTOP III/ENGOT-ov20. *J Clin Oncol* 2020;38(Suppl. 15):6000.

6A

In Patients with BRCA-negative and HRD-negative Epithelial Ovarian Cancer, Should Molecular Profiling be Routinely Done to Guide Adjuvant Therapy?

Yes

Ilaria Betella and Matteo Repetto

Debate

Undoubtedly, gynecological oncologists have witnessed a dramatic change in the landscape of epithelial ovarian cancer (EOC) management since the introduction of poly ADP-ribose polymerase inhibitors (PARPi) into adjuvant standard-of-care therapy in 2018. In this relatively short period, not only geneticists and molecular biologists, but all healthcare providers involved in EOC treatment had to expand their knowledge of cancer genetics and molecular profiling in order to acquire expertise to integrate the new clinical available tools in the appropriate management strategy. Since the advent of PARPi, which target cells with homologous recombination repair deficiency (HRD), including BRCA mutated cells, different HRD panels and assays have been investigated for predicting the response to PARPi. To date, there are two commercially available tests to assess HRD: Myriad myChoice®CDx and Foundation Medicine's Foundation Focus®CDx. Beside sequencing and evaluating large rearrangement of *BRCA1/2* genes, both these assays only analyze the phenotypic consequence on DNA of genomic instability, without identifying the specific causative gene alterations. Thus, further molecular profiling in BRCA-negative and HRD-negative EOCs is still worthy to guide adjuvant therapy [1].

Molecular profiling is not a new concept, if immunohistochemistry (IHC), Fluorescence In Situ Hybridization (FISH), Sanger sequencing or Quantitative Polymerase Chain Reaction (qPCR) are taken in consideration. However, all these techniques permit the identification of few specific alterations at a time. The advent of the Next-Generation Sequencing (NGS), which allows us to simultaneously examine millions of gene fragments and more broadly detect DNA mutations, copy number variations and gene fusions across the genome in only a few days and at affordable cost, represents a major breakthrough, allowing the routine use of comprehensive molecular profiling in clinical decision making [2].

The cornerstone in extensive genomic analysis in EOC was settled in 2011, with the publication of The Cancer Genome Atlas (TCGA). Methylation, messenger RNA (mRNA) and microRNA (miRNA) expression, and DNA copy number variations were tested as prognostic predictors in advanced high-grade serous (HGS) EOC, enabling the identification of four subtypes, namely differentiated, immunoreactive, mesenchymal, and proliferative. Moreover, the DNA exome sequencing and the pathway analysis not only identified that 50% of HGS-EOC harbor homologous recombination repair (HRR) defects and may benefit from PARPi, but also pinpointed other commonly deregulated pathways, including RB, RAS/PI3 K, FOXM1, and NOTCH, which are potential targets for therapeutic treatment. Furthermore, comparison with literature allowed identification of different mutation spectrums across distinct EOC histological subtypes: while HGS-EOCs harbor *TP53* and *BRCA* mutations in 96% and 22% of specimens respectively, clear-cell ovarian cancers show recurrent *ARID1A* and *PIK3CA* mutations and endometrioid ovarian tumors frequently have *CTNNB1*, *ARID1A*, and *PIK3CA* mutations [3].

Despite the obvious benefit of gaining a deeper understanding of tumor biology, the huge amount of data obtained from NGS panels may quickly overwhelm gynecological oncologists, increasing the risk of missing clinically valuable information. To overcome the complexity of interpreting the NGS data and providing timely results according to the clinical need, a number of precision medicine platforms have been developed to assist Molecular Tumor Boards (MTB) and oncologists. An example is OncoKb, a comprehensive and curated precision oncology knowledge base, which classifies the clinical actionability of mutations in levels ranging from 1, that identifies a biomarker for a Food and Drug Administration (FDA-) approved drug for that same indication, to 4, indicating a biomarker potentially predictive of response based on compelling biological evidence [4]. Specifically for EOC, as of October 2020, the OncoKb database identified 15 actionable genes (*NTRK1-2–3, AKT1, BRAF, CDK12, CDKN2A, FGFR1-2–3, KRAS, MET, MTOR, NF1 and PTEN*) and two actionable signatures, named Tumor Mutational Burden (TMB) and MicroSatellite Instability (MSI), in addition to *BRCA1* and *BRCA2* mutations. Among these 17 actionable alterations, MSI-high, TMB-high, and NTRK1-2–3 fusions are targets for FDA-approved therapies in EOC. Specifically, MSI-high, occurring in roughly 3% of HGS-EOC, is a genomic signature characterized by abundant nonsynonymous mutations and neoantigens, causing a high tumor mutational burden (TMB), conditions that predict sensibility to immunotherapy. NTRK1-2–3 fusions predict sensitivity to specific small-molecule inhibitors named Larotrectinib and Entrectinib [4]. As these alterations are relatively rare when considered singularly, routine use of an alteration-specific test might not be a viable strategy. Instead, NGS multiplexing allows us to simultaneously investigate several genes, cumulatively increasing the probability of finding at least one rare actionable mutation. Considering that the list of actionable alterations is progressively growing, routinely performing NGS in EOC can help in expanding therapeutic options for strategic management of patients.

Additionally, NGS panels represent clinically valuable prognostic tools. As a number of alterations have been linked to worse response to platinum salts and PARPi, for example *EMSY* and *CCNE1* amplifications [5], their early identification might predict drug resistance and avoid unnecessary costs and drug-associated morbidity. Indeed, in some countries, patients with cancer are required to pay a variable proportion of their medical bills leading sometimes even to bankruptcy, while in other countries public health resources are limited, requiring a cautious evaluation of the balance between advantages and risks of a specific therapy. Moreover, adjuvant therapy is responsible for a range of adverse events which, in drug-resistant disease, may worsen the patient's quality of life without improvement in prognosis. As such, extended NGS-derived information represents an additional instrument that can be adopted in oncological counseling to help patients making an aware choice.

Furthermore, tumor molecular profiling can favor patient enrollment in basket or umbrella clinical trials for testing the efficacy of new drugs against specific molecular targets. This achieves two purposes: on the one hand, it allows patients to access innovative tailored treatment with potential benefit; on the other hand, it helps fast-track evaluation and approval of tailored adjuvant therapies with improved efficacy and a more favorable toxicity profile [2].

Conclusion

In conclusion, molecular profiling should be routinely done in BRCA-negative HRD-negative EOC. Even though EOC guidelines do not recommend systematical NGS analysis at diagnosis yet, it effectively helps fulfill several purposes. Indeed, the use of extended molecular panels not only leads to greater understanding of tumor biology, but it also identifies alternative actionable alterations, predicts prognosis and/or drug resistance, and allows access to alteration-directed clinical trials with potential benefit for the patients.

References

1. Mirza MR, et al. The forefront of ovarian cancer therapy: update on PARP inhibitors. *Ann Oncol* 2020;31(9):1148–1159. https://doi.org/10.1016/j.annonc.2020.06.004

2. Berger MF, et al. The emerging clinical relevance of genomics in cancer medicine. *Nat Rev Clin Oncol* 2018;15:353–365. https://doi.org/10.1038/s41571-018-0002-6

3. Cancer Genome Atlas Research Network. Integrated genomic analyses of ovarian carcinoma. *Nature* 2011;474(7353):609–15. https://doi.org/10.1038/nature10166. Erratum in: *Nature* 2012;490(7419):298.

4. www.oncokb.org/ [last accessed October 18, 2022].

5. Konstantinopoulos PA, et al. Homologous recombination deficiency: exploiting the fundamental vulnerability of ovarian cancer. *Cancer Discov* 2015;5:1137–1154.

6B
In Patients with BRCA-negative and HRD-negative Epithelial Ovarian Cancer, Should Molecular Profiling be Routinely Done to Guide Adjuvant Therapy?
No

Raanan Alter and Ernst Lengyel

Debate

In the era of targeted medicine, the use of poly (ADP-ribose) polymerase (PARP) inhibitors in homologous recombination deficient (HRD) tumors has represented the first clinically actionable mutation in gynecologic malignancies. The dramatic results seen across multiple clinical trials completely changed the landscape of epithelial ovarian cancer (EOC) treatments in both primary and recurrent settings. For many, it has spawned hope that additional biomarkers would soon be discovered that could find similarly spectacular results in different patient populations. However, molecular profiling's efficacy in selecting targeted therapies and its economic practicality are difficult to justify.

Multigene panel testing using Next Generation Sequencing (NGS) for both germline and somatic mutations are now offered by dozens of companies and often tests for over 1000 different genetic mutations, insertions/deletions, copy number variations, and fusion/translocations. While these represent significant advances in molecular profiling technology and contribute to the overall understanding of ovarian cancer biology, their clinical utility is controversial. Up to 50% of patients will have HRD tumors and thus have the ability to be treated with a PARP inhibitor; however, the clinical relevance of NGS for treating the other half has not been at all established. As it turns out, the rate of matching an "actionable" mutation to a targeted therapy is quite low. In a 2020 National Cancer Institute (NCI) match trial analysis, only 75 out of 530 (14.2%) patients with EOC were paired with a targeted therapy [1]. In a 2019 study, Jae Lee et al. found that out of 84 EOC patients, 57 (67.9%) were determined to have an actionable mutation; out of which only seven patients were matched to a targeted therapy [2]. Even those patients who had been matched to a therapy exhibited low response rates. In the MOSCATO-1 trial, 199 out of 1035 patients were paired to a targeted therapy, although only 22 (11% of the paired patients or 2.1% of the total patient population) achieved an objective response. In the published literature, clinically meaningful response rates for common targetable non-HRD mutations (*HER2/NEU*, *PI3 K*) range from 10–17%, which is similar to standard of care cytotoxic chemotherapies in the platinum-resistant setting.

Additionally, there is also data that suggests a significant discordance between commercial tests. In a 2017 study, Kuderer et al. compared two commercial NGS platforms on specimens from the same patients. They found a 22% concordance between the specimens and only nine of 36 targeted drugs were suggested by both tests [3]. While this discordance was thought to be attributed to tumor heterogeneity from different biopsy specimens or anatomic locations, this would question the overall utility of NGS from a single sample given that tumor heterogeneity can heavily influence results.

One must acknowledge the dramatic costs associated with these panels. The cost to patients for multigene panels ranges anywhere from $4000–$6500 [4]. While most insurances will provide coverage for these panels, that does not diminish the large cost incurred by our healthcare system for such a relatively low-yield product paired with aggressive direct-to-consumer advertising by companies. Furthermore, the mutations found in NGS may lead to the prescribing of off-label targeted therapy which can be extremely costly (>$100,000 per year of therapy) and has not been shown to provide improvements in response rates, progression-free survival or overall survival over traditional cytotoxic chemotherapy regimens. In a recent cost utility model, Wallbillich et al. found that treatments with targeted therapies were projected to have a mean cost of $90,271 with 0.71 quality-adjusted life years (QALY), compared with standard of care therapies which would cost $74,926 and 0.68 QALYs resulting in an incremental cost-effectiveness ratio (ICER) of over $470,000 per QALY [5]. In fact, in a sensitivity analysis, the genomic strategy never became cost effective even when the genomic testing was free, as the driver of cost-effectiveness lay in the high price per cycle of targeted therapies.

Conclusion

In summary, while the remarkable technological advances and the results seen in the treatment of HRD tumors with PARP inhibitors are impressive, we do not recommend the routine molecular profiling of EOC patients. The concordance between NGS platforms is disappointingly low, the actionability of mutations is low, and the subsequent response rates remain unchanged.

Ordering molecular testing can also generate a false sense of hope among our patients that a novel or targeted therapy may be an option, when for almost all of these patients, such options are not available. To this end, in an European Society for Medical Oncology (ESMO) Precision Medicine Working Group analysis in 2020, the writing group felt that the use of multigene NGS is justified, but cautions against larger panels on the basis that the overall cost of the strategy must be considered. We would argue that beyond testing for BRCA and HRD, molecular profiling for epithelial ovarian cancer should only be performed in the clinical trial setting or for research purposes.

References

1. Flaherty KT, et al. Molecular landscape and actionable alterations in a genomically guided cancer clinical trial: National Cancer Institute Molecular Analysis for Therapy Choice (NCI-MATCH). *J Clin Oncol* 2020;38(33):3883–3894.

2. Lee YJ, et al. Integrating a next generation sequencing panel into clinical practice in ovarian cancer. *Yonsei Med J* 2019;60(10):914–923.

3. Kuderer NM, et al. Comparison of 2 commercially available next-generation

sequencing platforms in oncology. *JAMA Oncol* 2017;3(7):996–998.

4. Haunschild CE, et al. The current landscape of molecular profiling in the treatment of epithelial ovarian cancer. *Gynecol Oncol* 2020;160(1):333–345.

5. Wallbillich JJ, et al. A personalized paradigm in the treatment of platinum-resistant ovarian cancer: a cost utility analysis of genomic-based versus cytotoxic therapy. *Gynecol Oncol* 2016;142(1):144–149.

Is MEK Inhibitor Therapy the Best Treatment Recommendation for Low-Grade Serous Ovarian Cancer Patients at First Relapse?

Yes

Rachel N. Grisham

Debate

Patients with recurrent low-grade serous ovarian cancer have multiple options for treatment: chemotherapy with or without bevacizumab, bevacizumab alone, or endocrine therapy with Lupron, tamoxifen, or aromatase inhibitors. While all of these are viable and appropriate options, recently reported data regarding the activity of MEK inhibitors in recurrent low-grade serous ovarian cancer has shown that MEK inhibitors are a key treatment option that should be considered at time of first recurrence in all patients with low-grade serous ovarian cancer.

There has been considerable interest in the use of MEK inhibitors for the treatment of low-grade serous ovarian cancer for over a decade, since the molecular profile of low-grade serous ovarian cancer was first characterized as most commonly displaying alterations affecting the Mitogen Activated Pathway Kinase (MAPK) pathway. Approximately a third of patients with recurrent low-grade serous ovarian cancer harbor *KRAS* mutations, while additional patients display fewer common alterations affecting components of the MAPK pathway, such as in the *BRAF*, *NF1*, and *MAPK1* genes [1,2].

The first prospective clinical trial examining the use of single agent MEK inhibitor in recurrent low-grade serous ovarian cancer (GOG 0239), treated women with recurrent measurable disease with single agent selumetinib (AZD6244) until progression of disease or intolerable toxicity. Patients had a median of three prior lines of chemotherapy. The study showed a promising objective response rate of 15%. No correlation was found between presence of *KRAS* or *BRAF* mutation and response to therapy; however, sufficient DNA was available for analysis in only 34/52 (65%) of evaluable patients [3].

Subsequently, two randomized phase III studies were performed comparing use of single-agent MEK inhibitor to standard of care, in patients with recurrent measurable low-grade serous ovarian cancer [4,5]. The GOG 0281 phase II/III study of the MEK inhibitor trametinib versus physician's choice of chemotherapy or endocrine therapy in patients with recurrent disease and unlimited prior lines of chemotherapy found a significant difference in median progression-free survival (PFS) with trametinib (13 months) versus physician's choice of chemotherapy (7.2 months; HR=0.48; p<0.001). The overall response rate (ORR) was 26% and 6.2% for trametinib and physician's choice, respectively (p < 0.0001) [4]. The MILO/ENGOT-ov11 study was a phase III study of the MEK inhibitor binimetinib versus physician's choice of chemotherapy in patients with recurrent low-grade serous ovarian cancer and up to three prior lines of chemotherapy. Although the study was discontinued early based on an interim analysis revealing that the PFS hazard ratio crossed the predefined futility boundary, an updated analysis indicated a median PFS of 10.4 months for binimetinib versus 11.5 months for physician's choice (HR=1.15; p=0.748), and an ORR of 24% in both arms of the study. Notably, for patients treated with binimetinib, the ORR and median PFS in the *KRAS* mutant group (ORR=44%; median PFS=17.7 months) were significantly better than in the *KRAS* wild-type group (ORR=19%; median PFS=10.8 months) (p=.006) [5] indicating that patients with *KRAS* mutation may be most likely to respond to MEK inhibitor treatment.

Based on the above results, trametinib is now National Comprehensive Cancer Network (NCCN) compendium listed for the treatment of recurrent low-grade serous ovarian cancer, and combination studies seeking to further enhance efficacy both for MEK inhibitor-naïve patients, and for patients following progression on MEK inhibition, are ongoing. While MEK inhibitors have shown clear efficacy in the treatment of recurrent low-grade serous ovarian cancer, these agents also cause considerable toxicity, with rash, diarrhea, edema, and ocular toxicity all commonly observed. In many cases, these toxicities are most pronounced within the first three months of starting treatment and can be more significant than the toxicities most frequently seen with chemotherapy, bevacizumab, or endocrine therapies. These associated toxicities can lead to dose interruptions and dose reductions, causing decreased dose intensity that translates into a missed opportunity for optimal response and control of disease. MEK inhibitors are therefore best administered early in the disease course, at time of first relapse, when patients generally have the best performance status and are most likely to be able to tolerate continuous therapy without dose reduction.

A particular concern in patients with recurrent low-grade serous ovarian cancer is the risk of small bowel or large bowel obstruction, as this is frequently a consequence of progressive disease. All of the currently Food and Drug Administration (FDA)-approved MEK inhibitors (trametinib, binimetinib, and cobimetinib) are oral drugs which require gastrointestinal absorption. Unfortunately, patients with progressive disease and bowel obstruction are not candidates for oral MEK inhibitors but can benefit from infusional chemotherapy and certain endocrine therapies such as fulvestrant. It is therefore important to give patients the opportunity to receive a MEK inhibitor earlier in their disease course before progressive symptoms may eliminate this option.

In making treatment decisions for patients, it is essential to perform somatic mutation testing at time of first recurrence or earlier, as the third of patients with *KRAS* mutations may derive the greatest benefit from treatment with MEK inhibitors, and should preferentially be treated with MEK inhibitors early in their disease course.

Conclusion

MEK inhibitors offer the best chance of response in the recurrent setting and should be considered for all patients with low-grade serous ovarian cancer at time of first recurrence. MEK inhibitors are associated with significant toxicity, which may result in dose reductions or early discontinuation of treatment in patients with multiple prior lines of therapy and more symptomatic disease. In addition, the need for oral administration may limit the ability to receive this important treatment in later line settings where patients are more likely to develop obstructive complications. Therefore, it is imperative to evaluate patients for potential treatment with MEK inhibitors at time of their first recurrence.

References

1. Grisham RN, et al. Extreme outlier analysis identifies occult mitogen-activated protein kinase pathway mutations in patients with low-grade serous ovarian cancer. *J Clin Oncol* 2015;33(34):4099–4105.

2. Grisham RN, et al. BRAF mutation is associated with early stage disease and improved outcome in patients with low-grade serous ovarian cancer. *Cancer* 2012;119(3):548–554.

3. Farley J, et al. Selumetinib in women with recurrent low-grade serous carcinoma of the ovary or peritoneum: an open-label, single-arm, phase 2 study. *Lancet Oncol* 2013;14(2):134–140.

4. Gershenson DM, et al. A randomized phase II/III study to assess the efficacy of trametinib in patients with recurrent or progressive low-grade serous ovarian or peritoneal cancer. *Ann Oncol* 2019;30(Suppl. 5):v851–v934.

5. Monk BJ, et al. MILO/ENGOT-ov11: binimetinib versus physician's choice chemotherapy in recurrent or persistent low-grade serous carcinomas of the ovary, fallopian tube, or primary peritoneum. *J Clin Oncol* 2020;2020:JCO2001164.

Is MEK Inhibitor Therapy the Best Treatment Recommendation for Low-Grade Serous Ovarian Cancer Patients at First Relapse?

No

David M. Gershenson

Debate

Low-grade serous carcinoma of the ovary/peritoneum (LGSOC) is a rare ovarian cancer characterized by younger age at diagnosis, relative chemoresistance, and prolonged overall survival compared to high-grade serous carcinoma. Like high-grade serous carcinoma, however, it is most frequently diagnosed in advanced stages, and over 70% of women relapse. The mitogen-activated protein kinase (MAPK) pathway plays a major role in the pathogenesis of LGSOC, with frequent mutations of *KRAS*, *NRAS*, and *BRAF*.

Early studies consistently indicated that LGSOC is relatively chemoresistant in the adjuvant, neoadjuvant, and recurrent settings – clearly signaling the need for novel therapies [1]. Once MEK inhibitors – orally bioavailable, non-ATP competitive, small molecule inhibitors of MEK 1/2 – were developed, it was natural to study them in LGSOC based on its biology. To date, three clinical trials of MEK inhibitors for recurrent LGSOC have been completed – two fully published and the third published only in abstract form thus far. In a phase II trial of selumetinib in recurrent LGSOC, the response rate was 15%; another 65% of patients had stable disease [2]. The median progression-free survival (PFS) was 11.0 months. However, there was no correlation between presence of *KRAS* or *BRAF* mutation in tumor tissue and objective response. The MEK inhibitor in low-grade serous ovarian cancer (MILO)/ENGOT-ov11 trial was a randomized trial of binimetinib versus physician's choice of chemotherapy (pegylated liposomal doxorubicin (PLD), weekly paclitaxel, or topotecan) in 341 patients [3]. Although the study was closed early based on interim analysis that revealed the PFS hazard ratio had crossed the predefined futility boundary, the updated response rate was 24% in both arms of the study, and the median PFS was 10.4 months for binimetinib versus 11.5 months for the chemotherapy arm (HR=1.15; p=0.748). Additionally, the response rate and median PFS in the *KRAS* mutant group were significantly better than in the *KRAS* wild-type group (response rate=44% vs. 19%; median PFS=17.7 months vs. 10.8 months). GOG 0281 was a phase II/III randomized trial of trametinib versus standard of care (physician's choice of one of five drugs – pegylated liposomal doxorubicin (PLD), weekly paclitaxel, topotecan, letrozole, and tamoxifen) in 260 women [4]. This trial was successful in meeting its primary end point, with a median PFS of 13.0 months versus 7.2 months for trametinib and standard of care, respectively (HR=0.48; p<0.001) as well as a better response rate for trametinib – 26% versus 6.2% (p<0.0001).

Mutational analysis associated with this trial is pending. The difference in the outcomes of the two latter trials is likely due in part to an unexpected higher response rate in the chemotherapy arm of MILO related to the lower number of prior regimens compared to the GOG 0281 trial.

Thus, MEK inhibitors clearly have demonstrated promising activity against recurrent LGSOC. However, they can be somewhat difficult to manage, especially for the neophyte, related to potential side effects. The most common side effects are skin rash, fatigue, gastrointestinal side effects, anemia, and hypertension. Rarer but potentially serious side effects include pneumonitis, retinal vein occlusion, and decreased ejection fraction or left ventricular dysfunction. In fact, in the MILO trial, 31% of women had adverse effects serious enough to lead to permanent discontinuation of binimetinib. In GOG 0281, the permanent discontinuation rate was 35%.

Since the majority of women with stage II–IV LGSOC will require salvage therapy at some point in their clinical course, comprehensive counseling regarding various treatments is essential. The good news is that there are several options. However, there is no standard of care related to precise sequencing of therapeutics in the recurrent setting. Options for treatment at first relapse include clinical trials, endocrine therapies (aromatase inhibitors, tamoxifen, fulvestrant, and leuprolide acetate), chemotherapy (platinum-based, pegylated liposomal doxorubicin, gemcitabine/cisplatin, weekly paclitaxel, topotecan, etc.), bevacizumab, and targeted agents (usually either MEK inhibitors or BRAF inhibitors).

Conclusion

The choice of therapy for first relapse of LGSOC – the focus of this debate – is based on several key factors, including type of primary therapy, efficacy and side effects of standard regimens, availability of clinical trials, and patient preferences. If a clinical trial is available, that is this author's preference. Off protocol, while a MEK inhibitor is an attractive option and should be included in discussion with the patient, it is not necessarily the first choice. This opinion is based on its therapeutic index relative to other options. First, not all women with relapse of LGSOC have received endocrine therapy – either monotherapy or maintenance therapy following chemotherapy – as part of their primary treatment. In such a case, the author's priority recommendation is an aromatase inhibitor. If aromatase inhibitor therapy has been included in a patient's primary therapy, then the author generally prioritizes initial options for first relapse, in no particular order, to platinum-based chemotherapy (especially if they have either never received it or if they are still platinum-sensitive), pegylated liposomal doxorubicin (PLD), bevacizumab-containing regimens (e.g., PLD/bevacizumab), or trametinib. For instance, the author will often recommend PLD at first relapse and consider trametinib at the time of second relapse. In the MILO trial, in which 42% of patients had received only one prior systemic regimen, the updated response rates for binimetinib and chemotherapy were both 24%. And, as noted, the permanent discontinuation rate of binimetinib was 31%. GOG 0281 included patients who were significantly more heavily pre-treated, with only 23% of patients receiving one prior line of systemic therapy. As noted, the response rate to trametinib and the median PFS were significantly better compared to the control arm. Is trametinib simply a more potent MEK inhibitor than binimetinib or does it really matter when in the course of treating recurrent LGSOC a MEK inhibitor is employed? There may be one caveat in choosing a regimen for first LGSOC relapse, and that is related to genomic profiling results. If a patient has a mutation in the

MAPK pathway, especially if a *KRAS* mutation, based on the preliminary findings of the MILO trial, should a MEK inhibitor be more seriously considered as the drug of choice for first relapse? The author believes that further study is required to answer this question.

References

1. Slomovitz B, et al. Low-grade serous ovarian cancer: state of the science. *Gynecol Oncol* 2020;156:715–725.

2. Farley J, et al. Selumetinib in women with recurrent low-grade serous carcinoma of the ovary or peritoneum: an open-label single-arm, phase 2 study. *Lancet Oncol* 2013;14:134–140.

3. Monk BJ, et al. MILO/ENGOT-ov11: binimetinib versus physician's choice chemotherapy in recurrent or persistent low-grade serous carcinomas of the ovary, fallopian tube, or primary peritoneum. *J Clin Oncol* 2020;38(32):3753–3762.

4. Gershenson DM, et al. A randomized phase II/III study to assess the efficacy of trametinib in patients with recurrent or progressive low-grade serous ovarian or peritoneal cancer. *Ann Oncol* 2019;30(Suppl. 5):v851–v934.

Should Stage IC Mucinous Ovarian Carcinoma be Managed by Observation or Adjuvant Chemotherapy?

Observation

Jason D. Wright[1]

Debate

Mucinous carcinomas of the ovary are a rare histologic subtype that account for approximately 3% of all newly diagnosed epithelial ovarian carcinomas [1]. Compared to serous carcinomas, mucinous tumors are more commonly diagnosed in younger women and are much more likely to present as early-stage tumors that are confined to the ovary.

Survival rates for stage I mucinous carcinomas are similar to high-grade serous carcinomas. In a population-based dataset, five-year survival was 81.5% for stage I mucinous tumors compared to 80.8% for high-grade serous carcinomas. Ten-year survival for women with stage I mucinous tumors is 67.9%. In contrast, advanced stage mucinous tumors are associated with inferior survival compared to serous carcinomas. Among women with stage III–IV tumors, five-year survival is 18.4% for mucinous carcinomas compared to 24.0% for high-grade serous carcinomas [2]. Interestingly, the percentage of women with mucinous ovarian carcinomas diagnosed at an early-stage appears to be increasing. From 2000 to 2016, there was a 1.5-fold increase in the percentage of women with mucinous carcinomas identified with stage I tumors, increasing from 50.5% to 75.6% during the time period [2].

Historically, early-stage mucinous carcinomas of the ovary have been treated in a similar manner to other histologic subtypes of epithelial ovarian cancer. For women with stage IC tumors, treatment would typically include surgical resection followed by adjuvant platinum- and taxane-based chemotherapy. However, there is growing recognition that individualized management of mucinous carcinomas may be warranted. In particular, evidence suggests that observation may be appropriate for stage IC mucinous ovarian carcinomas. First, the biologic underpinnings of mucinous carcinomas differ significantly from serous carcinomas and other epithelial ovarian tumors. Unlike serous tumors, mucinous tumors frequently harbor *KRAS* mutations which are identified in 40–65% of these neoplasms [1]. This mutational profile is similar to colorectal cancers. Second, mucinous carcinomas are poorly responsive to chemotherapy. Reviews of reports of women with ovarian cancer treated with first-line, platinum-based chemotherapy have consistently shown that response rates in women with mucinous tumors are much lower than in women with serous carcinomas, with response rates of 13–60% versus 64–87%, respectively [1]. The poor

---

[1] Dr. Wright has served as a consultant for Clovis Oncology and received research support from Merck.

response rates to platinum-based chemotherapy and biologic similarity of mucinous ovarian carcinomas to colorectal tumors has led many to advocate for treatment with 5-fluorouracil and gastrointestinal chemotherapy regimens when chemotherapy is utilized. Finally, data from large cohort studies and subgroup analyses from prospective trials have suggested that chemotherapy is not associated with improved survival for women with stage I mucinous ovarian carcinomas [3,4].

Prospective trials examining the value of adjuvant chemotherapy for women with stage IC mucinous carcinomas are largely lacking. A combined analysis of the International Collaborative Ovarian Neoplasm Trial 1 (ICON1) and Adjuvant ChemoTherapy in Ovarian Neoplasm Trial (ACTION) which randomized women with apparent early-stage ovarian cancer to either platinum-based adjuvant chemotherapy or observation included 180 women with mucinous ovarian carcinomas. Although this cohort included women with a wide variety of stages, it found no statistically significant association with use of adjuvant chemotherapy and overall survival [5].

Observational data and data from population-based tumor registries have also failed to demonstrate a benefit for chemotherapy for women with stage I mucinous ovarian carcinoma [3,4]. In an analysis of 4811 women with stage I mucinous ovarian carcinoma recorded in the National Cancer Data Base, adjuvant chemotherapy was utilized in 20.2% of women with stage IA/IB tumors and in 60.2% of those with stage IC neoplasms. Use of chemotherapy was relatively stable over time. Within this cohort there was no association between chemotherapy use and survival for any patients with stage I neoplasms. For women with stage IA and IB tumors, five-year overall survival was 90.5% for women who did not receive chemotherapy compared to 88.1% for those who received chemotherapy. Similarly, for patients with stage IC carcinomas, five-year overall survival was 85.1% for women who had observation compared to 85.6% in those treated with adjuvant chemotherapy. These results were unchanged when stratified by tumor grade. In a sensitivity analysis including only patients who underwent lymphadenectomy (at least ten nodes removed) to exclude women with occult stage III disease the investigators also noted no beneficial effect of chemotherapy. In the cohort of women with stage IC tumors who underwent lymphadenectomy, five-year overall survival was 89.4% in patients who did not receive chemotherapy compared to 88.8% in those treated with chemotherapy [4].

Matsuo and colleagues performed a similar analysis using the National Cancer Data Base of women with stage IC mucinous carcinomas. The overall findings were similar, with no benefit in survival for chemotherapy. The investigators performed a rigorous series of sub-group analyses and confirmed that there was a lack of survival benefit for adjuvant chemotherapy regardless of age, tumor grade, stage IC sub-stage, or performance of lymphadenectomy. These investigators also performed a confirmatory analysis using population-based data from the National Cancer Institute's Surveillance, Epidemiology, and End Results database. Again, there was no association between adjuvant chemotherapy use and survival. In the validation cohort, adjuvant chemotherapy had no impact on seven-year cancer-specific survival (84.6% for chemotherapy vs. 88.3% for observation) or seven-year overall survival (77.1% for chemotherapy vs. 77.1% for observation) [3].

Conclusion

Improved understanding of the biology and natural history of mucinous ovarian carcinomas has led to changes in treatment recommendations for women with early-stage mucinous tumors. The National Comprehensive Cancer Network (NCCN) now considers either observation or systemic chemotherapy as appropriate for women with stage IC mucinous ovarian carcinomas [6]. Further, for those women treated with systemic therapy, either a platinum and taxane-based therapy or a gastrointestinal regimen including 5-fluorouracil/leucovorin and oxaliplatin or capecitabine/oxaliplatin are considered appropriate [6]. In sum, given the lack of data supporting chemotherapy for women with stage IC mucinous ovarian carcinomas, observation appears to be warranted in the majority of women.

References

1. Morice P, et al. Mucinous ovarian carcinoma. *N Engl J Med* 2019;380:1256–1266.

2. Matsuo K, et al. Evolving population-based statistics for rare epithelial ovarian cancers. *Gynecol Oncol* 2020;157:3–11.

3. Matsuo K, et al. Effectiveness of postoperative chemotherapy for stage IC mucinous ovarian cancer. *Gynecol Oncol* 2019;154:505–515.

4. Nasioudis D, et al. Adjuvant chemotherapy is not associated with a survival benefit for patients with early-stage mucinous ovarian carcinoma. *Gynecol Oncol* 2019;154:302–307.

5. Trimbos JB, et al. International Collaborative Ovarian Neoplasm trial 1 and Adjuvant ChemoTherapy In Ovarian Neoplasm trial: two parallel randomized phase III trials of adjuvant chemotherapy in patients with early-stage ovarian carcinoma. *J Natl Cancer Inst* 2003;95:105–112.

6. National Comprehensive Cancer Network. Ovarian Cancer Including Fallopian Tube and Primary Peritoneal Cancer. Version 2.2021. Available from: www.nccn.org/professionals/physician_gls/pdf/ovarian.pdf

Should Stage IC Mucinous Ovarian Carcinoma be Managed by Observation or Adjuvant Chemotherapy?

Adjuvant Chemotherapy

Yien Ning Sophia Wong and Jonathan A. Ledermann

Debate

Mucinous ovarian carcinomas (MOCs) are a rare subtype of epithelial ovarian cancer accounting for less than 10% of all epithelial ovarian cancers. Improvements in diagnosis have suggested that the incidence has been overestimated and the true incidence is less than 5% [1]. Adjuvant chemotherapy studies have included mucinous tumors and other less common types of epithelial ovarian cancers together with high-grade serous tumors, the most common subtype.

Sixty-five to eighty percent of mucinous ovarian cancers are diagnosed at an early stage and have an excellent prognosis compared to early-stage serous cancers. The standard treatment approach for stage I MOC is surgery and based upon the surgical and pathological staging, further adjuvant treatment may be needed. The International Federation of Gynecology and Obstetrics (FIGO) staging classification, last updated in 2018, defined substages of stage I ovarian cancers that are confined to the ovaries. In particular, tumor rupture – intraoperative (IC1) or preoperative (IC2), surface involvement by tumor cells or presence of malignant cells in the ascites or peritoneal washings (IC3) are the subcategories of stage IC [1]. Tumor rupture, whether intraoperative or preoperative, may become a risk factor for recurrence, regardless of the presence or absence of surface invasion, because it has the possibility of seeding recurrence in the peritoneal cavity. In the case of a large cystic mucinous tumor, preoperative or intraoperative rupture is a real possibility and contributes to the decision regarding the role of adjuvant chemotherapy to eliminate microscopic cells and prevent their further growth leading to recurrence of the disease.

There are few prospective large-scale randomized controlled trials (RCTs) comparing chemotherapy to observation in stage I ovarian cancers. The International Collaborative Ovarian Neoplasm 1 (ICON1) and EORTC-Adjuvant ChemoTherapy In Ovarian Neoplasm (ACTION) trials, together recruited over 900 patients who had surgery for early-stage ovarian cancer. Patients were randomly assigned to receive platinum-based adjuvant chemotherapy or observation until chemotherapy was indicated. This demonstrated that patients who received chemotherapy had an improved five-year overall survival (OS) with a hazard ratio (HR) of 0.67 (95% CI: 0.50–0.90; p=0.008), as well as an improved five-year recurrence-free survival with a HR of 0.64 (95% CI: 0.50–0.82; p=.001) [2]. It is worth noting that nearly 20% of patients (n=180) had a mucinous tumor. Although confidence intervals were wide for all subgroups, the HR in favor of chemotherapy for mucinous tumors was no less favorable than any of the other subgroups, including the serous subtype [2].

Currently, several guidelines worldwide recommend all patients with high-risk early-stage epithelial ovarian cancer should receive adjuvant chemotherapy, regardless of histology. However, it is worth noting that only a fraction of patients with MOCs were included in these large clinical trials. For example, only 7% of patients had MOCs in ICON3, which assessed the addition of paclitaxel to carboplatin-based chemotherapy; while only 2–6% of patients had MOCs in recent studies such as ICON7 and GOG 218, which assessed the addition of bevacizumab to standard carboplatin and paclitaxel chemotherapy [1]. Therefore, whilst robust RCTs are lacking to guide the management of MOCs, this "one-size-fits-all" approach is obsolete and is not evidence based.

Given that MOCs are distinctly different biologically and clinically compared to the other epithelial histological subtypes, it is crucial to evaluate MOCs as a separate entity. Several studies have shown that advanced MOCs respond poorly to platinum and taxane chemotherapy and have a worse prognosis to other histologies, in part due to inherent platinum resistance [1]. Large RCTs have used platinum-based chemotherapy as the backbone treatment in epithelial ovarian cancer, making it more difficult to ascertain the true benefit of chemotherapy in patients with early-stage MOCs. Interestingly, MOCs share many similarities with gastrointestinal (GI) adenocarcinomas and there is preclinical evidence to support a GI-based approach in the management of this unique group, with platinum-resistant in vitro and in vivo models exhibiting responses to 5-FU and oxaliplatin [1].

In one of the largest retrospective studies, Richardson and colleagues [3] looked at over 2000 patients from the National Cancer Database from 2004 to 2014 with stage I MOCs, including 1362 (67%) with stage IA/IB disease, 598 (29%) with stage IC disease, and 81 (4%) with stage I disease not otherwise specified. A total of 737 patients (36%) received adjuvant chemotherapy in this cohort. A nomogram was used to stratify between low- and high-risk groups which included age, stage, presence of lympho-vascular invasion, malignant ascites and grade. Patients with a score of higher than 93 were put into a high-risk group. Whilst there was no difference in survival in the low-risk group with or without adjuvant chemotherapy, the authors found that in the high-risk patients (n=405), chemotherapy was associated with an improvement in ten-year OS of 23% (74% vs. 51%). Patients in the high-risk group not treated with adjuvant chemotherapy had a 58% increased risk of death (HR=1.58, 95% CI: 1.05–2.38, p=0.03) and worse survival relative to those treated with adjuvant chemotherapy. The likelihood ratio test showed an interaction between higher patient risk score and increasing survival benefit from chemotherapy (p=0.02).

In contrast, another large database study from the United States that included patients with stage I mucinous ovarian cancer did not show a survival benefit associated with chemotherapy, regardless of the substage of disease [4,5]. However, when compared to Richardson et al.'s study, these analyses only reported five-year rather than ten-year survival data, and did not consider any prognostic index that might guide clinicians in deciding who may benefit from chemotherapy. The type of chemotherapy may impact on survival and none of these large database studies reported which chemotherapy regimens were used.

Conclusion

Taken together, there is evidence for the use of adjuvant chemotherapy in stage IC MOCs, particularly in those in a high-risk group. Continued national and international collaborative efforts are needed to collect high-quality data and to conduct meaningful clinical trials to find better treatments that will help guide clinicians to improve the outcome of this unique subset of patients.

References

1. Crane EK, et al. Early stage mucinous ovarian cancer: a review. *Gynecol Oncol* 2018;149(3):598–604.

2. Trimbos JB, et al. International Collaborative Ovarian Neoplasm trial 1 and Adjuvant ChemoTherapy In Ovarian Neoplasm trial: two parallel randomized phase III trials of adjuvant chemotherapy in patients with early-stage ovarian carcinoma. *J Natl Cancer Inst* 2003;95(2):105–112.

3. Richardson MT, et al. Long-term survival outcomes of stage I mucinous ovarian cancer – A clinical calculator predictive of chemotherapy benefit. *Gynecol Oncol* 2020;159(1):118–128.

4. Nasioudis D, et al. Adjuvant chemotherapy is not associated with a survival benefit for patients with early stage mucinous ovarian carcinoma. *Gynecol Oncol* 2019;154(2):302–307.

5. Matsuo K, et al. Effectiveness of postoperative chemotherapy for stage IC mucinous ovarian cancer. *Gynecol Oncol* 2019;154(3):505–515.

9A How Many Cycles of Adjuvant Chemotherapy Should be Administered to Patients with High-risk Stage I Epithelial Ovarian Cancer?

Three Cycles

Annalisa Garbi, Eleonora Zaccarelli, and Federica Tomao

Debate

High-risk stage I ovarian cancer (OC) encompass clear cell and grade 3 tumors according to European Society of Medical Oncology-European Society of Gynaecological Oncology (ESMO–ESGO) consensus conference recommendations [1]. Carboplatin in monotherapy for six cycles or the combination of carboplatin and paclitaxel for a minimum of three cycles are available options for adjuvant treatment adhering to ESMO–ESGO guidelines [1].

A Cochrane systematic review evaluated the role of adjuvant chemotherapy for early-stage tumors, demonstrating that platinum-based chemotherapy after an optimal staging surgery is effective in significantly prolonging long-term overall survival (OS) and progression-free survival (PFS) [2].

Particularly, a long-term survival update from the two most important randomized clinical trials (ICON1 and ACTION) included in the meta-analysis described a benefit in terms of OS (HR=0.67, 95% CI: 0.50–0.90; p=.008) and in terms of recurrence-free survival (RFS) (HR=0.64, 95% CI: 0.50–0.82; p=.001) for women considered at high-risk of recurrence (stage IA grade 3, IB, or IC, grade 2 or 3, any clear cell tumors and un-optimally staged tumours) who received chemotherapy. The chemotherapy administered in the ICON1 and ACTION trials consisted of a variety of platinum-based regimens with heterogynous number of cycles, thus being inconclusive to establish the optimal duration of treatment.

Scientific evidence comparing three versus six cycles are limited to retrospective analysis and few data are available from prospective studies about the comparison of monotherapy versus combination regimen and shorter versus longer treatment.

GOG-157 clinical trial randomized patients with early-stage tumors to receive three versus six cycles of adjuvant chemotherapy with carboplatin and paclitaxel administered every three weeks [3]. This study found that longer treatment was not associated with a significant reduction in recurrence risk (HR for PFS adjusted for stage and grade: 0.76, 95% CI: 0.512–1.13, p=0.19; HR for OS: 1.02, 95% CI: 0.662–1.57, p=0.9), but resulted in significant increased toxicity (neurotoxicity, granulocytopenia, and anemia). A post-hoc analysis of the same trial (GOG 157) [4] revealed that longer adjuvant therapy was associated with a significant reduction in recurrence risk for serous tumors, but not for nonserous tumors, suggesting that three cycles of chemotherapy could be considered to treat nonserous tumors.

Prendergast et al. retrospectively compared six versus three cycles of adjuvant platinum-based chemotherapy with or without taxane in early-stage ovarian clear cell carcinoma with 90% receiving combination therapy. The longer treatment was not associated to survival benefit. Subgroup analysis of surgically staged patients also showed no difference in survival between three versus six cycles of chemotherapy [5].

Conclusion

In conclusion, on the basis of these data, three cycles of carboplatin plus paclitaxel represents an effective strategy to reduce the probability of recurrence in high-risk early-stage OC patients, especially in nonserous tumors. Notably, three cycles compared with six cycles of carboplatin and paclitaxel do not significantly alter the recurrence rate in high-risk OC, but six cycles are associated with more toxicity.

Nevertheless, further studies are needed to better define the duration of treatment. Moreover, in the era of personalized medicine, molecular characteristics of tumors could help in the therapeutic decision-making process. Finally, the advent of genomic characterization is continuously changing our knowledge about peculiarities and differences among single histotype that might influence the response to standard medical treatment. This would make adjuvant treatment personalized in terms of duration and schedule, according to molecular characteristics.

References

1. Colombo N, et al. ESMO-ESGO Ovarian Cancer Consensus Conference Working Group. ESMO-ESGO consensus conference recommendations on ovarian cancer: pathology and molecular biology, early and advanced stages, borderline tumours and recurrent disease. *Ann Oncol* 2019;30 (5):672–705.

2. Lawrie TA, et al. Adjuvant (post-surgery) chemotherapy for early stage epithelial ovarian cancer. *Cochrane Database Syst Rev* 2015;12:CD004706.

3. Bell J, et al. Randomized phase III trial of three versus six cycles of adjuvant carboplatin and paclitaxel in early stage epithelial ovarian carcinoma: a Gynecologic Oncology Group study. *Gynecol Oncol* 2006;102:432–439.

4. Chan JK, et al. The potential benefit of 6 vs. 3 cycles of chemotherapy in subsets of women with early-stage high-risk epithelial ovarian cancer: an exploratory analysis of a Gynecologic Oncology Group study. *Gynecol Oncol* 2010;116:301–306.

5. Prendergast H, et al, Three versus six cycles of adjuvant platinum-based chemotherapy in early stage clear cell ovarian carcinoma – A multi-institutional cohort. *Gynecol Oncol* 2017;144:274–278.

Debate

How Many Cycles of Adjuvant Chemotherapy Should be Administered to Patients with High-risk Stage I Epithelial Ovarian Cancer?

Six Cycles

John K. Chan and Daniel S. Kapp

Debate

Early-stage Ovarian Cancer Treatment Indications and Controversies

Based on a systematic review of clinical trials, chemotherapy is currently recommended in all early stages of disease after surgical staging except those with stage IA–B, grade 2 disease [1]. However, the number of cycles of adjuvant chemotherapy remains controversial.

Prospective Randomized Trial: Interpretations and Statistical Considerations

The Gynecologic Oncology Group conducted a randomized phase III trial of three versus six cycles of adjuvant carboplatin and paclitaxel in early-stage epithelial ovarian carcinoma. Of 427 patients with surgically staged IA grade 3, IB grade 3, clear cell, IC and completely resected stage II disease, it was reported that "the recurrence rate for 6 cycles was 24% *lower* (hazard ratio [HR]: 0.761; 95% confidence interval [CI]: 0.51–1.13, p=0.18), and the estimated probability of recurrence within 5 years was 20.1% (6 cycles) versus 25.4% (3 cycles)" [2]. It was concluded that "compared to 3 cycles, 6 cycles of [chemotherapy] do not *significantly* alter the recurrence rate." The statistical design of GOG-157 aimed to achieve an 85% chance of finding that the additional three cycles regimen as active if it decreased the recurrence rate by 50%. It is likely that the power analysis in this trial design may have been overly optimistic [3].

Exploratory Analysis Results

An exploratory analysis was performed to identify any subgroups of patients within the GOG-157 trial who might have benefited from six cycles of treatment [4]. The results demonstrated that those with serous tumors had a significantly higher recurrence-free survival after six versus three cycles (82.7% vs. 60.4%). However, no significant improvements in recurrence-free survival (RFS) were noted in those with nonserous cancers. Statisticians caution clinical researchers on the perils of subset analyses to guide treatment;

in particular they warn of dangers in reporting on a lack of benefit in subgroups in a clinical trial showing an overall benefit. On the other hand, it is unclear if there is more validity in subset analysis demonstrating a benefit in a subgroup of patients in an overall negative clinical trial as shown in this current exploratory analysis. Obviously, the results of this current study are based on an exploratory analysis, and only a randomized clinical trial comparing three versus six cycles of chemotherapy in serous ovarian cancer patients can definitively confirm these preliminary findings. However, with the knowledge that it is not feasible to conduct a randomized trial on uncommon diseases such as that in early-stage epithelial ovarian cancer, clinicians are compelled to make decisions based on limited scientific evidence. It is then important to carefully consider these options for each individual patient, weighing the potential risk of toxicities and consequence of recurrence.

Consequences of Recurrent Early-stage Cancer

It is important to avoid under treatment of women with early-stage high-risk ovarian cancer who have a high likelihood of cure. In fact, the survival after recurrence of early-stage disease is poor and comparable to those with recurrent advanced-stage disease; both with a median survival of only 24 months [5]. Thus, as oncologists, we have an important role in helping patients to make sound decisions and to ensure that they feel comfortable that they made the best possible choice to avoid future decisional regret or remorse.

Toxicity of Six Cycles Compared to Three Cycles?

It was clear that compared to three cycles, those who had six cycles of chemotherapy had significantly higher grade 3 and 4 neurotoxicity (2% vs. 11%) and grade 4 granulocytopenia (52% vs. 66%). Nevertheless, the additional treatment did not result in any worsening of thrombocytopenia, gastrointestinal, renal, alopecia, ototoxicity, infection, fever, allergy, or myalgia. Although there were no formal studies on the patient-reported outcome, it is unlikely that the additional three cycles of chemotherapy significantly affected their overall quality of life.

Consensus Guidelines and Adoption of Early-stage Disease in Ovarian Cancer Trials

Based on the results seen in advanced disease, platinum-based chemotherapy has been adopted for use in early-stage disease. Accepted practice in the UK NICE 2011 clinical guideline on ovarian cancer states that adjuvant chemotherapy with six cycles of adjuvant chemotherapy should be offered to women with stage IC disease or more. Other countries including Canada (Alberta consensus) and the United States (NCCN guidelines) have also recommended a minimum of three cycles and up to six cycles, particularly in those with serous histology.

Clinical Evidence of Advantages of Six Cycles of Treatment and Beyond in Advanced Disease

Over the last few years, a number of clinical trials in advanced ovarian cancer have demonstrated a significant advantage of extended treatment with maintenance therapy using anti-vascular or Poly (ADP-ribose) polymerase inhibition for up to three years.

Clearly, it is not our intent to adopt maintenance strategies in early-stage disease, but it is important to highlight the trends in treatment and maintenance of advanced cancer and the potential implications toward more cycles or maintenance strategies, possibly in stage II high-risk disease.

Adoption of Cycles in Real World and Future Clinical Trials

Since early-stage ovarian cancer trials may not feasible due to low accrual and lack statistical power in design, most cooperative groups have included high-risk early ovarian cancer patients in the phase III randomized trials in advanced ovarian cancer. For example, clinical trial researchers have incorporated these high-risk early-stage ovarian cancer patients into advanced-stage cancer trials with regimens that contain six cycles of chemotherapy. This strategy has been adopted by the U.S. NRG Gynecologic Oncology Group (GOG-261 – stage I–IV carcinosarcoma of uterus or ovary) and in Europe, Gynaecological Cancer Intergroup (GCIG) trial, Arbeitsgemeinschaft für Gynäkologische Onkologie (AGO) OVAR-9, and the GCIG-EORTC trials.

Conclusion

Recognizing that it is important to individualize treatment based on risk factors and the tolerance of therapy, we advise administration of paclitaxel plus carboplatin for six cycles for all early-stage ovarian cancer patients.

References

1. Lawrie TA, et al. Adjuvant (post-surgery) chemotherapy for early stage epithelial ovarian cancer. *Cochrane Database Syst Rev* 2015;;2015(12):CD004706. https://doi.org/10.1002/14651858.CD004706.pub5

2. Bell J, et al. Gynecologic Oncology Group. Randomized phase III trial of three versus six cycles of adjuvant carboplatin and paclitaxel in early stage epithelial ovarian carcinoma: a Gynecologic Oncology Group study. *Gynecol Oncol* 2006;102(3):432–439. https://doi.org/10.1016/j.ygyno.2006.06.013

3. Vergote I, et al. Treatment of patients with early epithelial ovarian cancer. *Curr Opin Oncol* 2003;15(6):452–455. https://doi.org/10.1097/00001622-200311000-00008

4. Chan JK, et al. The potential benefit of 6 vs. 3 cycles of chemotherapy in subsets of women with early-stage high-risk epithelial ovarian cancer: an exploratory analysis of a Gynecologic Oncology Group study. *Gynecol Oncol* 2010;116(3):301–306. https://doi.org/10.1016/j.ygyno.2009.10.073

5. Chan JK, et al. Survival after recurrence in early-stage high-risk epithelial ovarian cancer: a Gynecologic Oncology Group study. *Gynecol Oncol* 2010;116(3):307–311. https://doi.org/10.1016/j.ygyno.2009.10.074

10A Patients with Advanced Ovarian Cancer who are 75 Years Old and Above Should Routinely be Treated with Neoadjuvant Chemotherapy?

Yes

Michelle Davis and Ursula Matulonis

Debate

A combination of surgical cytoreduction and chemotherapy has been the foundation of treatment for newly diagnosed advanced-stage ovarian cancer since the 1930s. However, elderly patients remain at risk for undertreatment of advanced ovarian cancer. United States national registry studies have demonstrated that elderly women with ovarian cancer are less likely to complete combination therapy because of their inability to tolerate therapy or medical complications of receiving that therapy. Approximately 20% of patients with ovarian cancer are above 75 years of age. The probability of dying from ovarian cancer increases with increasing age; however, some studies suggest that when elderly women receive optimal therapy, outcomes are equivalent to younger counterparts. The question remains, how to ensure optimal therapy and best manage women with ovarian cancer over the age of 75?

While it is agreed upon that complete cytoreduction to no visible disease (i.e., R0) as well as six cycles of platinum- and taxane-based chemotherapy is the preferred treatment for newly diagnosed advanced-stage ovarian cancer, the optimal sequencing of treatment has been debated. To date, there have been three multi-center international randomized controlled trials (RCTs) (EORTC-GCG, CHORUS, JCOG 0602) and two international single institution RCTs (the Scorpion trial and Chekman et al.) comparing primary cytoreductive surgery (PCS) followed by platinum-based chemotherapy to neoadjuvant chemotherapy (NACT) with interval cytoreductive surgery. All these studies showed equivalency of PCS versus NACT. The TRUST trial which included only surgical centers with high rates (>50%) of complete cytoreduction is awaiting results. In a Cochrane review which evaluated 1952 articles, a meta-analysis was performed with the five above RCTs. In a pooled analysis of 1713 patients, there was no difference in progression-free survival (PFS) (HR=1.02, 95% CI: 0.92–1.13) or overall survival (OS) (HR=1.06; 95% CI: 0.94–1.19) between NACT and PCS [1]. Surgical morbidity and quality-of-life outcomes were reported inconsistently; however, pooled data from available studies show a significant reduction in serious advance events (SAE) grade 3+ with NACT, most prominently, infection. Perhaps most importantly, there was a reduction in 30-day mortality in all five RCTs reported at 0.4% (NACT) versus 3.1% in PCS (RR=0.18;

95% CI: 0.06–0.54) [1]. This equates to 31 deaths per 1000 patients with PCS compared to six per 1000 patients following interval cytoreduction surgery. While some observational studies have favored PCS, these data remain limited by selection bias. The highest level of evidence to date suggests equivalent oncologic outcomes with PCS and NACT with a reduction in perioperative morbidity and mortality with NACT.

There are no randomized trials that address the role for NACT versus PCS specifically in an elderly patient population. Of the available RCTs, only two include patients above75 years of age, and the SCORPION trial specifically excluded patients over 75 years. In a subgroup analysis by age, there was no difference in OS for patients 70 years or above (20% with PCS vs. 18% for NACT) with similar rate of receipt of both surgery and chemotherapy [1]. In a study by Melamed et al., comparing regions with high adoption of NACT to low adoption regions as controls, adoption of NACT led to a reduction in mortality at three years over time compared to no change in mortality among low-adopter regions [2]. In regions where NACT increased, there was a reduction in 30- and 90-day mortality as well as a higher rate of receipt of both surgery and chemotherapy [2]. In another paper by the same group, older age was a significant factor associated with increased utilization of NACT. This suggests that triaging higher risk, elderly patients to NACT can reduce morbidity and improve rates of optimal therapy which may explain the benefit of NACT in these data, more reflective of true practice.

For an elderly patient population, consideration of co-morbidities and treatment-related SAEs is critical to minimize harm. Thrall et al. evaluated 30-day postoperative mortality from the Surveillance Epidemiology, End Results (SEER) database in ovarian cancer patients over the age of 65 (just under half of patients were above 75 years of age) [3]. Each increasing year of age was associated with a 7.5% increased risk of 30-day mortality (95% CI: 1.06–1.10). Patients who received NACT had a 70% lower 30-day postoperative mortality compared to PCS (1.8% vs. 6.1%, p<0.001) and in the adjusted model this remained significant (RR=0.37, 95% CI: 0.17–0.83) [3]. They concluded that all women age 75+ with stage IV disease and women age 75+ with Stage III disease and a Charleson Comorbidity Index score of 1+ comprised the highest risk group with a 12.7% average 30-day mortality. Several tools have sought to predict treatment morbidity in the elderly; however, no clear superior tool has emerged [4]. Neither the Preoperative Assessment of Cancer in the Elderly (PACE) study evaluating patients with solid tumors nor NRG CC-002 evaluating patients above70 years of age with ovarian cancer found an association between preoperative assessment tools and major postoperative complications. However, a single institution retrospective study utilizing the frailty index (FI) did demonstrate an association between frailty and postoperative morbidity and mortality [5]. It is unclear in this study the percentage of patients above 75 years of age that were considered frail, but there is a statistically significant increase in age (mean 67.8 years) among frail patients and age remains an independent predictor of mortality [5]. While frailty is an important area of ongoing investigation, increasing age, consistently across studies, is predictive of increased morbidity and mortality with treatment.

Conclusion

Based on these data, all patients over the age of 75 with a single medical co-morbidity are at high risk for treatment morbidity and the highest risk for postoperative death. Treatment with NACT can minimize these risks without compromising oncologic outcomes based on randomized clinical trial data. In the treatment of women above 75 years of age with ovarian cancer, the goal should be to maximize receipt of optimal therapy while minimizing SAEs, to which they are more susceptible. Patients with advanced ovarian cancer who are 75 years old and older should routinely be treated with NACT.

References

1. Coleridge SL, et al. Chemotherapy versus surgery for initial treatment in advanced ovarian epithelial cancer. *Cochrane Database Syst Rev* 2019;10:CD005343. https://doi.org/10.1002/14651858.CD005343.pub4

2. Melamed A, et al. Effect of adoption of neoadjuvant chemotherapy for advanced ovarian cancer on all-cause mortality: quasi-experimental study. *Br Med J* 2018;360:5463.

3. Thrall MM, et al. Thirty-day mortality after primary cytoreductive surgery for advanced ovarian cancer in the elderly. *Obstet Gynecol* 2011;118(3):537–547. https://doi.org/10.1097/AOG.0b013e31822a6d56

4. Tew W. Ovarian cancer in the older woman. *J Geriatr Oncol* 2016;7(5):354–361.

5. Kumar A, et al. Functional not chronologic age: frailty index predicts outcomes in advanced ovarian cancer. *Gynecol Oncol* 2017;147(1):104–109.

10B Patients with Advanced Ovarian Cancer who are 75 Years Old and Above Should Routinely be Treated with Neoadjuvant Chemotherapy?

No

Olga T. Filippova and William P. Tew

Debate

When choosing between primary debulking surgery (PDS) or neoadjuvant chemotherapy (NACT) for upfront treatment of women with advanced-stage ovarian cancer, we must balance two opposing approaches. On one hand is the "optimize survival" approach, with all four large randomized studies – CHORUS, EORTC 55971, SCORPION, and JGOG 0602 – showing the longest survival in women treated with PDS in whom complete gross resection was achieved [1,2]. On the other hand is the "do minimal harm" view, as it is well known that NACT followed by interval debulking surgery systematically leads to fewer postoperative complications [1,2]. Therefore, the real question that should be posed is how do we safely maximize the number of women above 75 years of age who are treated with PDS, thus allowing them the survival benefit, without undue morbidity. Instead of an "all or nothing" approach, we propose the following ways to select appropriate PDS candidates, and reserve NACT for those not meeting these criteria.

First and foremost, we must stop using chronological age alone for selection of upfront treatment, and instead must transition to evaluating a patient's functional age. Not only is ageism a source of significant bias, many studies have shown that age alone is a poor predictor of a patient's physiologic reserve. Several reliable, objective, and easy-to-use tools for accessing function have been introduced, and should be used for all women, not just patients ≥75 years of age. Frailty is defined as a decrease in physiologic reserve beyond that expected with aging alone. While the geriatric assessment continues to be the most comprehensive evaluation of frailty and the gold standard supported by international societies, several frailty indices are available with similar predictive value and can be easily incorporated into daily clinical practice [3]. With the use of these tools, we propose that all women identified as vulnerable, regardless of age, should routinely be treated with NACT.

We must also not forget that older women, especially vulnerable women, are commonly not included in randomized trials, making it difficult to extrapolate the findings of these studies to the older cohort. While both CHORUS and EORTC 55971 did not have age restrictions and included octogenarians, they are a minority of the cohort and their outcomes were not reported separately [1]. Additionally, it is not possible to judge the functional status of older, or any, women included in these two studies. On the other hand, the two most recent trials, SCORPION and JGOG 0602, had an upper age cut-off at 75 years [1,2]. Since JGOG 0602 was the first trial that was not able to demonstrate the noninferiority of NACT [2], we do not know if the lack of this noninferiority holds in the older population. We must not take the lack of data as evidence of a lack of benefit. All eyes are now on the International Trial on Radical Upfront Surgery in Advanced Ovarian Cancer (TRUST), which not only includes all women 18 and older, but focuses on surgical quality. We must also acknowledge that the optimal chemotherapy regimen for older women is yet to be determined. EWOC-1, a trial investigating single-agent carboplatin, and carboplatin with either weekly or every three-week paclitaxel in women 70 or older, was closed early, as the survival of the carboplatin-only arm was found to be significantly worse [4]. GOG 273 aimed at evaluating chemotherapy tolerance based on pre-treatment instrumental activities of daily living, and showed that performance status was not as good a predictor as functional status [5]. These two studies are a step in the right direction toward evaluating our "standard" treatments in the vulnerable and frail population.

The question of PDS versus NACT must be discussed in the setting of the latest developments for the treatment of ovarian cancer. Novel therapeutics, such as vascular endothelial growth factor (VEGF) and poly (ADP-ribose) polymerase (PARP) inhibitors, have been developed for use in the postoperative or maintenance phase of treatment. While the use of bevacizumab is common in the NACT setting in Europe, it is not approved for this indication in the United States. All novel therapies must be studied in the older population to determine benefit, and more importantly, tolerance.

Conclusion

In summary, we believe that it is time to stop framing the question as "PDS vs. NACT" and instead start focusing on how to identify and safely maximize the number of women treated with PDS during which optimal or complete resection is achieved, resulting in the longest survival, as well as how to identify women in whom the morbidity of PDS is too high and thus NACT is the better upfront approach. NACT should only be the approach in those unfit for PDS or those with truly unresectable disease, not just older women. Just because a treatment is not inferior does not mean it is superior. An "all or nothing" approach is never the best answer, especially in the older, commonly more vulnerable, population.

References

1. Long Roche K, et al. Practical guidelines for trial to neoadjuvant chemotherapy in advanced ovarian cancer: big risk, big reward . . . or too much risk? *Gynecol Oncol* 2020;157:561–562.

2. Onda T, et al. Comparison or survival between primary debulking surgery and neoadjuvant chemotherapy for stage III/IV ovarian, tubal and peritoneal cancers in phase III randomized trial. *Eur J Cancer* 2020;130:114–125.

3. Wright AA, et al. Neoadjuvant chemotherapy for newly diagnosed, advanced ovarian cancer: Society of Gynecologic Oncology and American Society of Clinical Oncology Clinical Practice Guideline. *Gynecol Oncol* 2016;143:3–15.

4. Falandry C, et al. EWOC-1: a randomized trial to evaluate the feasibility of three different first-line chemotherapy regimens for vulnerable elderly with ovarian cancer (OC): a GCIG-ENGOT-GINECO study. *J Clin Oncol* 2019;37S:ASCO #5508.

5. von Gruenigen VE, et al. Chemotherapy completion in elderly women with ovarian, primary peritoneal or fallopian tube cancer – an NRG oncology/Gynecologic Oncology Group study. *Gynecol Oncol* 2017;144(3):459–467.

11A

Should an Attempt at Aggressive Cytoreduction be Made for all Surgical Candidates with Advanced Ovarian Cancer prior to Treatment with Adjuvant Chemotherapy?

Yes

Sven Mahner, Anca Chelariu-Raicu,
and Fabian Trillsch

Debate

The extent of residual disease following upfront cytoreductive surgery for stage III–IV ovarian cancer is one of the strongest prognostic factors for progression-free and overall survival. Currently, there are two approaches proposed in order to achieve minimal residual disease: primary debulking surgery (PDS) and neoadjuvant chemotherapy (NACT) followed by interval debulking surgery. In the last decade, the field has developed a greater understanding of both approaches and more importantly, several prospective randomized trials were designed to address the question of which patients are most or least likely to benefit from primary debulking surgery versus neoadjuvant chemotherapy.

In this context, two randomized controlled trials showed that neoadjuvant chemotherapy followed by interval cytoreductive surgery can be a suitable therapeutic approach in patients with comorbidities and high tumor burden, especially when full cytoreductive surgery is not feasible. While there is general consensus regarding the group of patients who will be triaged directly for palliative chemotherapy, there is still debate over the remaining surgical candidates, including the patients with whom complete gross resection can be achieved and patients who will be left with residual tumor. Our objective here is to state the rationale for PDS as the primary treatment in this heterogeneous group of surgical candidates with advanced ovarian cancer. To demonstrate our perspective, we will discuss topics such as the surgical management, systemic therapy, and the biology of ovarian cancer.

It is widely accepted that the maximal surgical effort towards complete gross resection yields the best clinical outcome [1]. In specialized gynecologic cancer centers, the rate of macroscopic complete resection ranges from 50% to 70% [2]. Contrarily, some studies have reported a rate of less than 20% [3], with factors such as patient selection or lack of surgical qualification or infrastructure potentially contributing to the low resection rate. In this context, intraoperative findings preventing complete resection in some cancer centers, including diffuse carcinomatosis, tumor involvement of the pancreas or the truncus celiacus, or central or multisegmental liver metastasis, are not reliably diagnosed before surgery. Therefore, complete resection in these patients could be impaired by a lack of expertise in more sophisticated surgical techniques such as diaphragmatic stripping, splenectomy, distal pancreatectomy, resection of porta hepatis, or partial liver resection.

Clear evidence is available demonstrating that ovarian cancer is a disease with distinct molecular abnormalities, including *TP53, BRCA1/2,* and mutations in homologous recombination [4]. Furthermore, others have observed that recurring tumors have substantial heterogeneity due to multiple spontaneous genetic and epigenetic events. This dynamic tumor phenotype results in emerging drug resistance in almost every patient, even though some of these patients initially responded to the platinum-based chemotherapy. One explanation might be that the initial response of ovarian cancer to chemotherapy initiates clonal selection of resistant cells to platinum or other therapies. These cellular events might result in the reduced overall survival of 45.2% in patients with residual tumors greater than 10 mm in diameter compared to 65.8% in patients who underwent complete resection or a debulking surgery with a residual tumor of less than 10 mm in diameter [1].

In contrast to other solid tumors being treated with NACT, ovarian cancer still remains a disease best treated by upfront surgery, especially since patients receiving NACT rarely respond completely. Furthermore, previous studies clearly show a benefit in patients after treatment with PDS followed by chemotherapy. One large retrospective meta-analysis suggested that early initiation of first-line chemotherapy following surgical resection might improve overall survival [5]. Given the purpose of removing as much tumor as possible in order to augment the effectiveness of subsequent chemotherapy and maintenance, changing the treatment sequence by introducing NACT before surgery for patients with advanced ovarian cancer calls previous studies into question [1, 5]. Furthermore, a subgroup of patients diagnosed with advanced-stage ovarian cancer are usually symptomatic with very large masses, and may have a partial bowel obstruction. Therefore, these patients require immediate attention, so that front-line NACT would be not appropriate due to the required interval for the chemotherapy to be effective.

Conclusion

In summary, several aspects favor upfront cytoreduction. First, the complexity of cytoreductive surgery performed for ovarian cancer plays an important role in achieving complete resection. Since patients receiving NACT rarely respond completely and the molecular heterogeneity of ovarian cancer might play a role in drug resistance, systemic therapy is likely to be more effective in surgically debulked, chemotherapy-naïve patients. Therefore, the treatment sequence including primary cytoreductive surgery followed by early induction of chemotherapy might augment the effectiveness of chemotherapy. In the scenario of interval debulking surgery, given the fact that patients rarely attain pathologic complete response after NACT, its effectiveness might potentially be affected by the high tumor burden, since most patients are primarily diagnosed with advanced-stage ovarian cancer. Taken together, there is a strong rationale to support primary debulking for all surgical patients with advanced ovarian cancer. Nevertheless, the group of women triaged to be suitable for surgery is sometimes overestimated and the procedure is then abandoned due to intraoperative complications or technical issues preventing resection. Despite advanced radiologic images, it is still not possible to reliably preoperatively predict which patients will fall into this class.

To address these observations, an international collaboration of expert surgical centers for ovarian cancer initiated the prospectively randomized TRUST trial (NCT02828618), designed to evaluate the caliber of PDS as well as its relative benefit versus NACT [6]. In contrast with previous trials, the TRUST trial includes rigorous criteria in selecting patients with operable disease and on the other hand focuses on high volume centers with proven high complete resection rates at upfront debulking surgery for patient recruitment. In addition, this study will perform a systematic collection of biomaterials for translational research, to potentially identify markers to select patients for either PDS or NACT. The trial completed recruitment in 2019, is expected to report results in 2024, and may define the standard of care in regards to the optimal timing of primary debulking surgery in ovarian cancer.

References

1. du Bois A, et al. Role of surgical outcome as prognostic factor in advanced epithelial ovarian cancer: a combined exploratory analysis of 3 prospectively randomized phase 3 multicenter trials: by the Arbeitsgemeinschaft Gynaekologische Onkologie Studiengruppe Ovarialkarzinom (AGO-OVAR) and the Groupe d'Investigateurs Nationaux Pour les Etudes des Cancers de l'Ovaire (GINECO). *Cancer* 2009;115(6):1234–1244.

2. Woelber L, et al. Perioperative morbidity and outcome of secondary cytoreduction for recurrent epithelial ovarian cancer. *Eur J Surg Oncol* 2010;36 (6):583–588.

3. Vergote I, et al. Neoadjuvant chemotherapy versus debulking surgery in advanced tubo-ovarian cancers: pooled analysis of individual patient data from the EORTC 55971 and CHORUS trials. *Lancet Oncol* 2018;19(12):1680–1687.

4. Cancer Genome Atlas Research. Integrated genomic analyses of ovarian carcinoma. *Nature* 2011;474 (7353):609–615.

5. Mahner S, et al. Prognostic impact of the time interval between surgery and chemotherapy in advanced ovarian cancer: analysis of prospective randomised phase III trials. *Eur J Cancer* 2013;49(1):142–149.

6. Reuss A, et al. TRUST: Trial of Radical Upfront Surgical Therapy in advanced ovarian cancer (ENGOT ov33/AGO-OVAR OP7). *Int J Gynecol Cancer* 2019;29(8):1327–1331.

11B

Should an Attempt at Aggressive Cytoreduction be Made for all Surgical Candidates with Advanced Ovarian Cancer prior to Treatment with Adjuvant Chemotherapy?

No

Sean Kehoe and Jason Yap

Debate

Primary cytoreductive surgery [PCS] in ovarian cancer is an important therapeutic strategy. In early-stage disease, excision of all disease is relatively uncomplicated and affords cure for many patients, which is further increased in selected patients by the addition of adjuvant chemotherapy. However, in advanced disease, particularly in FIGO stage IIIC and IV, the surgical goal of PCS remains excision of all visible disease, but may require more extensive surgical procedures, such as splenectomy; bowel and liver resection; and diaphragmatic stripping. The average age at diagnosis of women with ovarian cancer is 65 years, and at least a quarter of those are over 75-year-olds. Naturally, underlying medical co-morbidities increase with age; rendering many patients unsuitable for extensive surgery and even those selected may experience a protected period of postoperative recovery, delaying commencement of chemotherapy with potential impact on outcome [1]. Recently, one center which achieves high rates of macroscopic clearance at primary surgery, reported that 17% of the patients initially deemed suitable for primary surgery were in fact operated on after Neo-Adjuvant ChemoTherapy (NACT) [2]. Hence, despite with the best of intentions, stating "attempt at aggressive cytoreduction should be made for all surgical candidates with advanced ovarian cancer prior to treatment with adjuvant chemotherapy," the reality is different.

The role of PCS and NACT in advanced ovarian cancer has generated widespread discussion and predictably divided opinion. Focusing on the two pivotal randomized controlled trials (RCTs), the findings were that both PCS and NACT had similar survival outcomes, but morbidities significantly reduced in NACT [3,4]. However, advocates of PCS were quick to unpick the potential bias in these RCTs, namely that the studies recruited a bias study population; there was a lack of standardization in surgical skills;

and that NACT is associated with more "resistant disease," rendering surgery more difficult. The "bias study population" is interesting. Arguably, patients who agree to become involved in trials are to some extent subjected to "self- selection bias." Taken to its logical conclusion, trials are "inherently biased" as patients in trials rarely reflect all patients treated in the health service, and, thus, let's abandon trials altogether! A more recent example of rebuttal of a trial that challenged "standard care" is the Laparoscopic Approach to Cervical Cancer (LACC) study for early cervical cancer where rebuttals occurred even before peer-reviewed publication [5]. Nevertheless, when the outcomes of the clinical trials befit the practice already deemed "standard of care," these studies often go unchallenged.

A major issue with debates on PCS versus NACT is the inability to "fight fire with fire." If an RCT is the evidence base, then ideally this should be refuted or challenged by evidence from another RCT. But such studies are unavailable, so there is an element of imbalance in the debate. However, finally the first attempt at a prospective RCT has commenced exploring the value of PCS in advanced ovarian cancer, the TRUST trial, which aims to standardize the surgical component of the study, and the results are keenly awaited. But remember in the TRUST trial – it is likely not all those recruited will totally reflect the entire population of women with advanced ovarian cancer.

We now recognize the complexities of the disease called "ovarian cancer" or maybe it is more accurate to say: what we believed in the past as correct is now proven wrong. It is now accepted that most, if not all, high-grade serous carcinomas arise from the distal end of the fallopian tubes, which has major implications for screening and detecting earlier stage disease. Mucinous tumors, once deemed common, have been shown to be mainly metastatic from the gastro-intestinal tract. We categorize diseases into type 1 and 2, the latter more chemo-sensitive, more mutational aberrations, and more aggressive in nature. Equally, evidence continues to accumulate on the mutational heterogeneity of high-grade serous cancers, depending where the biopsy is taken. These evolutionary advances in knowledge are welcomed and permit exploration of potential novel therapeutic strategies. But the important point is that in advanced disease, a single approach as suggested in the title seems somewhat simplistic when dealing with such a complex disease.

Conclusion

So where are we now? It is time to consider cessation of the debate and focus on other matters. Irrespective of the outcomes in the TRUST trial, we need systems to identify the preferable primary therapy for each patient – which could be either PCS or NACT or some novel approaches for others, rather than "a one size fits all" approach. We should endeavor to avoid "open and close" operations and identify those where, following long extensive surgery and chemotherapy, relapse early after completion of treatment – and develop alternative therapeutic strategies. Do we need to reconsider our chemotherapeutic approach – do all patients require six cycles of chemotherapy – should it be less or more? Should treatment strategies be switched after three cycles in those patients with limited response? Or should the circulating cells or tumor mutational profiles guide treatment? Research in this and other areas is required, as the reality remains that few patients with advanced disease achieve a "cure," as defined by surviving ten years from diagnosis.

A final thought, what would have happened if by some statistical quirk the two trials had shown that PCS was preferable to NACT? Could it be possible that the studies would have been hailed as excellent, unbiased, well-constructed and with the appropriate patient group? A thought for reflection?

References

1. Gemma Searle, et al. Prolonged interruption of chemotherapy in patients undergoing delayed debulking surgery for advanced high-grade serous ovarian cancer is associated with a worse prognosis. *Gynecol Oncol* 2020;158(1):54–58. https://doi.org/10.1016/j.ygyno.2020.04.048

2. Straubhar AM, et al. A multimodality triage algorithm to improve cytoreductive outcomes in patients undergoing primary debulking surgery for advanced ovarian cancer: a Memorial Sloan Kettering Cancer Center team ovary initiative. *Gynecol Oncol* 2020;158(3):608–613.

3. Vergote I, et al. European Organization for Research and Treatment of Cancer-Gynaecological Cancer Group; NCIC Clinical Trials Group. Neoadjuvant chemotherapy or primary surgery in stage IIIC or IV ovarian cancer. *N Engl J Med* 2010;363(10):943–953.

4. Kehoe S, et al. Primary chemotherapy versus primary surgery for newly diagnosed advanced ovarian cancer (CHORUS): an open-label, randomized, controlled, non-inferiority trial. *Lancet* 2015;386 (9990):249–257.

5. Ramirez PT, et al. Minimally invasive versus abdominal radical hysterectomy for cervical cancer. *N Engl J Med* 2018;379 (20):1895–1904. https://doi.org/10.1056/NEJMoa1806395

Should Minimally Invasive Modalities be Routinely/Uniformly Utilized for Assessment of Resectability prior to Attempted Primary Debulking in Patients with Advanced Ovarian Cancer?

Yes

Juliet E. Wolford and Robert E. Bristow

Debate

Ovarian cancer, though not the most common gynecologic malignancy, remains the deadliest. The lethality attributed to its aggressive nature, nondescript symptomatology, and absence of effective screening, has resulted in 85% of the population diagnosed at an advanced stage with widespread disease at time of presentation. Standard treatment for advanced ovarian cancer is a complete or a "so-called" optimal cytoreductive surgery (no gross versus <1 cm of residual disease) followed by a platinum-based chemotherapy doublet, except in those patients where it is thought that a primary cytoreductive surgery would not be possible. In these patients there is determined to be a high risk of perioperative morbidity and mortality based on functional status, preexisting medical co-morbidities, and/or the amount or location of disease burden limiting the ability to achieve a complete cytoreductive surgery. Those patients are given neoadjuvant chemotherapy with a plan to then proceed with an interval debulking surgery if there is a satisfactory response to chemotherapy. Often, the widespread extent of the disease is not known until the time of surgery, despite standard axial imaging. There have been numerous previous studies done to determine if standard CT imaging can predict feasibility of a primary optimal cytoreductive surgery but thus far, results have been inconsistent and as of yet there is no accurate standard in place for determining potential resectability. As a result, many gynecologic oncologists have adopted the use of diagnostic laparoscopy prior to deciding to proceed with an exploratory laparotomy in order to determine feasibility of cytoreduction. In newly diagnosed ovarian cancer patients where axial imaging is inconclusive for determining resectability potential, as it often is, we routinely perform diagnostic laparoscopy for several reasons. Although it adds time to the start of the case, it can spare patients from an invasive open procedure if they are deemed to not be able to undergo an optimal cytoreductive procedure. Thus, avoiding recovery from a procedure associated with more pain, a higher risk of infection, costlier hospital stays, and a potential cause of delay in starting chemotherapy which could have a significant impact on their overall survival.

In 2019, there was a Cochrane review analyzing the data to determine the accuracy of this exact question. At the time, there were 18 studies, evaluating a total of 1563 women who underwent laparoscopy to identify the feasibility of optimal cytoreductive surgery. They found across the included trials that 16–73% of patients on laparoscopic assessment were considered to have extensive disease excluding the attempt of an exploratory laparotomy. While the remaining patients who had been deemed as resectable by laparoscopy, 54–96% ultimately had a complete cytoreductive surgery to no gross residual disease and 69–100% had an optimal cytoreductive surgery with <1 cm of residual cancer at the conclusion of the case. Unfortunately, only two of the studies included laparotomy despite findings on laparoscopy (thus a reference standard) to provide data that could be analyzed for sensitivity or specificity, indicating verification bias of the other included studies. Importantly though, there were no false positives identified, in other words: there were no patients that were deemed unresectable by laparoscopic criteria and then were able to be completely or optimally debulked [1]. Accordingly, the authors suggested that diagnostic laparoscopy offers benefit to determining the extent of disease at the time of surgery.

The Cochrane analysis was unable to complete a meta-analysis as there was marked heterogeneity across trials. The two studies that included the reference standard were by Fagotti et al., which led to a laparoscopic scoring system in order to provide standardization [2,3]. The Fagotti system calculates a predictive index value (PIV) to estimate the achievability of optimal cytoreduction. The variables in this system include the presence of the following at the time of laparoscopy: peritoneal carcinomatosis, diaphragmatic carcinomatosis, mesenteric retraction, omental caking, gastric and/or bowel infiltration, and liver metastases. In a pilot study, it was found that a high score (greater than 8) was associated with prediction of a suboptimal cytoreductive procedure with a positive predictive value of 100% and a negative predicative value of 70% [4]. To validate the findings and to prove the reproducibility of the findings at other institutions, the Olympia-MITO13 trial was implemented to assess the applicability of the laparoscopic scoring algorithm across multiple institutions. The most difficult assessment to achieve on laparoscopy was mesenteric root retraction, but overall the study did find an accuracy rate of 80% or greater across the sites included for determining disease extent [5].

Conclusion

Laparoscopy has known limitations. It adds operative time; also, the surgeon is unable to completely visualize all areas of concern, which could limit ability to perform a complete or optimal cytoreductive surgery. Thus, there will still be patients that will have a laparotomy that may not be able to have a complete or optimal cytoreductive surgery once completely assessed open. However, we have concluded that with a step-wise, multimodal approach, the benefits outweigh the drawbacks of proceeding with laparoscopy. Patients should be assessed carefully for concerning symptomatology and functional status. Images should be reviewed thoroughly to assess if there are any clear indicators of an unsuccessful cytoreductive procedure, such as liver parenchymal disease, lung metastases, or obvious large tumor implants seen at the celiac axis or porta hepatis.

Once it is confirmed that the patient can proceed with an operative assessment, the procedure starts with a laparoscopic approach to determine disease extent. If the patient is deemed appropriate for laparotomy, at that time we proceed will a small (10 cm) incision to assess the abdomen and pelvis with palpation before proceeding with a full incision from xiphoid to pubis. Laparoscopy has minimal associated complications as compared to open laparotomy, with complications related to the initial access into the peritoneal cavity as being less than 1% [6].

In addition, there are many other known advantages to MIS approach versus laparotomy, such as decreases in hospital stay length, postoperative pain, wound infection rates, and healing time. Furthermore, at the time of laparoscopy, directed biopsies of tumor tissue can be obtained for a more definitive diagnosis and further somatic tumor testing. The time added with laparoscopy is minimal, often only 15–20 minutes. When you consider the addition of laparoscopy can spare patients from an open procedure with associated increased costs secondary to unnecessary hospital stays, as well as increased morbidity that could potentially delay the initiation of their neoadjuvant chemotherapy, we feel that the added time and potential need for further exploration are small disadvantages when considerable benefit is acheived.

References

1. Vrie Rvan de et al. Laparoscopy for diagnosing resectability of disease in women with advanced ovarian cancer. *Cochrane Database Syst Rev* 2019;3: CD009786. https://doi.org/10.1002/14651858.CD009786.pub3

2. Fagotti A, et al. Role of laparoscopy to assess the chance of optimal cytoreductive surgery in advanced ovarian cancer: a pilot study. *Gynecol Oncol* 2005;96(3):729–735. https://doi.org/10.1016/j.ygyno.2004.11.031

3. Fagotti A, et al. Prospective validation of a laparoscopic predictive model for optimal cytoreduction in advanced ovarian carcinoma. *Am J Obstet Gynecol* 2008;199(6):642.e1–642.e6. https://doi.org/10.1016/j.ajog.2008.06.052

4. Fagotti A, et al. A laparoscopy-based score to predict surgical outcome in patients with advanced ovarian carcinoma: a pilot study. *Ann Surg Oncol* 2006;13(8):1156–1161. https://doi.org/10.1245/ASO.2006.08.021

5. Fagotti A, et al. A multicentric trial (Olympia–MITO 13) on the accuracy of laparoscopy to assess peritoneal spread in ovarian cancer. *Am J Obstet Gynecol* 2013;209(5):462.e1–462.e11. https://doi.org/10.1016/j.ajog.2013.07.016

6. Jansen FW, et al. Complications of laparoscopy: an inquiry about closed- versus open-entry technique. *Am J Obstet Gynecol* 2004;190(3):634–638. https://doi.org/10.1016/j.ajog.2003.09.035

12B

Should Laparoscopic Modalities be Routinely Utilized for Assessment of Resectability prior to Attempted Primary Debulking in Patients with Advanced Ovarian Cancer?

No

Beverly Long and William A. Cliby

Debate

Routine laparoscopy is increasingly being used to assess resectability of ovarian cancer prior to laparotomy for primary debulking. Laparoscopic scoring algorithms are designed to triage patients to primary debulking surgery or neoadjuvant chemotherapy and reduce the number of unsuccessful primary debulking attempts. However, we do not recommend routine laparoscopy prior to debulking surgery for the following reasons: additional operative time and risk associated with laparoscopy, inaccuracy of laparoscopy compared to palpation, lack of validated or reproducible laparoscopic scoring algorithms, limited improvement compared to CT scan alone to predict suboptimal debulking, and excellent outcomes with the use of small laparotomy [1], CT scan, and careful patient selection.

Laparoscopy can immediately precede a planned laparotomy or be performed as a separate procedure. A separate procedure does provide final histologic results prior to laparotomy and may allow for more precise operating room planning. However, it also adds an additional anesthetic risk, a small but definite surgical risk, and a high risk of port-site implantation when done separately. When performed immediately prior to laparotomy, laparoscopy adds additional equipment and time to an already complex procedure. In a single institution study of one laparoscopic algorithm, laparoscopic assessment required a median of 37 minutes and was associated with a 2% risk of gastrointestinal trocar injury in addition to a lengthy debulking operation [2].

Notwithstanding, laparoscopy could be justified if laparoscopic assessment consistently prevented laparotomy in patients destined for suboptimal debulking. Laparoscopy is excellent for detection of miliary disease but is relatively fruitless for the common barriers to successful debulking. Lesser sac disease, upper abdominal lymphadenopathy, mesenteric involvement, and porta hepatis disease is not well characterized by laparoscopy and is better assessed by preoperative CT scan and intraoperative palpation. The findings of mesenteric retraction or bowel immobility are subjective and impossible to evaluate adequately in the setting of a large omental cake. In the prospective, multi-center Olympia-MITO 13 trial, mesenteric retraction was not evaluable in over 25% of cases [3]. Multiple studies also report adhesions and extensive disease as barriers to accurate laparoscopic assessment. In our experience, a small laparotomy is superior to laparoscopy, as it allows palpation of areas that may be difficult or impossible to access laparoscopically, such as the root of the mesentery, celiac axis, porta hepatis, lesser sac, pelvis, and spleen with lower risk of viscus injury or port site metastases

Scoring algorithms have been developed to standardize laparoscopic assessment. The scoring system published by Fagotti et al. is the most widely used [3]. However, by using scoring systems that are additive rather than exclusionary, most laparoscopic algorithms inappropriately equate "surgical resectability" with "surgical complexity." For instance, mesenteric retraction (disease at the root of the mesentery or extensive mesenteric disease) typically precludes optimal cytoreduction even in the absence of other scoring criteria. Still, in the Fagotti algorithm this factor is given equal weight to other findings, including liver surface implants, stomach infiltration, diaphragmatic carcinomatosis, and omental cake, which while adding operative time and requiring specialized expertise, are not barriers to successful debulking. While a high score correlates with increased surgical complexity, it should not preclude primary debulking surgery in a fit surgical candidate. With appropriate patient selection, aggressive debulking procedures can be safely performed and are associated with higher rates of optimal cytoreduction and ovarian cancer survival. Because laparoscopic scoring algorithms do not account for patient factors, they may not be valid for fit patients who would tolerate complex surgery and may not be useful for frail patients who would benefit from neoadjuvant chemotherapy and a less complex procedure.

Laparoscopic scoring algorithms cannot account for varying levels of surgical experience and resources among gynecologic oncologists. Data from the Mayo Clinic demonstrated higher disease-specific survival in patients whose surgeons more frequently performed radical procedures. Chi et al. reported higher rates of optimal debulking when extensive upper abdominal procedures were systematically incorporated into their department's surgical approach. Because thresholds for resectability vary by surgeon, institution, and time period, laparoscopic algorithms are impossible to widely validate or standardize. While one could argue laparoscopy could be used to triage patients to centers of excellence, there does not appear to be enthusiasm for that.

Most importantly, laparoscopic assessment may not improve sensitivity for sub-optimal debulking compared to a preoperative CT scan. Laparoscopy cannot replace preoperative imaging, since parenchymal liver metastases, pleural metastases, and upper abdominal lymphadenopathy cannot be assessed laparoscopically and may significantly alter the treatment approach. Some CT findings may rule out optimal debulking without the need for surgery. Multiple CT-based algorithms have been developed to predict suboptimal or incomplete cytoreduction preoperatively. Many of these models compare favorably to the Fagotti score, predicting incomplete cytoreduction with an accuracy of 65–75%. A CT-based model proposed by the group at Memorial Sloan Kettering to predict gross residual disease was recently validated by the Mayo clinic and further reduces the value of laparoscopy [4].

Despite advances in preoperative imaging, surgical exploration will always play a role in assessment of resectability. Intraoperative palpation through a small laparotomy incision overcomes most of the challenges associated with laparoscopic scoring. In a European study, resectability assessment via mini-laparotomy demonstrated improved positive predictive value (89% vs. 60%) and equivalent negative predictive value (both 100%) compared to a Fagotti score cut-off ≥8. Median time from incision to complete assessment was only 10 minutes [1], and this method carries a lower risk of aborted debulking and port site implants. This approach, combined with a novel, evidence-based triage algorithm, produced excellent surgical and long-term outcomes in a recent study from the Mayo Clinic. This suggests that a multi-modality approach, incorporating patient performance status, nutrition status, CT findings, and intraoperative assessment, can predict optimal cytoreduction without undue surgical morbidity [5]. The fact that routine laparoscopy was not performed in this cohort demonstrates that superior outcomes can be achieved without the use of laparoscopy.

Conclusion

In summary, patient selection for ovarian cancer surgery is complex and requires consideration of multiple patient, surgeon, and disease-related factors. In our experience, routine laparoscopy is not the optimal method to assess resectability of ovarian cancer due to the need for additional operating room time and equipment, inability to assess common barriers to optimal debulking, poor sensitivity and reproducibility, and little to no improvement over CT scan alone. A multi-modality approach can appropriately triage patients without the need for routine laparoscopy.

References

1. Sircar S, et al. Mini-laparotomy in advanced ovarian cancer. *Gynecol Surg* 2011;9:179–183.

2. Fleming N, et al. Laparoscopic algorithm to triage the timing of tumor reductive surgery in advanced ovarian cancer. *Obstet Gynecol* 2018;132(3):545–554.

3. Fagotti A, et al. A multicentric trial (Olympia-MITO 13) on the accuracy of laparoscopy to assess peritoneal spread in ovarian cancer. *Am J Obstet Gynecol* 2013;209(5):462.e1–462.e11.90

4. Kumar A, et al. Models to predict outcomes after primary debulking surgery: independent validation of models to predict suboptimal cytoreduction and gross residual disease. *Gynecol Oncol* 2019;154 (1):72–76.

5. Narasimhulu DM, et al. Using an evidence-based triage algorithm to reduce 90-day mortality after primary debulking surgery for advanced epithelial ovarian cancer. *Gynecol Oncol* 2019;155 (1):58–62.

Should Enlarged Supradiaphragmatic Lymph Nodes be Routinely Removed during Debulking Surgery Procedures for Patients with Advanced Ovarian Cancer?

Yes

Annalisa Garbi and Vanna Zanagnolo

Debate

The goal of advanced ovarian cancer treatment is the achievement of a complete cytoreduction. Although the ideal timing of debulking surgery (primary vs. interval) is still under discussion, its primary aim is to remove all the macroscopically visible disease, since a complete cytoreduction is significantly associated with a better prognosis. According to the European Society of Gynaecological Oncology (ESGO) and to the American Society of Clinical Oncology (ASCO), an optimal cytoreduction is considered as no residual disease or microscopic residual disease. For this reason, increasingly complex procedures including the debulking of the upper abdomen have been implemented to achieve this goal. The positive impact of no residual disease has been observed even in patients with stage IV disease who would benefit from debulking surgery, requiring extensive upper abdominal procedures, if no or small residual is obtained [1].

Involvement of cardiophrenic lymph nodes (CPLNs), that qualifies as stage IVB disease, is quite common in advanced ovarian cancer and it is has been reported between 11–62% at preoperative CT scan. Cardiophrenic lymph nodes, also known as paracardiac or supradiaphgramatic lymph nodes, are located just above the diaphragm, and are easily reached when the diaphragm is opened. Enlarged CPLNs could be predictive of massive diaphragmatic involvement, however they are not a contraindication to the attempt of cytoreductive surgery. The presence of pathological enlarged CPLNs is usually related to a worst prognosis and the presence of an extensive abdominal tumor burden. Furthermore, CPLNs' involvement predicts the presence of carcinomatosis of the upper abdomen in more than 90% of cases, and is associated with a reduced chance of a complete optimal abdominal surgical debulking [2]. Why should they be removed? Several surgical techniques have been described to remove CPLNs including video-assisted thoracoscopic surgery (VATS), subxiphoid, and transdiaphragmatic approaches. When performed by experienced surgeons in high-volume oncology centers, removal of CPLNs has been demonstrated feasible with no significant increase of surgical time and blood loss [3]. Postoperative surgical morbidity associated with CPLN removal has been reported as negligible or low and most likely related to diaphragmatic surgery than to the dissection of the CPLNs themselves [3]. Moreover, adding this procedure does not delay adjuvant chemotherapy [3]. The most frequent complication, in accordance to procedure involving the diaphragm, is an asymptomatic pleural effusion detected on postoperative imaging. CPLN removal in the case of absence of diaphragmatic involvement is controversial. However, it should be considered that in such an instance it would require only a small diaphragmatic incision and it's likely associated with much fewer complications compared to a procedure requiring a large diaphragmatic resection.

No consensus exists on the dimension cut-off to define enlarged CPLNs. Different criteria have been proposed starting from 5 mm in short axis (ESUR guidelines). Others suggested the 7 mm cut-off and even, more than 10 mm has been considered. The removal and histological evaluation of "enlarged" CPLNs will help define the best radiological cut-off. Moreover, such a finding could confirm the predictivity of diaphragmatic involvement also in patients with no evidence of disease at preoperative CT scan, and therefore the need of more extensive upper abdominal procedures in a potentially frail population. Literature data of patients with FIGO stage III ovarian cancer with enlarged CPLNs at preoperative imaging (CT scan or PET) show a significantly lower rate of optimal debulking surgery, a shorter disease-free interval, and worse overall survival (OS). Therefore, the presence (only radiological findings, not removed) of abnormal CPLNs appears to have a significant negative impact on OS, mostly, in patients with no gross residual disease (NGR) in the abdomen. The median OS of women with abnormal CPLNs (not removed) and NGR was similar to patients who had abdominal residual disease, losing the benefit of optimal abdominal surgery. Accordingly, in a recent study, Luger et al. confirmed that enlarged (not removed) CPLNs had a prognostic relevance for PFS (HR=2.02, 95% CI: 1.14–3.55, p=0.015) and OS (HR=2.46, IQR=1.54–3.93; p=0.0001); nonetheless these patients still benefit from complete intraabdominal tumor debulking in terms of PFS (HR=0.60, 95% CI: 0.38–0.94) and OS (HR=0.59, 95% CI: 0.35–0.82) [2]. The therapeutic role of resection of enlarged CPLNs is not clear yet. A recent study did not demonstrate a significant impact on survival of metastatic CPLNs removal. Nevertheless, these data are retrospective and with a low number of cases. A large multicentric series should be advocated if a prospective randomized trial is not feasible [4]. The presence of preoperative enlarged CPLNs left in place at the time of surgery has been associated with an increased risk of recurrence (81.5% in CPLNs positive vs. 57,4% in CPLNs negative); specifically with an increased risk of thoracic recurrence (CPLN, pleura, parenchyma) therefore limiting treatment options [5]. It can be argued that having left the CPLNs in place may have affected the pattern of relapse and therefore it could be seen as a factor in favor of their removal.

Conclusion

In conclusion, it is still unclear whether removal of suspicious CPLNs will improve the oncological outcomes when NGR is obtained, however, given the minimal surgical effort and the related low morbidity of such a procedure, that makes it feasible and safe, it seems reasonable to be implemented when indicated.

References

1. Ataseven B, et al. Impact of abdominal wall metastases on prognosis in epithelial ovarian cancer. *Int J Gynecol Cancer* 2016;26:1594–1600.

2. Luger AK, et al. Enlarged cardiophrenic lymph nodes predict disease involvement of the upper abdomen and the outcome of primary surgical debulking in advanced ovarian cancer. *Acta Obstet Gynecol Scand* 2020;99(8):1092–1099.

3. Cowan RA, et al. Feasibility, safety and clinical outcomes of cardiophrenic lymph node resection in advanced ovarian cancer. *Gynecol Oncol* 2017;147 (2):262–266.

4. Prader S, et al. Pattern and impact of metastatic cardiophrenic lymph nodes in advanced epithelial ovarian cancer. *Gynecol Oncol* 2019;152(1):76–81.

5. Larish A, et al. Recurrence patterns in=patients with abnormal cardiophrenic lymph nodes at ovarian cancer diagnosis. *Int J Gynecol Cancer* 2020;30(4):504–508.

13B

Should Enlarged Supradiaphragmatic Lymph Nodes be Routinely Removed during Debulking Surgery Procedures for Patients with Advanced Ovarian Cancer?

No

Javier F. Magrina, Kristina Butler, and Paul Magtibay

Debate

Background

Because complete abdominal cytoreduction improved survival in advanced epithelial ovarian carcinoma (EOC), there was great interest generated in evaluating whether complete extra-abdominal debulking, such as enlarged supradiaphragmatic nodes (ESDN), resulted in improved survival. Evidence suggests removal of ESDN at primary debulking does not improve survival [1–5].

Incidence, Sites, and Size of Enlarged Supradiaphragmatic Nodes

There is no agreement to what constitutes ESDN. We know ESDN are common in stage IIIC [1–3], but incidence varies according to the selected size and imaging modality. The detection rate is almost double with positron emission tomography (PET) (67–76%) [1,3,4] as compared to computed tomography (CT) (33–43%) [1,2]. Using a cut-off >10 mm on the short axis eliminates many patients with metabolically active nodes on PET because most are <10 mm [3]. Using the same cut-off on CT, only 11.1% have ESDN [5].

Most with ESDN have multiple nodal sites (cardiophrenic, parasternal, mediastinal, axillary, and subclavian) involved (76%) and only 14% are surgically accessible [3]. Forty-five percent of patients with ESDN have parenchymal metastases in the liver, spleen, pleura, or other extra-abdominal sites [5].

Not all ESDN are metastatic, only 67–94%, therefore routine removal is not advisable [4,6]. The size range of metastatic nodes is 0.3–2.9 cm [4,6], with a median of two positive nodes [6].

Patients with stage IV should be considered as a single group for therapeutic purposes regardless of the type and location of extra-abdominal metastases because their survival is similar regardless of the location of the extra-abdominal metastases [3,4,7]. In 124 stage IV patients, there was no significant difference in overall survival (OS) between 38 patients with parenchymal metastases (18 months), 28 with extra-abdominal enlarged nodes (16 months), and 58 with pleural effusions (21.5 months) (p=0.7085) [7].

Enlarged supradiaphragmatic nodes are best treated with primary chemotherapy (PC) (i.e., neoadjuvant) because it is effective for ESDN and their resection does not improve survival.

1. Primary chemotherapy has multiple benefits.
    (a) Primary chemotherapy identifies chemo-resistance and those unlikely to benefit from cytoreduction.
    (b) Enlarged supradiaphragmatic nodes are responsive to PC. A complete or partial response was observed in 96% of 97 patients (complete 83%; partial 13%). The rate of response had no impact on progression-free survival (PFS) (13.6 vs. 14.9 months, p=0.59) [3], suggesting removal would not provide survival benefit.
    (c) Isolated ESDN recurrences are rare, at 5% [4].
    (d) Recurrences are abdominal in 80–85%, and only 2.4% are associated with recurrence in ESDN [3,4,7].
2. Resection of ESDN does not improve survival.
    A complete abdominal and thoracic debulking (involving thoracic surgeons) in 25 patients, resulted in similar PFS (p=0.425) and OS (p=0.465,) as compared to complete abdominal debulking alone (n=151) [4].
3. There is no survival difference in stage IIIC with or without ESDN.
    The median survival of 92 patients with ESDN was similar to 120 patients without ESDN (45 vs. 50 months, p=0.09) [2]. Among 176 patients there was no difference in PFS (p=0.671) or OS (p=0.525) for patients with or without ESDN [4].
    Additionally, among 136 patients with complete abdominal debulking and enlarged cardiophrenic nodes there was no significant difference in OS as compared to patients without ESDN (38.4 vs. 69.6 months, p=0.08) [5].
4. Survival with single versus multiple sites of ESDN are similar.
    In eight patients with a single cardiophrenic site, there was no difference in PFS (p=0.22) or OS (p=0.56) versus 42 patients with multiple sites of ESDN [4].

What Should the Extent of Surgery be with Enlarged Supradiaphragmatic Nodes?

The most influential factor in stage IVB survival is a complete abdominal debulking [7]. Unfortunately, it is uncommon in stage IVB because these patients have more advanced abdominal disease than stage IIIC, usually with ascites, subdiaphragmatic carcinomatosis, and high CA-125 [1,3,6,7].

Conclusion

In conclusion, because complete resection of extra-abdominal metastases does not improve survival, it is hypothesized that stage IVB is a surrogate of aggressive tumor biology which will persist regardless of the extent of resection.

Is there ever an Indication for Resection of Enlarged Supradiaphragmatic Nodes?

Consider a rare patient with a single site of ESDN, surgically accessible, persistent after primary chemotherapy, and with no residual abdominal disease after completion of an interval debulking. This represents a site of unresponsive nodal disease for which there may be an indication.

References

1. Hynninen J, et al. FDG PET/CT in staging of advanced epithelial ovarian cancer: frequency of supradiaphragmatic lymph node metastasis challenges the traditional pattern of disease spread. *Gynecol Oncol* 2012;126(1):64–68. https://doi.org/10.1016/j.ygyno.2012.04.023

2. Kolev V, et al. Prognostic significance of supradiaphragmatic lymphadenopathy identified on preoperative computed tomography scan in patients undergoing primary cytoreduction for advanced epithelial ovarian cancer. *Int J Gynecol Cancer* 2010;20(6):979–984. https://doi.org/10.1111/IGC.0b013e3181e833f5

3. Laasik M, et al. Behavior of FDG-avid supradiaphragmatic lymph nodes in PET/CT throughout primary therapy in advanced serous epithelial ovarian cancer: a prospective study. *Cancer Imaging* 2019;19(1):27. https://doi.org/10.1186/s40644-019-0215-7

4. Lee IO, et al. Prognostic significance of supradiaphragmatic lymph node metastasis detected by (18)F-FDG PET/CT in advanced epithelial ovarian cancer. *BMC Cancer* 2018;18(1):1165. https://doi.org/10.1186/s12885-018-5067-1

5. Mert I, et al. Clinical significance of enlarged cardiophrenic lymph nodes in advanced ovarian cancer: implications for survival. *Gynecol Oncol* 2018;148(1):68–73. https://doi.org/10.1016/j.ygyno.2017.10.024

6. Cowan RA, et al. Feasibility, safety and clinical outcomes of cardiophrenic lymph node resection in advanced ovarian cancer. *Gynecol Oncol* 2017;147(2):262–266. https://doi.org/10.1016/j.ygyno.2017.09.001

7. Jamieson A, et al. Subtypes of stage IV ovarian cancer; response to treatment and patterns of disease recurrence. *Gynecol Oncol* 2017;146(2):273–278. https://doi.org/10.1016/j.ygyno.2017.05.023

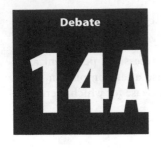

Debate

14A

Is there a Role for Hyperthermic Intraperitoneal Chemotherapy in Front-line Therapy for Ovarian Cancer?

Yes

S. Lot Aronson, Gabe S. Sonke, and Willemien J. van Driel

Debate

Introduction

Ovarian cancer is the leading cause of mortality amongst gynecological cancers worldwide. Despite progress in therapeutic strategies and surgical techniques, long-term survival rates have not improved substantially over the last decades and remain poor. Standard treatment consists of cytoreductive surgery (CRS) and platinum- and taxane-based chemotherapy, followed by optional maintenance therapy with bevacizumab or poly-(ADP)-ribose polymerase (PARP) inhibitors. Although response rates to first-line therapy are high, ovarian cancer recurs in most patients within two years, for whom curative treatment is unavailable. In the search for new strategies, hyperthermic intraperitoneal chemotherapy (HIPEC) is a next step forward, targeting the predominant site of ovarian cancer metastases and recurrence: the peritoneum.

From Intraperitoneal Chemotherapy to Hyperthermic Intraperitoneal Chemotherapy

Advanced ovarian cancer is typically characterized by peritoneal dissemination, following the route of peritoneal fluid, whereas lymphatic and hematogenous spreading occurs less frequently. In 1955, Weisberger introduced intraperitoneal chemotherapy (IPC) for ovarian cancer. The rationale was to achieve higher concentrations of chemotherapeutics within the abdominal cavity, enhancing tumor deposit penetration, while limiting systemic toxic effects due to the physiologic peritoneal-plasma barrier. In this way, locoregional chemotherapy targets microscopic, poorly vascularized lesions on the peritoneal surface, which are relatively resistant to systemic therapy. The rationale was supported by extensive pharmacological data and a meta-analysis by Jaaback and others (2016), which showed significant long-term improvement of survival in patients with primary advanced ovarian cancer, who received intravenous paclitaxel plus intraperitoneal cisplatin [1]. As pharmacologic studies have shown limited penetration depth (0.5–3 mm) of cytotoxic agents into the tumor deposits, (near) complete CRS is a prerequisite for an optimal effect.

Improved outcome by IPC came at the expense of increased toxicity, catheter-related complications, and decreased quality of life, leading to premature termination of the regimen in more than half of patients. These factors, together with challenging patient selection and complex logistics, prevented IPC from becoming widely adopted. In an effort to avoid treatment intolerance encountered with IPC, the search for novel options for intraperitoneal chemotherapy administration continued.

Rationale for Hyperthermic Intraperitoneal Chemotherapy in Ovarian Cancer

Experience in the use of HIPEC for pseudomyxoma peritonei, peritoneal mesothelioma, and gastro-intestinal cancer has built up since the 1980s. The procedure of a single intraoperative intraperitoneal administration of heated chemotherapy has several clinical advantages over IPC. While formation of adhesions and fibrosis impairs the distribution of IPC in the adjuvant setting, HIPEC enables optimal distribution of cytotoxic agents within the abdominal cavity. Also, intraoperative administration avoids delay between cytoreduction and chemotherapy, which is known to significantly impact prognosis due to growth of residual cancer cells in the time interval [2]. Furthermore, a single administration avoids complications associated with repetitive administration over an indwelling catheter.

The rationale for addition of hyperthermia to IPC is based on several mechanisms [2,3]. First, hyperthermia has direct lethal effect selectively on malignant cells through heat-induced lysosomes, inhibition of oxidative metabolism, and selective vascular stasis. Second, hyperthermia leads to transient induction of homologous recombination deficiency that sensitizes tumor cells to chemotherapy that induces double-stranded DNA breaks. Third, hyperthermia increases penetration of chemotherapeutic agents into tumor deposits.

Clinical evidence for the benefit of HIPEC in ovarian cancer comes from the pivotal phase 3 OVHIPEC-1 trial and is supported by several observational studies that established safety and feasibility [4]. The OVHIPEC-1 trial by van Driel and others included patients with stage III primary epithelial ovarian cancer who underwent optimal or complete interval CRS [5]. Eligible patients had at least stable disease after three cycles of neo-adjuvant carboplatin and paclitaxel and were randomized during surgery to receive HIPEC with cisplatin or no additional intraoperative treatment. Sodium thiosulphate was administered to prevent nephrotoxicity. The trial showed a significant improvement in recurrence-free survival (10.7 vs. 14.2 months, HR=0.66 [0.50–0.87]) and overall survival (33.9 vs. 45.7 months, HR=0.67 [0.48–0.94]) with addition of HIPEC. The likelihood of complete CRS and bowel surgery was similar in both arms, indicating no difference in surgical quality. The higher number of ileo- or colostomies in the HIPEC group probably reflects surgeons' caution regarding anastomotic leakage after HIPEC as reported in early publications. However, the trial showed no important differences in postoperative complications or adverse events and HIPEC did not delay the reinitiation of adjuvant chemotherapy. Importantly, HIPEC did not adversely affect quality of life and cost-effectiveness analysis indicated that addition of HIPEC was cost-effective in the Netherlands and in countries with comparable healthcare systems [6].

Conclusion

Long-term survival of women with advanced ovarian cancer is poor and the peritoneum is the primary site of recurrence even after high-quality surgery in expert centers. HIPEC therefore specifically targets microscopic residual disease at the peritoneal surface after surgery. Mechanistic and pre-clinical data, early phase studies, and randomized evidence all support the conclusion that HIPEC improves survival in women after interval CRS for advanced ovarian cancer. Moreover, HIPEC is safe and cost-effective. Whether these advantages apply to women undergoing primary CRS is the topic of the ongoing international OVHIPEC-2 trial (NCT03772028). Several unanswered questions remain, regarding the administration procedure (temperature, dosing, duration, open vs. closed technique), the additive effect of hyperthermia, integration with subsequent treatment, and optimal patient selection. These knowledge gaps need more research, ultimately leading to a uniform protocol and adoption into routine care, with the aim of improving survival outcomes for women with advanced ovarian cancer.

References

1. Jaaback K, et al. Intraperitoneal chemotherapy for the initial management of primary epithelial ovarian cancer. *Cochrane Database Syst Rev* 2016;11:CD005340. https://doi.org/10.1002/14651858.cd005340.pub3

2. de Bree E, et al. Pharmacological principles of intraperitoneal and bidirectional chemotherapy. *Pleura Peritoneum* 2017;2:47–62.

3. González-Moreno S, et al. Hyperthermic intraperitoneal chemotherapy: rationale and technique. *World J Gastrointest Oncol* 2010;2:68–75.

4. Huo YR, et al. Hyperthermic intraperitoneal chemotherapy (HIPEC) and cytoreductive surgery (CRS) in ovarian cancer: a systematic review and meta-analysis. *Eur J Surg Oncol* 2015;41:1578–1589.

5. van Driel WJ, et al. Hyperthermic intraperitoneal chemotherapy in ovarian cancer. *N Engl J Med* 2018;378:1363–1364.

6. Koole SN, et al. Cost effectiveness of interval cytoreductive surgery with hyperthermic intraperitoneal chemotherapy in stage iii ovarian cancer on the basis of a randomized phase iii trial. *J Clin Oncol* 2019;37:2041–2050.

14B Is there a Role for Hyperthermic Intraperitoneal Chemotherapy in Front-line Therapy for Ovarian Cancer?

No

Richard Schwameis, Luis M. Chiva, and Philipp Harter

Debate

The hype around Hyperthermic IntraPEritoneal Chemotherapy (HIPEC) started roughly two decades ago when a randomized trial comparing surgery and HIPEC versus palliative chemotherapy only in patients with colon cancer showed favorable results [1]. The prognostic differences were limited to patients with complete resection, suggesting that surgery played the main role. Unfortunately, there was no surgery-alone arm. Nevertheless, based upon these data, some clinicians commenced adding HIPEC to cytoreductive surgery for a variety of malignancies including ovarian cancer (OC).

Currently in the management of OC, data from two prospective randomized controlled trials and several retrospective trials are available.

The OVHIPEC trial randomized 245 patients with FIGO stage III OC after three cycles of carboplatin and paclitaxel to either HIPEC with 75 mg/m^2 cisplatin or no HIPEC at the time of interval debulking surgery (IDS) [2]. Subsequently, all patients received three additional cycles of chemotherapy. Notably, this study showed a significant benefit in progression-free survival (PFS) (14.2 vs. 10.7 months, p=0.003) and overall survival (OS) (45.7 vs. 33.9 months, p=0.02).

Although publicized very prominently, this study was the target of multiple criticisms. First, the statistical plan was changed, while the study was already ongoing. In detail, the statistical calculations were based upon the assumption that patients in the standard treatment arm would have a PFS of 18 months and that by adding HIPEC an increase of 50% (18 to 24 months) could be achieved. Accordingly, a sample size calculation revealed 280 patients would be necessary to detect a hazard ratio of 1.5 with a 0.05 two-sided significance level and a power of 80%. However, when the study recruited slowly, the sample size was simply reduced to 240 patients. Furthermore, both study arms performed significantly worse in terms of PFS than expected, which also reduced statistical validity.

Second, when comparing the original study protocol with the published paper, different time points of study inclusion and randomization can be identified. While the protocol initially allowed participant inclusion and randomization only prior to any treatment, this was changed in an amendment to the protocol allowing randomization also just before IDS.

Therefore, there is a possibility that the timing of randomization might have biased the surgeons performing the IDS in favor of the HIPEC arm. Unfortunately, the number of patients randomized at the different time points was not reported.

Third, the limited number of 245 patients might have led to possible biases. For example, regarding the OS statistics, the difference in death events was only 15 patients. Unfortunately, patients were not stratified according to important factors such as tumor grade, *BRCA* status or histologic type and therefore an imbalance of patients with histologic types favoring the HIPEC arm occurred.

Fourth, patient recruitment took more than nine years, resulting in only three randomized patients per center per year. Within this time period treatment of OC changed significantly (introduction of bevacizumab and PARP-inhibitors). This might have had a significant impact, as other studies have shown a dramatically reduced benefit from intraperitoneal chemotherapy in the era of bevacizumab treatment. Furthermore, study center and surgeon selection were arbitrary without thorough quality assurance and no information was given about the surgeon's qualifications. Notably, in the largest participating center (National Cancer Institute Amsterdam, n=105) no significant beneficial effect of HIPEC was observed. A beneficial effect of HIPEC was only observed in smaller centers, including only 18 to 36 patients.

In addition, further points of criticism include incomplete reporting of HIPEC-associated adverse events and toxicities, a missing general strategy of patient allocation to either primary debulking surgery (PDS) or IDS and a remarkably high rate for colostomy in the HIPEC arm.

Interestingly, Lim et al. also conducted a prospective randomized trial investigating the impact of HIPEC in OC. This study included 184 patients with FIGO stage III and IV OC undergoing PDS or IDS [3]. Patients were eligible if residual disease was <1 cm. In the control arm, patients received intravenous chemotherapy, while patients in the study arm received additional HIPEC using cisplatin 75 mg/m^2. This study showed similar five-year PFS rates (HIPEC arm: 20.9%; control arm: 16.0%, p=n.s.) and five-year OS rates (HIPEC arm: 51.0%, control arm: 49.4%, p=n.s.) in both arms, respectively. In direct comparison and in contrast to the OVHIPEC trial, patients of the IDS subgroup showed similar PFS and OS rates (PFS: 20 vs. 19 months; OS: 54 and 51 months, for HIPEC and control arm, respectively).Recently, the trial was published after a longer follow up confirming the results in the ITT population, but now with a difference in IDS favoring HIPEC [Lim MC, Chang SJ, Park B, et al. Survival After Hyperthermic Intraperitoneal Chemotherapy and Primary or Interval Cytoreductive Surgery in Ovarian Cancer: A Randomized Clinical Trial. JAMA Surg. 2022 May 1;157(5):374-383]. However, the primary endpoint was changed and multiple questions regarding the methodology of analysis of the primary endpoint remain open [Harter P, Bogner G, Chiva L. Statement of the AGO Kommission Ovar, AGO Study Group, NOGGO, AGO Austria, Swiss AGO, BGOG, CEEGOG, and GEICO Regarding the Use of Hyperthermic Intraperitoneal Chemotherapy (HIPEC) in Epithelial Ovarian Cancer. Le Bulletin du Cancer 2023 (accepted)

Additional evidence is provided by a prospective randomized trial in relapsed OC that included 98 patients undergoing secondary cytoreductive surgery. In this study, HIPEC did not shown any impact on perioperative morbidity, PFS, or OS [4].

Admittedly, there are retrospective trials showing a benefit of HIPEC in OC. A recent systematic review included 22 trials and data from more than 1450 patients. This review summarized the information on 493 patients that were treated with HIPEC in the first-line setting and of 957 patients at secondary debulking surgery. This review failed to show a survival benefit and hence concluded that the use of HIPEC cannot be recognized as a standard of care in ovarian cancer [5].

A randomized trial evaluating the role of HIPEC at primary debulking surgery in primary OC (NCT03772028) is currently ongoing. However, we must be cautious that the story of HIPEC in OC may follow a similar path to that of HIPEC in colorectal cancer. Initially there was a trial showing a benefit (Verwaal et al.), however subsequently there have been several prospective phase III trials failing to show a survival benefit of HIPEC, but in contrast, more toxicity in the experimental arms [6,7,8].

Conclusion

In summary, there are insufficient data to support HIPEC in primary or relapsed ovarian cancer. Furthermore, the possibility of a detrimental effect has still not been completely evaluated nor ruled out.

References

1. Verwaal VJ, et al. Randomized trial of cytoreduction and hyperthermic intraperitoneal chemotherapy versus systemic chemotherapy and palliative surgery in patients with peritoneal carcinomatosis of colorectal cancer. *J Clin Oncol* 2003;21(20):3737–3743.

2. van Driel WJ, et al. Hyperthermic intraperitoneal chemotherapy in ovarian cancer. *N Engl J Med* 2018;378(3):230–240.

3. Lim MC, et al. Randomized trial of hyperthermic intraperitoneal chemotherapy (HIPEC) in women with primary advanced peritoneal, ovarian, and tubal cancer. *J Clin Oncol* 2017;35(15,Suppl.): meeting abstract.

4. Zivanovic O, et al. Secondary cytoreduction and carboplatin hyperthermic intraperitoneal chemotherapy for platinum-sensitive recurrent ovarian cancer: an MSK Team Ovary Phase II Study. *J Clin Oncol* 2021;39(23):2594–2604.

5. Chiva LM, et al. A critical appraisal of hyperthermic intraperitoneal chemotherapy (HIPEC) in the treatment of advanced and recurrent ovarian cancer. *Gynecol Oncol* 2015;136(1):130–135.

6. Quénet F, et al. Cytoreductive surgery plus hyperthermic intraperitoneal chemotherapy versus cytoreductive surgery alone for colorectal peritoneal metastases (PRODIGE 7): a multicentre, randomised, open-label, phase 3 trial. *Lancet Oncol* 2021;22(2):256–266.

7. Goéré D, et al. Second-look surgery plus hyperthermic intraperitoneal chemotherapy versus surveillance in patients at high risk of developing colorectal peritoneal metastases (PROPHYLOCHIP-PRODIGE 15): a randomised, phase 3 study. *Lancet Oncol* 2020;21(9):1147–1154.

8. Klaver CEL, et al. Adjuvant hyperthermic intraperitoneal chemotherapy in patients with locally advanced colon cancer (COLOPEC): a multicentre, open-label, randomised trial. *Lancet Gastroenterol Hepatol* 2019;4(10):761–770.

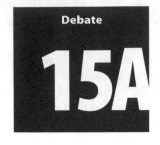

Debate

15A Is there a Role for Intraperitoneal Chemotherapy after Optimal Cytoreduction of Ovarian Cancer?

Yes

Molly Morton, Tiffany Y. Sia, Laura M. Chambers, Roberto Vargas, and Robert Debernardo

Debate

Epithelial ovarian cancer (EOC) is a leading cause of cancer-related death in women. Patients diagnosed with advanced EOC often present with disease throughout the peritoneal cavity, and surgical cytoreduction in combination with platinum- and taxane-based chemotherapy are the backbone of initial treatment. Unfortunately, recurrence is common and is typically associated with carcinomatosis, ascites, and worsening performance status. Once this occurs, treatments are palliative in nature and outcomes are predicated upon response to subsequent lines of chemotherapy, so long as the patient can continue to tolerate the cytotoxic treatments.

The rationale for administering chemotherapy directly into the peritoneal cavity is supported by pharmacokinetic data as well as clinical evidence from both retrospective and randomized clinical trials. Intraperitoneal (IP) administration of chemotherapy overcomes the plasma-peritoneal barrier and directly treats peritoneal surfaces involved with metastatic implants, allowing for a 20-fold higher drug concentration to be delivered directly to the peritoneum and ovarian cancer implants compared to the plasma, sparing systemic exposure to high concentrations of the drug.

With these principles in mind, several studies were developed to investigate the safety and efficacy of IP therapy in treating EOC. In GOG114, patients with stage III EOC were randomized to either a standard regimen of IV cisplatin and IV paclitaxel (135 mg/m^2 over 24 hours) or high-dose IV carboplatin (AUC 9) for two cycles followed by the 24-hour IV paclitaxel regimen and IP cisplatin [1]. Eligible patients had stage III disease and had undergone optimal debulking (<1 cm residual disease). Patients in the IP arm had improved PFS (28 vs. 22 months, p=0.01) and OS (63 vs. 52 months, p=0.05). Critics of the study attributed the benefit to the treatment regimen's differences, as the IP group received higher doses and additional cycles [1]. Furthermore, 18% of patients in the IP arm received ≤2 cycles of IP therapy due to toxicity.

In a landmark study by Armstrong et al., GOG172 randomized patients with stage III disease to either IV cisplatin and IV paclitaxel or IV paclitaxel with IP cisplatin (100 mg/m^2)

and IP paclitaxel after undergoing optimal debulking [2]. As in GOG114, the paclitaxel administration was over 24 hours. In patients treated with IP chemotherapy, significant improvements in PFS (23.8 vs. 18.3 months, p=0.05) and OS were observed (65.6 vs. 49.7 months, p=0.03). Importantly, patients were assessed with an intention to treat analysis, and the treatment effect was preserved despite fewer patients completing the regimen due to toxicity and difficulty with treatment administration, with only 42% of patients in the IP cohort completing treatment. A subsequent analysis found that aberrant tumor BRCA1 expression was an independent prognostic factor for median OS in women receiving IP therapy (84 months IP vs. 47 months IV), suggesting a role of *BRCA1* expression as a biomarker for response [3].

In an exploratory analysis of GOG114 and GOG172 with a median follow-up of 10.7 years, Tewari et al. confirmed the long-term benefits of IP chemotherapy, demonstrating an improvement in overall survival of 61.8 months in patients treated with IP chemotherapy compared to 51.4 months for IV therapy (p<0.05) [4]. Similarly, IP therapy was associated with a 21% reduced risk of progression and 23% reduced risk of death. Notably, in this analysis, the risk of death decreased by 12% for each IP cycle administered (p<0.001). Multivariate analysis demonstrated that patients with clear cell and mucinous ovarian cancer, gross residual disease, and fewer IP chemotherapy cycles had worse OS.

Across all of these studies, patients who received IP chemotherapy had increased frequency of G3/4 toxicities, including leukopenia, fatigue, thrombocytopenia, and gastrointestinal, neurologic, and renal adverse events. Although the reported quality of life in GOG172 was decreased in patients who received IP chemotherapy prior to cycle four and immediately after treatment, no differences were observed one year after completion of IP therapy [2]. Furthermore, administration of IP therapy posed logistical challenges for physicians and hospital systems, often requiring long administration times and inpatient stays. For these reasons, many providers were hesitant to offer IP therapy despite a clear improvement in PFS and OS across multiple randomized trials.

To address these concerns, modifications to the GOG172 protocol were made and ultimately evaluated in GOG252. In this phase III trial, women with stage II through IV EOC were randomized to one of three arms: dose dense IV paclitaxel and IV carboplatin (IV carboplatin), dose dense IV paclitaxel and IP carboplatin (IP carboplatin), or a modification of the original IP arm of GOG172 using IV paclitaxel (135 mg/m^2 over three hours) in combination with IP paclitaxel and a lower dose of IP cisplatin (75 mg/m^2) (IP cisplatin) [5]. All arms included bevacizumab. The investigators found no difference in median PFS between the three arms (24.9, 27.4, and 26.2 months, respectively). Subgroup analyses of patients with optimal cytoreduction or no residual disease failed to show a difference between arms. Additionally, median OS did not differ between groups (75.5, 78.9, and 72.9 months, respectively) [5]. The IP arms suffered higher rates of serious infections and abdominal discomfort, and the IP cisplatin arm suffered increased rates of grade 3 or worse hypertension as well as neurotoxicity. Critics of the study mention that use of bevacizumab resulted in excellent PFS and OS in all subgroups, making it difficult to analyze smaller differences in outcome between groups.

To further define the benefit of IP therapy without bevacizumab, the Intraperitoneal Therapy for Ovarian Cancer with Carboplatin (iPocc) trial randomized women with stage II to IV EOC to IV dose dense paclitaxel in combination with either IP carboplatin or IV carboplatin, without bevacizumab. Unlike previous trials, the study included women with residual disease, with 55% of enrolled patients with residual disease >2 cm after initial surgery. The investigators found a PFS benefit with IP chemotherapy (23.5 months vs. 20.7 months), though median OS did not differ between groups (64.9 vs. 64.0 months) [6]. Rates of adverse events were similar between the two arms except for catheter-related infections which were more prevalent in the IP arm.

Conclusion

In conclusion, IP therapy should be considered in all patients following optimal cytoreduction for stage III ovarian cancer who are not candidates to receive bevacizumab. Although IP therapy is complicated to administer and has been associated with increased toxicity, its usage provides a durable PFS and OS benefit in EOC treatment which may be secondary to the improved control of abdominopelvic disease. Further research must be performed to elucidate biomarkers to predict improved response to IP therapy such as homologous recombination deficiency status. Furthermore, as PARP inhibitor maintenance has become part of upfront management of EOC, further work needs to be done to evaluate its combination with IP chemotherapy.

References

1. Markman M, et al. Phase III trial of standard-dose intravenous cisplatin plus paclitaxel versus moderately high-dose carboplatin followed by intravenous paclitaxel and intraperitoneal cisplatin in small-volume stage III ovarian carcinoma: an intergroup study of the Gynecologic Oncology Group, Southwestern Oncology Group, and Eastern Cooperative Oncology Group. J Clin Oncol 2001;19(4):1001–1007. https://doi.org/10.1200/JCO.2001.19.4.1001

2. Armstrong DK, et al. Intraperitoneal cisplatin and paclitaxel in ovarian cancer. N Engl J Med 2006;354(1):34–43. https://doi.org/10.1056/NEJMoa052985

3. Lesnock JL, et al. BRCA1 expression and improved survival in ovarian cancer patients treated with intraperitoneal cisplatin and paclitaxel: a Gynecologic Oncology Group Study. Br J Cancer 2013;108(6):1231–1237. https://doi.org/10.1038/bjc.2013.70

4. Tewari D, et al. Long-term survival advantage and prognostic factors associated with intraperitoneal chemotherapy treatment in advanced ovarian cancer: a gynecologic oncology group study. J Clin Oncol 2015;33(13):1460–1466. https://doi.org/10.1200/JCO.2014.55.9898

5. Walker JL, et al. Randomized trial of intravenous versus intraperitoneal chemotherapy plus bevacizumab in advanced ovarian carcinoma: an NRG Oncology/Gynecologic Oncology Groups study. J Clin Oncol 2019;37(16):1380–1390. https://doi.org/10.1200/JCO.18.01548

6. Fujiwara K, et al. A randomized phase 3 trial of intraperitoneal versus intravenous carboplatin with dose-dense weekly paclitaxel in patients with ovarian, fallopian tube, or primary peritoneal carcinoma (a GOTIC-001/JGOG-3019/GCIG, iPoccTrial). Presented at the 2022 SGO Annual Meeting on Womens' Cancer; March 18–21, 2022; Phoenix, AZ. Abstract 241.

15B Is there a Role for Intraperitoneal Chemotherapy after Optimal Cytoreduction of Ovarian Cancer?

No

Angeles Alvarez Secord and Laura J. Havrilesky

Debate

Intraperitoneal (IP) chemotherapy for women with optimally cytoreduced advanced ovarian, tubal, and peritoneal cancer is a therapeutic relic and no longer has a role in the current treatment of ovarian cancer. IP refers to the delivery of unheated chemotherapy into the peritoneal cavity through a catheter connected to a surgically implanted port. To establish our position against IP therapy, we argue that historical IP therapy survival outcomes are not relevant in the current era of biologic therapy, demonstrate that IP therapy is too toxic, and examine the challenging and costly logistics of delivering IP therapy.

The rationale for IP therapy is based on a favorable pharmacokinetic profile, direct intraperitoneal drug delivery, and prolonged systemic exposure [1]. Historically, IP therapy was supported by multiple randomized trials and an independent meta-analysis [1] demonstrating improved progression-free survival (PFS) and/or overall survival (OS) outcomes compared to intravenous (IV) chemotherapy alone. A National Cancer Institute alert reported that IP therapy was associated with approximately 22% reduction in the risk of death (HR=0.79, 95% CI: 0.70–0.89) [1]. Furthermore, an ancillary analysis reported that IP therapy conferred the longest survival outcomes, beyond ten years, of any ovarian cancer study [2]. Based on these studies, we were strong proponents of IP therapy and routinely administered this treatment to our patients. However, the irrefutable negative results from GOG0252, a randomized phase III clinical trial evaluating IV and IP chemotherapy with bevacizumab in women with ovarian cancer, clearly illustrated that IP therapy is not relevant in the current era of biologic therapy [3]. GOG0252 included 1560 participants randomized to 21-day cycles of IV paclitaxel weekly + IV carboplatin versus IV paclitaxel weekly + IP carboplatin versus IV paclitaxel day 1 + IP cisplatin day 2 + IP paclitaxel day 8. The IP arms were developed to be more tolerable than the proven but toxic GOG0172 IP regimen. Of note, bevacizumab every three weeks was included in each arm, concurrent with chemotherapy and followed by 16 maintenance cycles. The median PFS was similar in each group: 24.9 months in the IV arm, 27.4 months in the IV/IP carboplatin arm, and 26.2 months in the IV/IP cisplatin arm. At the time of analysis, 51% of patients had died and median OS was similar (75.5, 78.9, and 72.9 months, respectively).

Despite the improvement in drug delivery and pharmacokinetic advantages, IP therapy at tolerable doses does not translate to improved survival outcomes in the modern therapeutic ovarian cancer landscape that increasingly includes maintenance regimens.

Intraperitoneal therapy is too toxic; this has always been a barrier to its widespread adoption due to catheter-related issues, increased adverse effects due to IP administration, and increased chemotherapy-induced toxicity. In GOG0172, 33% had catheter-related complications including infection (n=21), blockage (n=9), leak (n=3), access issues (n=5), and vaginal drainage of IP fluid (n=1). Another 27 women discontinued IP therapy due to possible catheter issues including abdominal pain (n=4), bowel complications (n=4), and refusal (n=19). Women who received IP chemotherapy were more likely to experience $\geq$ grade 3 toxicities including leukopenia (76% vs. 64%, $p<0.001$), thrombocytopenia (12% vs. 4%, $p<0.001$), fatigue (18% vs. 4%, $p=0.02$), gastrointestinal (46% vs. 24%, $p<0.001$), infection (16% vs. 6%, $p<0.001$), hepatic (3% vs. <1%, $p=0.05$), renal (7% vs. 2%, $p=0.03$), neurologic (19% vs. 9%, $p<0.001$), and abdominal pain (11% vs. 1%, $p<0.001$) compared to IV [1]. Moreover, the "less toxic" GOG0252 IP regimens remained more toxic than IV therapy, with significantly more $\geq$ grade 3 infections (~17% vs. 10.2%), $p=0.008$). The IP cisplatin group had higher frequency of $\geq$ grade 3 hypertension (18.7% vs. 11.4%, $p<0.001$), $\geq$ grade 3 nausea/vomiting (10.8% vs. 4.7%, $p<0.001$), and $\geq$ grade 2 CNS toxicity (2% vs. 0.8%, $p=0.58$) [3]. Importantly, Wright et al. reported that IP therapy toxicity and complications for IP chemotherapy were higher in the general population than reported in clinical trials, leading to a higher frequency of emergency room visits and hospitalization [4]. Furthermore, in GOG0172 and GOG0252, IP therapy demonstrated significantly worse quality of life (QoL) during therapy, extending up to one year [1,3]. In GOG0172, sensory neuropathy was more likely to persist and be more severe in the IP cohort. Previously, many justified the worse toxicity and QoL related to IP therapy with improved survival outcomes. However, the negative PFS findings from GOG0252 have nullified that justification. IP therapy yields increased frequency and severity of toxicity and impairs QoL without significantly enhancing survival outcomes.

Finally, IP therapy is challenging and costly to deliver. IP therapy implementation has always been difficult and often not feasible in community centers. Specific nursing skills are required for port management and chemotherapy administration, and infusion times are increased compared to conventional IV therapy. Even at the height of its popularity, IP therapy remained underutilized at approximately 15%; and was only 41% at National Comprehensive Cancer Centers [4], likely due to logistical barriers. The most effective IP regimen was also costly due to the inpatient portion. Our group used a decision model to compare the cost-effectiveness of IV carboplatin and paclitaxel, IV cisplatin and paclitaxel, and IV/IP paclitaxel and cisplatin. Compared with IV outpatient therapy, inpatient IP cisplatin/paclitaxel therapy was not cost-effective, with an incremental cost-effectiveness ratio of $180,022 per quality-adjusted life year saved at a seven-year time horizon. We predicted that an outpatient IV/IP paclitaxel cisplatin would be cost-effective if proven as effective as the inpatient regimen [5]. GOG0252 subsequently incorporated a less costly outpatient IP regimen, but unfortunately the effectiveness vanished.

Conclusion

In conclusion, despite four decades of research expended evaluating IP chemotherapy, the data demonstrate that front-line IP therapy does not have a role in the current management of ovarian cancer. These conclusions are drawn from the lack of survival improvement reported in the GOG0252 trial, lack of relevance in an era of biologic therapy with bevacizumab and PARPi, higher rate of toxicity associated with IP therapy, worse QoL conferred by IP therapy, and costly challenges to delivery.

References

1. NCI alert (2006). Available from: https://w ayback.archive-it.org/org-350/20211101182 949/https://www.nlm.nih.gov/databases/ale rts/ovarian_ip_chemo.html

2. Tewari D, et al. Long-term survival advantage and prognostic factors associated with intraperitoneal chemotherapy treatment in advanced ovarian cancer: a gynecologic oncology group study. *J Clin Oncol* 2015;33:1460–1466.

3. Walker JL, et al. Randomized trial of intravenous versus intraperitoneal chemotherapy plus bevacizumab in advanced ovarian carcinoma.*J Clin Oncol* 2019;37(16):1380–1390. https://doi.org/10 .1200/JCO.18.01568

4. Wright JD, et al. Utilization and toxicity of alternative delivery methods of adjuvant chemotherapy for ovarian cancer. *Obstet Gynecol* 2016;127 (6):985–991.

5. Havrilesky LJ, et al. Gynecologic Oncology Group. Cost effectiveness of intraperitoneal compared with intravenous chemotherapy for women with optimally resected stage III ovarian cancer: a Gynecologic Oncology Group study. *J Clin Oncol* 2008;26 (25):4144–4450.

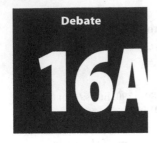

What is the Best Front-line Maintenance Therapy for HRD-positive Ovarian Cancer?

Single-agent PARP Inhibitor

Antonio González-Martín

Debate

High-grade serous ovarian cancer (HGSOC) is the most frequent epithelial ovarian cancer representing up to 85% of the patients with advanced disease (FIGO III–IV). Biologically, almost all the patients harbor a TP53 mutation, and approximately 50% are deficient in the homologous recombination (HR) system for DNA double-strand break repairs. This molecular feature explains the sensitivity of HGSOC to DNA damaging agents, like platinum analogs, and poly ADP ribose polymerase (PARP) inhibitors that induce synthetic lethality in cells with HR deficiency. The most frequent cause of HR deficiency is inactivating mutation in the BRCA 1 or 2 gene, which is detected in the germline in about 15–18% of patients, and exclusively in the tumor in an additional 5–7% of patients.

Maintenance therapy with oral PARP inhibitors (PARPi) has been demonstrated to significantly expand the progression-free survival of patients with advanced HGSOC in response to front-line platinum-based chemotherapy [1–4]. SOLO-1, PRIMA/ENGOT-OV26/GOG-3012, and PAOLA-1 /ENGOT-OV25 trials achieved their primary endpoint of PFS determined in the intent to treat population, leading to health authorities' approvals that have revolutionized the landscape of front-line ovarian cancer. In addition, there are three more studies, ATHENA-MONO/GOG-3020/ENGOT-OV45, PRIME and VELIA that provide more evidence of the effectiveness of PARPi in front-line maintenance therapy [4-6]. Albeit positive results in the global population, veliparib and rucaparib were not submitted to filing and are not available in the clinic.

Importantly, the significant benefit achieved with PARPi maintenance on PFS is highly dependent on the status of BRCA and HR identified as genomic instability by Myriad MyChoice, with the highest difference in outcome observed in patients with BRCA mutated tumors and patients with BRCA wild type but HR-deficient tumors which are the focus of this controversy. In patients with HR-proficient tumors only niraparib showed benefit but of less magnitude.

Currently, three options have been approved for patients with BRCAmut tumors (olaparib, niraparib, or olaparib-bevacizumab) and only two options for patients with BRCAwt/HRD tumors (niraparib or olaparib and bevacizumab). The reason for the controversy we are discussing in this chapter is the lack of evidence from randomized trials comparing single-agent PARPi versus PARP combined with bevacizumab. Both strategies have shown similar benefits in terms of hazard ratio, but medians are not comparable due to the different patient populations included and the different tumor assessment schedule. Nevertheless, several arguments in favor of the single-agent PARPi option can be argued:

- There is no clear evidence indicating that bevacizumab added to PARPi could improve the outcome of HR-deficient tumors. The SOLO-1 and PAOLA-1 trials have recently shown a clinically meaningful benefit in overall survival (OS) at 7 and 5 years, in the BRCA mut and HR-deficient population (regardless of BRCAmut status), respectively [7,8]. However, we still do not have the OS outcome of the niraparib monotherapy trials in patients with BRCAwt, but HR-deficient tumors [3, 5]. On the other hand, a matched indirect comparison of individual data of SOLO-1 patients and patients with BRCAmut tumors from PAOLA-1 has indicated a potential additive effect. However, this analysis compares events of two trials in which the frequency of tumor assessment was different by protocol, every 12 weeks in SOLO-1 and every 24 weeks in PAOLA-1 [9]. In addition, the role of bevacizumab alone in BRCAmut patients is not clear. In the exploratory analysis of the GOG-218 trial, the HR for the BRCA1mut population was 0.82 (95% CI: 0.55–1.21) and for BRCA2mut was 1.10 (95% CI: 0.61–2.01), and it could only be concluded that a benefit cannot be ruled out [10]. Fortunately, two ENGOT planned randomized clinical trials comparing niraparib with niraparib plus bevacizumab, NIRVANA/ENGOT-OV63 and AGO-OVAR 28/ ENGOT-OV57 trials, will probably clarify this controversy.
- The controversy of single-agent PARPi versus the combination of PARPi and bevacizumab leads to the debate of using biological agents as maintenance concurrently or sequentially. There is no doubt that PARPi should be used in front-line, in patients with HRD tumors, based on the increment of overall survival mentioned above. However, bevacizumab can be used in the front-line and the recurrent setting, both in patients for whom platinum is an option or not with the same HR. Unfortunately, many patients with stage III–IV will relapse. If both agents (bevacizumab and PARPi) were used in the front line, they would not have options for maintenance in the relapse. For this reason, there is a need for intensive biomarker research that could help us in identifying patients that may be cured within front-line with the combination of bevacizumab and PARPi. In the meantime, for many patients, sequential use of maintenance options is probably the most efficient approach. In addition, for some health systems, the cost of the double combination may be unaffordable, and sequential use of maintenance therapy will be preferred.
- The benefit of PARPi in patients with HR deficient (BRCAmut or BRCAwt) tumors is unprecedented, durable over time and improves the OS, as shown by the long-term follow-up of the SOLO-1 and PAOLA-1 trials [7,8]. This intervention may change the natural history of the disease in many patients, and, for this reason, the physicians should be adequately trained in the management of toxicity associated with these new agents to keep the patients on treatment for the whole duration of maintenance, preventing permanent therapy interruption. In this regard, physicians should be aware that the discontinuation rate due to adverse events of PARPi inhibitors is around 2%, but reaches 20% with the combination of olaparib and bevacizumab [1,2].

Conclusion

In summary, the combination of PARPi and bevacizumab in patients with HR-deficient (BRCAmut or BRCAwt) tumors has produced revolutionary data. Still, the additional benefit of bevacizumab added to single-agent PARP inhibitors has not yet been demonstrated and, for most patients, single-agent PARPi should be considered the preferred option.

References

1. Moore K, et al. Maintenance olaparib in patients with newly diagnosed advanced ovarian cancer. *N Engl J Med* 2018;379 (26):2495–2505.

2. Ray-Coquard I, et al. Olaparib plus bevacizumab as first-line maintenance in ovarian cancer. *N Engl J Med* 2019;381:2416–2428.

3. González-Martín A, et al. PRIMA/ ENGOT-OV26/GOG-3012 Investigators. Niraparib in patients with newly diagnosed advanced ovarian cancer. *N Engl J Med* 2019;381(25):2391–2402.

4. Monk BJ, Parkinson C, Lim MC et al. A Randomized, Phase III Trial to Evaluate Rucaparib Monotherapy as Maintenance Treatment in Patients With Newly Diagnosed Ovarian Cancer (ATHENA-MONO/GOG-3020/ENGOT-ov45). J Clin Oncol. 2022 Dec 1;40(34):3952–3964.

5. Ning Li, Jianqing Zhu, Rutie Yin et al. Efficacy and safety of niraparib as maintenance treatment in patients with newly diagnosed advanced ovarian cancer using an individualized starting dose (PRIME Study): A randomized, double-blind, placebo-controlled, phase 3 trial (LBA 5), Gynecologic Oncology, 2022; 166 (S1): 50-S51.

6. Coleman RL, et al. Veliparib with first-line chemotherapy and as maintenance therapy in ovarian cancer. *N Engl J Med* 2019;381 (25):2403–2415.

7. DiSilvestro P, Banerjee S, Colombo N et al. Overall Survival With Maintenance Olaparib at a 7-Year Follow-Up in Patients With Newly Diagnosed Advanced Ovarian Cancer and a BRCA Mutation: The SOLO1/GOG 3004 Trial. J Clin Oncol. 2023 Jan 20;41(3):609–617.

8. I.L. Ray-Coquard, A. Leary, S. Pignata, et al. LBA29 Final overall survival (OS) results from the phase III PAOLA-1/ ENGOT-ov25 trial evaluating maintenance olaparib (ola) plus bevacizumab (bev) in patients (pts) with newly diagnosed advanced ovarian cancer (AOC). Annals of Oncology, 2022; 33 (s7): S1396–S1397.

9. Vergote I, Ray-Coquard I, Anderson DM et al. Population-adjusted indirect treatment comparison of the SOLO1 and PAOLA-1/ ENGOT-ov25 trials evaluating maintenance olaparib or bevacizumab or the combination of both in newly diagnosed, advanced BRCA-mutated ovarian cancer. Eur J Cancer. 2021 Nov;157:415–423.

10. Norquist BM, et al. Mutations in homologous recombination genes and outcomes in ovarian carcinoma patients in GOG 218: an NRG Oncology/Gynecologic Oncology Group Study. *Clin Cancer Res* 2018;24(4):777–783.

What is the Best Front-line Maintenance Therapy for HRD-positive Ovarian Cancer?

16B

Bevacizumab plus PARP inhibitor

Hélène Vanacker, Olivia Le Saux, and Isabelle Ray-Coquard

Debate

Epithelial high-grade ovarian carcinomas (HGOCs) have an overall poor prognosis due to frequent presentation in advanced stage, rapid clinical evolution, and an over 70% risk of relapse following completion of surgery and platinum-based chemotherapy. Two classes of targeted therapies have aimed at improving these outcomes. (1) Bevacizumab was approved in 2010 for front-line treatment and maintenance in all FIGO stages III–IV. Consequently, standard therapy in the front-line setting has (until recently) included debulking surgery and chemotherapy, with or without bevacizumab. Although in some countries bevacizumab has been restricted to women at high risk for progression (stage IV/stage III with residual disease, upfront inoperable stage III), the progression-free survival (PFS) benefit is also observed in patients with no residual disease [1]. (2) The poly(ADP-ribose) polymerases (PARP) inhibitors (PARPi), are oral targeted agents exploiting the particular biology of HGOC. Indeed, at least half of HGOCs are characterized by a defect in DNA repair, especially through homologous-recombination repair deficiency (HRD). So HRD signatures have been developed to capture the HRD-positive phenotype even in those patients and tumors that don't have a BRCA mutation.

The efficacy of PARPi over placebo was consistently demonstrated in the platinum-responsive front-line setting (SOLO1 and PRIMA/VELIA trials [2–4]), where PARPi showed a differential benefit across different subgroups by biomarker status (BRCA+/HRD+/HRD-). Indeed, the reduction in the risk of disease progression/death was consistently over 60% in patients with BRCA mutations, between 35–50% in the HRD-positive-wildtype BRCA population, as compared to less than 35% in HRD- tumors. However, all these trials tested PARPi as single agent maintenance *versus* placebo. Only the PAOLA-1 trial [5] tested a front-line double maintenance with bevacizumab + the PARPi olaparib, compared to a single active agent bevacizumab/placebo maintenance control arm. The trial was positive for the primary end point (PFS on ITT analysis) with a HR=0.59 (95% CI: 0.49–0.72), for the bevacizumab + olaparib over bevacizumab + placebo.

Therefore, for patients who are possible candidates for bevacizumab (absence of medical contraindications or access/availability issues), we support the use of bevacizumab + PARPi in front-line maintenance therapy for HRD-positive HGOC. We feel the double

Frontline maintenance in PRIMA, SOLO-1 and PAOLA-1 trials :primary analysis :median PFS (months)

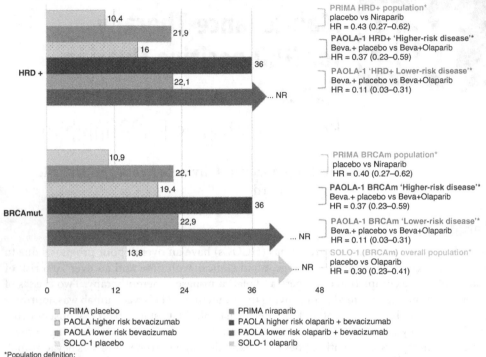

*Population definition:
PRIMA inclusion criteria: FIGO stage IV or III with upfront surgery and residual disease or neoadjuvant-chemotherapy (NACT), in CR/PR to platinum based CT
SOLO-1 inclusion criteria: BRCA-mutation and FIGO stage IV or III with upfront or interval surgery and platinum-based CT, in CR/PR/NED to platinum based CT
PAOLA-1 'Higher-risk disease' subgroup: FIGO stage IV or III with upfront surgery and residual disease or NACT, in NED/CR/PR to platinum-based + bevacizumab CT
PAOLA-1 'Lower-risk disease' subgroup: FIGO stage III receiving primary debulking surgery with no residual disease in NED/CR/PR to platinum-based + bevacizumab CT
Abbreviation CR complete response, NED: Non evidence of disease, PR partial response

Figure 16B.1 Front-line maintenance in PRIMA, SOLO-1, and PAOLA-1 trials; primary analysis PFS (months).

maintenance approach offers the greatest efficacy, highest potential for cure, with a good safety profile and cost-effectiveness.

The association of bevacizumab + olaparib maintenance brought a never-reached efficacy in the HRD-positive subgroup in the PAOLA-1 trial (Figure 16B.1). The pre-specified exploratory analyses revealed a significant and meaningful PFS improvement for patients with BRCA mutation (HR=0.31, 95% CI: 0.20–0.47), as well as in HRD-positive/BRCA wild type population (HR=0.43, 95% CI: 0.28–0.46), with 20 months of absolute benefit in median PFS. Of note, the population of PAOLA-1 was not selected based on surgical outcome or highest platinum-sensitivity (Ca125 could be elevated at inclusion) resulting in only 20% of patients in both arms having a complete response to first-line therapy. All patients had first-line treatment including bevacizumab with chemotherapy.

An additive effect of the antiangiogenic agent to PARPi seems supported by the population-adjusted indirect comparison (PAIC) of PAOLA-1 and SOLO1 population recently published [6] highlighting a 30% reduction in the risk of progression with bevacizumab + olaparib compared to olaparib alone. The combination of olaparib +

bevacizumab reached a higher and long-lasting PFS benefit compared to olaparib alone, bevacizumab alone or placebo, with a three-year progression-free rate (PFR) of 75.2%, 60%, 57%, and 27% respectively. Furthermore, the exploratory analysis of PAOLA-1 in the higher risk group (FIGO stage IV or stage III disease with upfront surgery and residual disease or neoadjuvant-chemotherapy), reached a median PFS of 36 months with the combination compared to 15.9 months with bevacizumab alone. In a comparable population, PRIMA reported a median PFS of 20.9 months for niraparib alone versus 10.4 months with placebo (Figure 16B.1). Similarly, in patients with clinically lower-risk disease from PAOLA-1, HRD-positive population benefitted from bevacizumab + olaparib with an impressive HR=0.15 over bevacizumab, translating into a rate of 90% of patients still progression free at two years with the combination. Hence, in both higher- or lower-risk disease, the front-line combination maintenance is an important therapeutic window for patients with BRCA and/or HRD-positive disease. Interestingly, such additive effect is also supported by data in the relapsed setting where a superiority of the combination antiangiogenic + PARPi in PFS, ORR, and OS (for over PARPi monotherapy have been reported, particularly in the HRD + wtBRCA population.

The association is safe, since those two drugs have no overlapping adverse events (AEs). The safety profile for the olaparib + bevacizumab arm was generally similar to that observed in previous trials, with no increase of myelodysplastic syndromes, nor increase in bevacizumab toxicity including all-grade or severe hypertension [5].

Playing all the best cards first may be the optimum approach for the whole course of patients with this disease! Analyses of PFS2 (survival on subsequent therapy following progression on front-line therapy), were significantly longer in the HRD-positive population treated with olaparib + bevacizumab compared to bevacizumab, The final overall survival (OS) data strenghtenned the clinically meaningfull improvement of first line olaparib = bevacizumab over bevacizumab in HRD-positive population witha median OS of 65.5 vs 48.5 months (HR 0.62 95% CI: 0.45-0.85), even with a high proportion of patients receiving a parp-inhibitor post progression (45.7% in the whole population of control arm) (Ray-Coquard, ESMO 2022). Moreover, the PAICS analyses of SOLO1 and PALOA-1 underline a superior efficacy in terms of long-term progression-free rate and suggest that a significant proportion of patients do not relapse after long-term follow-up and may even be cured [6].

The cost-effectiveness of bevacizumab + PARPi maintenance and HRD-testing is a legitimate concern. Recent cost-effectiveness analyses reported that combination maintenance is in fact cost-effective in the case of *BRCA*-mutated and HRD-positive population, due to their particular PFS benefit. Bevacizumab is much more cost-effective in first-line treatment as compared to relapse. Finally, the cost of HRD-testing may be lowered by the development of institutional testing and/or improved market access for commercially available assays.

Conclusion

Hence, our opinions are based on trends from currently available data on population-matched analysis and subgroup analyses. All PFS, PFS2 ans OS data demonstrated a significant and clinically meaningfull improvment for bevacizumab + olaparib over bevacizumab as fist line treatement even with a high proportion of subsequent PARPi which may convince the scientific community. Overall, consistent with the FDA and EMA 2020's recommendations, we definitely support the combination of bevacizumab and PARPi for front-line maintenance for all eligible patients with HRD-positive advanced-HGOC.

References

1. González Martín A, et al. Exploratory outcome analyses according to stage and/or residual disease in the ICON7 trial of carboplatin and paclitaxel with or without bevacizumab for newly diagnosed ovarian cancer. *Gynecol Oncol* 2019;152:53–60.

2. González-Martín A, et al. Niraparib in patients with newly diagnosed advanced ovarian cancer. *N Engl J Med* 2019;381:2391–2402.

3. Coleman RL, et al. Veliparib with first-line chemotherapy and as maintenance therapy in ovarian cancer. *N Engl J Med* 2019;381:2403–2415.

4. Moore K, et al. Maintenance olaparib in patients with newly diagnosed advanced ovarian cancer. *N Engl J Med* 2018;379:2495–2505.

5. Ray-Coquard I, et al. Olaparib plus bevacizumab as first-line maintenance in ovarian cancer. *N Engl J Med* 2019;381:2416–2428.

6. Vergote I, et al. Population-adjusted indirect treatment comparison of the SOLO1 and PAOLA-1/ENGOT-ov25 trials evaluating maintenance olaparib or bevacizumab or the combination of both in newly diagnosed, advanced BRCA-mutated ovarian cancer. *Eur J Cancer* 2021;157:415–423. https://doi.org/10.1016/j.ejca.2021.08.023

When is the Best Time to Use PARP Inhibitors for Maintenance?
Front-line

Duaa H. Al-Rawi, Karen Cadoo, and Roisin
O'Cearbhaill

Debate

The development and use of poly(ADP-ribose) polymerase inhibitors (PARPi) in advanced ovarian cancer (OC) have been an incredible clinical breakthrough. PARPi are FDA-approved as front-line maintenance for *BRCA1-/2*-associated (olaparib or niraparib), homologous recombination deficient (HRD) (niraparib or olaparib with bevacizumab), and homologous recombination proficient (HRP) (niraparib) advanced-stage high-grade ovarian cancer (HGOC). Along with a third PARPi, rucaparib, they are also approved following recurrence as both maintenance and treatment. Here we advocate for PARPi as front-line maintenance for *BRCA1-/2*-associated (germline or somatic) and HRD tumors. We also discuss our recommendations for patients with HRP tumors.

BRCA1 and BRCA2 are DNA damage signaling proteins fundamentally important for HR-dependent repair. HRD cells are particularly sensitive to certain chemotherapeutics such as platinum-based therapies; combined loss of the HR repair mechanism and PARP results in synthetic lethality. HRD cells upregulate PARP1 and critically depend on PARP for DNA replication. A commercially available assay called Myriad myChoice®CDx utilizes a genomic signature that combines loss of heterozygosity (LOH), telomeric allelic imbalance, and large-scale state transitions loss to identify patients with HRD tumors (beyond *BRCA1/2)* that may respond to PARPi.

SOLO1, PAOLA, and PRIMA examined PARPi switch maintenance after response to front-line platinum-based therapy. SOLO1, a double-blinded, placebo-controlled, randomized trial (RCT) in patients with *BRCA1-/2*-associated HGOC compared two years of olaparib with placebo. An improved three-year median progression-free survival (mPFS) of 60% versus 27% (HR=0.30) was observed with olaparib [1]. PAOLA, a RCT comparing front-line maintenance olaparib plus bevacizumab with bevacizumab alone in advanced-stage OC, demonstrated a mPFS of 37.2 months versus 21.7 months in the germline *BRCA1/2* subset; 28.1 months versus 16.6 months in the HRD subset (by Myriad myChoice®CDx); and 16.6 months versus 16.2 months in the HRP subset [2]. PRIMA compared up to three years of niraparib with placebo in a higher risk group of patients who responded to front-line platinum. The mPFS was 22.1 months versus 10.9 months in the germline *BRCA1/2* subset; 21.1 months versus 10.4 months in the HRD subset; and 8.1 months versus 5.4 months in the HRP subset [3]. Taken together, these RCTs demonstrate strong evidence of benefit in patients with germline or somatic *BRCA1/2* mutated and

HRD tumors. In PRIMA there was also a statistically significant but less compelling benefit in patients with HRP tumors but no such benefit was seen in PAOLA1. Adverse effects included fatigue, nausea, thrombocytopenia (more common with niraparib) anemia and a rare (1–3%) but lethal risk of myelodysplastic syndrome or acute myeloid leukemia (MDS/AML) across PARPi.

Several studies have examined PARPi in later lines of therapy. Patients continued PARPi/placebo until disease progression or toxicity. In SOLO2 olaparib was studied as post-platinum maintenance in patients with BRCA1-/2-associated platinum-sensitive OC who had received at least two lines of platinum-based therapies. Study 19 enrolled all comers with high-grade serous OC and at least two prior therapies to olaparib treatment. A recent update to SOLO2 [4] at median follow-up of 65.7 months, showed a median overall survival (OS) 51.7 and 38.8 months in the olaparib maintenance versus placebo groups. This represented a nonsignificant but clinically meaningful difference despite 38% of the placebo group receiving subsequent PARPi. In the subgroup analysis, OS was reduced in patients who had received incremental numbers of prior therapies (56.3 months, 41.5 months, and 43.6 months in patients with two, three, four prior lines of treatment, respectively). Alarmingly, 8% of patients in the olaparib group versus 4% in the placebo group developed MDS/AML. These data posit three interesting observations; the first is that there appears to be a reduction in the benefit from olaparib in patients who had received more than two prior lines of treatment, arguing towards moving olaparib into earlier lines of therapy for patients with BRCA1-/2-associated ovarian cancer; the second is that the duration of benefit appears to extend beyond the conventional two years of olaparib given as front-line maintenance; and finally the risk of leukemogenesis in BRCA1-/2-associated OC appears to be augmented by receipt of PARPi later in the disease course.

ARIEL2 assessed rucaparib in HGOC of all genetic backgrounds (HRD was character-ized by LOH on FoundationOne®CDX). NOVA, a RCT of niraparib maintenance versus placebo in patients who had responded to second- or greater-line platinum-based therapy included all genetic backgrounds [5]. QUADRA investigated niraparib treatment after at least three prior lines of treatment and not necessarily platinum-sensitive. NOVA reported a mPFS of 21 months versus 5.5 months in BRCA1-/2-associated tumors; 12.9 months versus 5.5 months in HRD tumors (Myriad myChoice®CDx); and 6.9 months versus 3.8 months in HRP tumors [5]. Interestingly, 20% of the HRP subgroup derived >18 months benefit from niraparib maintenance.

To date, no trial has compared front-line PARPi maintenance to a later line of therapy. However, if we extrapolate from SOLO2, in BRCA1/2 patients, there was a reduction in response to PARPi between patients who received three or more lines compared to two lines of prior therapy. Furthermore, the prolonged PFS noted in the front-line maintenance trials may ultimately translate into enhanced survival and proffer more cures. These bolster an argument towards moving PARPi to the front-line. The data and the benefit in patients with HRP tumors are less compelling. We would argue that PARPi could be better reserved for later line treatment in this patient subgroup based on the prolonged benefit in patients with HRP tumors and low MDS/AML rate noted in NOVA trial. Interestingly, ARIEL2 compared biopsies from patients at initial surgery and prior to receiving PARPi and noted apparent rare changes in HR status between the initial and pre-PARPi biopsies. In addition to preselection for patients with platinum-responsive disease the conversion of tumors from HRP to HRD maybe explain the prolonged benefit observed in the HRP patient subset in the NOVA trial. We anticipate that further refinement of biomarkers of PARPi response will better identify patients most likely to benefit from PARPi.

Conclusion

In conclusion, we favor utilizing PARPi in the front-line maintenance setting for patients with *BRCA1-/2*-associated and HRD tumors given the profound PFS benefit noted in the SOLO1, PAOLA1, and PRIMA trials. Further refinement of biomarkers of PARPi response are needed to better identify patients who are most likely to derive benefit.

References

1. Moore K, et al. Maintenance olaparib in patients with newly diagnosed advanced ovarian cancer. *N Engl J Med* 2018;379 (26):2495–2505.

2. Ray-Coquard I, et al. Olaparib plus bevacizumab as first-line maintenance in ovarian cancer. *N Engl J Med* 2019;381 (25):2416–2428.

3. Gonzalez-Martin A, et al. Niraparib in patients with newly diagnosed advanced ovarian cancer. *N Engl J Med* 2019;381 (25):2391–2402.

4. Poveda A, et al. Olaparib tablets as maintenance therapy in patients with platinum-sensitive relapsed ovarian cancer and a BRCA1/2 mutation (SOLO2/ENGOT-Ov21): a final analysis of a double-blind, randomised, placebo-controlled, phase 3 trial. *Lancet Oncol* 2021;22(5):620–631.

5. Moore KN, et al. Niraparib monotherapy for late-line treatment of ovarian cancer (QUADRA): a multicentre, open-label, single-arm, phase 2 trial. *Lancet Oncol* 2019;20(5):636–648.

Debate

17B When is the Best Time to Use PARP Inhibitors for Maintenance?

First Recurrence

Alvin Jun Xing Lee and Jonathan A. Ledermann

Debate

Poly ADP ribose polymerase (PARP) inhibitors have led to a step change in the management of advanced ovarian cancer following the first approval of these inhibitors in 2014. PARP is an enzyme needed for DNA repair and its inhibition results in the accumulation of single-strand DNA breaks. PARP inhibitors were initially hypothesized to have maximum efficacy in ovarian cancer with BRCA1/2 mutations or homologous recombination (HR) deficiency (HRD) given the role of these pathways in repairing double-stranded DNA breaks. The accumulation of both single-strand and double-strand breaks would result in synthetic lethality and preferential cancer cell cytotoxicity with BCRA1/2 mutations and HRD being a predictive biomarker of response. Here we present data that patients with recurrent ovarian cancer will benefit from PARP inhibitors, given as maintenance therapy irrespective of BRCA or HR status. This has been shown with olaparib, niraparib, and rucaparib; all three PARP inhibitors are licensed for the treatment of recurrent ovarian cancer following a response to platinum-based therapy in both BRCA-mutant and wild-type patients.

Two studies with olaparib demonstrate PFS and OS benefits in patients regardless of BRCA mutations. Study 19] was a randomized, placebo-controlled, phase II trial to evaluate maintenance treatment with olaparib in patients with platinum-sensitive, relapsed, high-grade serous ovarian cancer who had received two or more platinum-based regimens and had had a partial or complete response to their most recent platinum-based regimen. The study met its primary endpoint of improved median PFS (mPFS) in the overall population (8.4 vs. 4.8 months, Hazard Ratio (HR)=0.35, 95% Confidence Interval (CI): 0.25–0.49), BRCA mutant population (11.2 vs. 4.3 months, HR=0.18, 95% CI: 0.10–0.31) and BRCA wild-type patients (7.4 vs. 5.5 months, HR=0.54, 95% CI: 0.34–0.85). Long-term follow-up data in Study 19 [2] demonstrates an OS advantage following olaparib treatment (HR=0.73, 95% CI: 0.55–0.95) irrespective of BRCA1/2 mutation status. Thirty-two patients (24%) received maintenance olaparib for over two years with 15 (11%) receiving olaparib for over six years. SOLO2 [3] was an international, multicentre, double-blind, randomized, placebo-controlled, phase III trial evaluating olaparib in patients with recurrent ovarian cancer who received at least two lines of chemotherapy previously with an aim to evaluate the tablet formulation of olaparib and to confirm the efficacy in BRCA mutated ovarian cancer. The median PFS for olaparib was 19.1 months and 5.5 months with placebo (HR=0.30, 95% CI: 0.22–0.41). The final OS data for SOLO2 demonstrated a long-term benefit with olaparib versus placebo with an OS HR of 0.74 (95% CI: 0.54–1.00) unadjusted for the 38% of patients in the placebo arm who subsequently received a PARPA inhibitor. At five years,

42.1% of olaparib patients were alive compared to 33.2% of patients receiving placebo. Again, a prolonged benefit was seen in some patients with 22% of patients continuing on olaparib after five years compared with 9% on placebo.

Homologous recombination deficiency testing was performed in NOVA and ARIEL3 trials in which niraparib and rucaparib respectively were given following platinum-based therapy for recurrent ovarian cancer, and which confirmed a benefit of PARP inhibitors in patients who do not have BRCA mutations. In NOVA [4] women were stratified into germline BRCA (gBRCA) mutant and non-gBRCA groups. The non-gBRCA group was further divided into HRD-positive (according to the Myriad myChoice HRD test) and HRD-negative. Niraparib treatment improved PFS versus placebo in patients with mutant gBRCA (21.0 vs. 5.5 months, HR=0.27, 95% CI: 0.17–0.41), in the HRD-positive non-gBRCA cohort (12.9 vs. 3.8 months, HR=0.38, 95% CI: 0.24–0.59), and in the HRD negative group (6.9 vs. 3.8 months, HR=0.58, 95% CI: 0.36–0.92). The ARIEL3 [5] trial used the T5 NGS assay (Foundation Medicine) to determine HRD status, based on a loss of genomic heterozygosity (LOH). An improvement in the median PFS was seen following rucaparib versus placebo in patients with tumor BRCA mutations, 16.6 versus 5.4 months (HR=0.23, 95% CI: 0.16–0.34), in the LOH-high cohort 13.6 versus 5.4 months (HR=0.32, 95% CI: 0.24–0.42), and in those with an LOH-low score, 6.7 versus 5.4 months (HR=0.58, 95% CI: 0.40–0.85).

Following the success of these agents in recurrent ovarian cancer, the concept of switch maintenance after chemotherapy was tested in the first-line setting. The three trials using this approach were SOLO1 in which olaparib or placebo was given to patients with a BRCA mutation, and two trials that enrolled a broader group of patients in response to or not progressing after first-line treatment. They were PRIMA, comparing niraparib and placebo, and PAOLA-1, in which olaparib or placebo was added to bevacizumab maintenance.

As we can see from these front-line studies, PARP inhibitors should not be used in first-line maintenance for all patients. In particular, PAOLA-1 showed no benefit in the HRD-negative/unknown population with a mPFS of 16.9 versus 16.0 months (HR=0.92, 95% CI: 0.72–1.17). Whilst some benefit was seen among this group in the PRIMA trial, it should be noted that the population differed from PAOLA-1 in so far as all patients had demonstrated a response to platinum-based therapy to enter the study. This confirms that as in the case of patients with recurrent disease, the absence of HRD does not preclude a benefit from PARP inhibitors, and that a response to platinum remains an important selection criterion for benefit.

The key issue with front-line trials is how long patients benefit from a PARP inhibitor. For this progression, rates are important, as failure of a front-line PARP inhibitor currently precludes its use at relapse. In the non-BRCA mutated groups, particularly those with HR proficiency, the failure rate was high. About 50% of patients progressed within 16 months of randomization in PAOLA-1 and in PRIMA, 50% had progressed within about eight months from diagnosis. Even among the BRCA wild-type HRD-positive group, 48% were not free of progression at 24 months. Until survival data are seen, and in particular the outcome data from patients who cross over to a PARP inhibitor at relapse, the question whether non-BRCA-mutated patients might derive a greater benefit from the use of a PARP inhibitor at relapse remains open. PFS2 is the time from randomization to second disease progression or death. This is increasingly been used as a surrogate for OS in oncology clinical trials. In PAOLA-1, the median PFS2 in the HRD-negative/unknown groups was 26.3 versus 28.1 months for olaparib/bevacizumab versus placebo/bevacizumab (HR=0.98, 95% CI: 0.77–1.27), suggesting that there is unlikely to be an OS benefit from using PARP inhibitors upfront in HRD-negative patients. Given the PFS1 and PFS2 data, and that bevacizumab is a widely available maintenance option following first-line chemotherapy in stage IV ovarian cancer, patients with HRD-negative disease may derive the most benefit from bevacizumab maintenance in the first-line followed by PARP inhibitors at first recurrence.

Conclusion

In conclusion, PARP inhibitors are widely approved for use as maintenance after the first recurrence and patients benefit regardless of BRCA or HRD status. There is a long-term PFS and OS benefit with some patients remaining on treatment beyond five years. Until there is clear evidence that patients given PARP inhibitors after first-line treatment rather than at recurrence live longer, the value of offering PARP inhibitors to all patients in the first-line setting remains uncertain.

References

1. Ledermann J, et al. Olaparib maintenance therapy in platinum-sensitive relapsed ovarian cancer. *N Engl J Med* 2012;366 (15):1382–1392.

2. Friedlander M, et al. Long-term efficacy, tolerability and overall survival in patients with platinum-sensitive, recurrent high-grade serous ovarian cancer treated with maintenance olaparib capsules following response to chemotherapy. *Br J Cancer* 2018;119(9):1075–1085.

3. Pujade-Lauraine E, et al. Olaparib tablets as maintenance therapy in patients with platinum-sensitive, relapsed ovarian cancer

and a BRCA1/2 mutation (SOLO2/ ENGOT-Ov21): a double-blind, randomised, placebo-controlled, phase 3 trial. *Lancet Oncol* 2017;18(9):1274–1284.

4. Mirza MR, et al. Niraparib maintenance therapy in platinum-sensitive, recurrent ovarian cancer. *N Engl J Med* 2016;375 (22):2154–2164.

5. Coleman RL, et al. Rucaparib maintenance treatment for recurrent ovarian carcinoma after response to platinum therapy (ARIEL3): a randomised, double-blind, placebo-controlled, phase 3 trial. *Lancet* 2017;390(10106):1949–1961.

What is the best front-line maintenance therapy for optimally debulked HRD-negative advanced epithelial ovarian cancer? Bevacizumab

Krishnansu S. Tewari

Debate

The biology of high-grade serous ovarian carcinoma encourages early dissemination through activation of pro-angiogenic pathways [1]. Vascular endothelial growth factor (VEGF) has been recognized as a key promoter of tumor angiogenesis and disease progression in this disease [1]. Over the past decade VEGF has also emerged as an important therapeutic target. Nine phase 3 randomized clinical trials have each met their primary endpoint with a statistically significant and clinically meaningful improvement in progression-free survival (PFS) through the incorporation of bevacizumab or other anti-angiogenic molecules as compared to chemotherapy alone and/or placebo [1]. Five of these trials studied the efficacy and tolerability of the anti-VEGF fully humanized monoclonal antibody, bevacizumab, and have directly led to US FDA approval and European Medicines Agency approval of this agent for women with newly diagnosed disease, platinum-sensitive relapsing disease, and platinum-resistant recurrent ovarian carcinoma [1].

Specifically, for patients with newly diagnosed advanced disease, in Gynecologic Oncology Group protocol 0218, the integration of bevacizumab (15 mg/kg) with systemic platinum- and taxane-based chemotherapy (beginning with cycle #2 following cytoreductive surgery) and continuing as a maintenance monotherapy (15 mg/kg q21d) confers a 5.8 month (18.2 vs. 12.8 months) improvement in PFS compared to chemotherapy alone: stratified HR for progression or death 0.62; 95% CI: 0.52–0.75, two-sided $p<0.0001$ [2]. At a median follow-up of 102.9 months and 375 deaths in the control arm, the final analysis of overall survival did not attribute a survival benefit to bevacizumab [3].

In the ICON7 randomized trial of front-line bevacizumab, a survival benefit was observed in an exploratory analysis of a high-risk subgroup (i.e., suboptimal stage III and any stage IV) [1]. Although the placebo-controlled GOG-0218 was unable to validate the European trials findings, the observed 10-month relative survival benefit (42.8 vs. 32.6 months) suggests that bevacizumab, when administered with and following chemotherapy, may be beneficial for patients with stage IV disease by producing median survival rates that approximate those observed with the more favorable stage III tumors [3].

All of the studies with bevacizumab were conducted in unselected patients. Because validated serum and/or tissue factors that predict activity of anti-angiogenics have remained elusive, enrolment in GOG-0218 was not enriched for a specific biomarker. Accordingly, the label granted by the US FDA on June 13, 2018 is for all patients with advanced disease who do not have a contraindication to bevacizumab [1]. Black Box Warnings for bevacizumab include wound healing, hemorrhage and gastrointestinal wall disruption; while potentially catastrophic, bowel perforation has been largely avoided by withholding drugs to patients with signs (physical or radiographic) or symptoms of small bowel obstruction or known inflammatory bowel disease [1].

Poly-ADP-polymerase 1 inhibitors (PARPi) have also been developed as effective maintenance strategies for newly diagnosed ovarian carcinoma, particularly the high-grade serous histologic subtype. Because PARPi(s) prevent single-strand annealing of DNA, they are most effective in tumors with homologous recombination deficiency (HRD). Importantly, exploitation by PARPi(s) of the inability of HRD+ tumors to repair double-strand DNA breaks leads to conversion of single-strand breaks to lethal double-strand breaks with subsequent collapse at the replication fork.

Based on an astonishing PFS benefit observed among patients with HRD+ BRCA-mutated (somatic or germline) tumors receiving maintenance therapy with olaparib in the phase 3 randomized placebo-controlled SOLO-1 trial (NCT01844986), this agent was approved by the US FDA on December 19, 2018 for primary maintenance therapy in this population. Five-year follow-up data from this trial has demonstrated that olaparib continues to reduce the risk of disease progression or death compared to placebo (median 56.0 vs. 13.8 months) by 67% (HR=0.33, 95% CI: 0.25–0.43) with 48.3% of patients remaining disease-free compared with 20.5% of patients on placebo [1]. Based on the phase 3 randomized PAOLA-1 trial (NCT02477644), on May 8, 2020 the FDA expanded the indication of olaparib to include its combination with bevacizumab for first-line maintenance treatment of patients with advanced HRD+ disease defined by either a deleterious or suspected deleterious *BRCA* mutation and/or genomic instability according to Myriad's myChoice assay cut-off of ≥ 42. The rationale of combining anti-VEGF therapy with PARPi is based on in vitro data which indicates that hypoxia may induce a BRCA-like phenotype.

PARPi(s) were designed to target HRD+ tumors and there is no argument that the data in the HRD+ *BRCA*-mutated and HRD+ *BRCA*-wild type subpopulations are compelling. A third randomized phase 3 trial, PRIMA (NCT02655016), studied maintenance therapy with the PARPi, niraparib, and also demonstrated a PFS benefit in the overall intent-to-treat population (HR=0.62, 95% CI: 0.50–0.76) [4]. Although exploratory analyses demonstrated the treatment benefit was most pronounced in patients with somatic BRCA mutations (HR=0.40, 95% CI: 0.27–0.62), followed by BRCA-wild type HRD+ tumors (HR=0.50, 95% CI: 0.30–0.83), the FDA approved niraparib (200 mg daily) for primary maintenance therapy for all-comers, regardless of molecular signature. Although niraparib reduced the risk of disease progression or death by 32% (HR=0.68, 95% CI: 0.49–0.94) among patients with homologous recombination-proficient (HR-proficient) tumors, these data are based on *pre-specified exploratory analyses*, i.e., essentially a post-hoc retrospective study embedded within PRIMA!

The field continues to advance and now in the third decade of the twenty-first century, every patient with newly diagnosed advanced epithelial ovarian cancer should undergo genetic counseling, genetic testing and when applicable tumor HRD testing. All patients should be offered maintenance therapy, and for those with HR-proficient tumors, the choices are between bevacizumab and niraparib. While the HR(s) are somewhat similar (0.62 in GOG-0218 and 0.68 in PRIMA), certainly the prospectively derived median PFS of 18.2 months associated with bevacizumab maintenance in the non-enriched population of

GOG-0218 should resonate more strongly than the retrospectively derived median PFS of 8.1 months associated with niraparib in the HR-proficient subpopulation of PRIMA. Thus, because the Devil's in the details, there is no need to invoke the tired phrase of how cross-trial comparisons are never valid. The FDA's approval of niraparib for all-comers, fails to provide clinical guidance, and has only created confusion.

Perhaps another reason to argue in favor of bevacizumab maintenance therapy lies in the opportunity to realize the potential of immunotherapy in this disease. Ovarian carcinomas are relatively cold (i.e., non-immunogenic), and thus far the activity of checkpoint inhibition when administered as a monotherapy has been disappointing. However, because VEGF has immunosuppressive effects in the tumor microenvironment where it inhibits T-cell and dendritic cell function and reduces T-cell trafficking and infiltration into the tumor bed [5], there is great interest in the possibility of additive or synergistic effects when VEGF blockade is combined with immunotherapy. This hypothesis is particularly relevant and applicable to the HR-proficient subgroups that lack the immunostimulatory neoantigens generated through HRD-associated mutations including *BRCA*.

Conclusion

To summarize, bevacizumab is the appropriate maintenance therapy for women with HR-proficient ovarian carcinoma who have responded to platinum- and taxane-based systemic therapy. Unlike the findings concerning the HR-proficient subpopulation in PRIMA, the data supporting bevacizumab arrive through *prospective analysis* and may even be associated with a survival benefit among women with stage IV disease. The inconvenience of a 30-minute intravenous infusion every three weeks pales when framed against the potential for grade 3–4 anemia and thrombocytopenia associated with niraparib (as well as the 1–2% risk of potentially fatal myelodysplastic syndrome!). As stated earlier, the risk factors for gastrointestinal wall disruption with bevacizumab have been identified. Consequently, bevacizumab is the safer and more efficacious option. And that, as they say, is that.

References

1. Tewari KS, et al. Chapter 77: Ovarian cancer. In: DeVita VT, Lawrence TS, Rosenberg SA (Eds.), *DeVita, Hellman, and Rosenberg's Cancer: Principles & Practice of Oncology* (11th edn.). Philadelphia, PA: Lippincott Williams & Wilkins; 2019.

2. Burger RA, et al. Incorporation of bevacizumab in the primary treatment of ovarian cancer. *N Engl J Med* 2011;365:2473–2483.

3. Tewari KS, et al. Final overall survival of a randomized trial of bevacizumab for primary treatment of ovarian cancer. *J Clin Oncol* 2019;37:2317–2328.

4. González-Martín A, et al. Niraparib in patients with newly diagnosed advanced ovarian cancer. *N Engl J Med* 2019;381:2391–2402.

5. Yi M, et al. Synergistic effect of immune checkpoint blockade and anti-angiogenesis in cancer treatment. *Mol Cancer* 2019;18:60.

Debate

18B

What is the best front-line maintenance therapy for optimally debulked HRD-negative advanced epithelial ovarian cancer?

PARP Inhibitor

Francisco Grau, Lorena Fariñas-Madrid, and Ana Oaknin

Debate

The integrated genomic analysis of high-grade serous ovarian cancer carried out by The Cancer Genome Atlas Research Network (TCGA) identified two large subgroups of patients, those harboring homologous recombination (HR) deficiency (50%), characterized by genetic and epigenetic alterations of HR genes, most commonly the *BRCA1* and *BRCA2* genes, and those with an intact HR pathway, enriched in *Cyclin E1* (*CCNE1*) amplifications. These HR-proficient tumors are associated with inferior survival outcomes and poorer response to PARP inhibitors (PARPi), in comparison with HR-deficient tumors [1,2].

Currently, two of the most used commercially available assays to test HR-deficiency status, Myriad myChoice CDx and the Foundation Medicine's FoundationFocus CDx, are challenged by the reliable identification of HR-proficient tumors. Thus, some of those tumors identified as HR-proficient by using these tests, contrary to expectations, may be responsive to PARPi, as they may retain a certain degree of HR deficiency. This might explain why both phase 3 trials, NOVA and ARIEL3 [3,4], assessing niraparib and rucaparib respectively, in the platinum-sensitive recurrent disease setting, demonstrated a significant improvement in PFS in the HR-proficient/LOH-low subgroups (HR=0.58, p=0.02, and HR=0.58, p<0.001, respectively) . Similarly, PRIMA trial showed that the HRD-negative population had statistically significant PFS benefit from niraparib (HR=0.68; 95% CI: 0.492–0.944), in the first-line setting. Due to all that, and until the development of an accurate test determining HR-proficiency, the HR-negative status may not preclude from using PARPi in this subpopulation of advanced ovarian cancer.

Although PRIMA trial was run in high-risk "all-comers" advanced ovarian cancer population, namely suboptimally primary debulked stage III, stage III under neoadjuvant chemotherapy, and any stage IV ovarian cancer, patients included in this trial were highly platinum-sensitive, as 69% of the population achieved a complete response to platinum-based chemotherapy which may predict significant benefit from PARP inhibition. Thus, using niraparib as maintenance treatment after a documented good response to platinum-based chemotherapy in the first-line setting may still be an option.

From the perspective of optimizing the long-term sequential therapeutical strategy of the HR-proficient patients, the administration of PARPi in the first-line setting may represent an acceptable approach, even in comparison with the use of bevacizumab, which demonstrated a meaningful PFS benefit even in those patients with no residual disease [5,6]. HR-proficient patients represent a poor-prognosis population, with high probability of relapse within the first six months after finishing first-line chemotherapy. Besides, following disease recurrence, a response to subsequent platinum-based chemotherapy is mandatory for receiving maintenance PARPi. Therefore, the first-line setting may be the only opportunity for these patients to receive PARPi and provides the opportunity to delay the onset of primary resistance to platinum. Conversely, the use of bevacizumab could be postponed to the second-line based on data for patients with platinum-sensitive relapsed disease and to the second- or third-line for platinum-resistant relapse [7,8].

Conclusion

In conclusion, HR-proficient advanced ovarian cancer population represents a relevant unmet clinical need, in urgent need for novel therapeutical approaches to offer better outcomes. In this regard, PARPi may still be an appropriate alternative treatment in this subgroup.

References

1. Ray-Coquard I, et al. Olaparib plus bevacizumab as first-line maintenance in ovarian cancer. *N Engl J Med* 2019;381 (25):2416–2428.

2. González-Martín A, et al. Niraparib in patients with newly diagnosed advanced ovarian cancer. *N Engl J Med* 2019;381 (25):2391–2402.

3. Mirza MR, et al. Niraparib maintenance therapy in platinum-sensitive, recurrent ovarian cancer. *N Engl J Med* 2016;375 (22):2154–2164.

4. Ledermann JA, et al. Rucaparib for patients with platinum-sensitive, recurrent ovarian carcinoma (ARIEL3): post-progression outcomes and updated safety results from a randomised, placebo-controlled, phase 3 trial. *Lancet Oncol* 2020;21(5):710–722.

5. Burger RA, et al. Incorporation of bevacizumab in the primary treatment of ovarian cancer. *N Engl J Med* 2011 29;365 (26):2473–2483.

6. González Martín A, et al. Exploratory outcome analyses according to stage and/or residual disease in the ICON7 trial of carboplatin and paclitaxel with or without bevacizumab for newly diagnosed ovarian cancer. *Gynecol Oncol* 2019;152(1):53–60.

7. Aghajanian C, et al. OCEANS: a randomized, double-blind, placebo-controlled phase III trial of chemotherapy with or without bevacizumab in patients with platinum-sensitive recurrent epithelial ovarian, primary peritoneal, or fallopian tube cancer. *J Clin Oncol* 2012;30(17):2039–2045.

8. Pujade Lauraine E, et al.Bevacizumab combined with chemotherapy for platinum-resistant recurrent ovarian cancer: the AURELIA open-label randomized phase III trial. *J Clin Oncol* 2014;32(13):1302–1308.

What is the Optimal Therapeutic Option for Platinum-resistant Recurrent Ovarian Cancer

Single-agent Chemotherapy

David F. Cantú de León, Daniel Flores Alatriste, and Milagros Pérez Quintanilla

Debate

Platinum resistance is a very common event during the natural history of epithelial ovarian cancer (EOC); it is more prevalent as the number of treatment lines are given to patients, is multifactorial, and evolves during time. Intrinsic platinum resistance is present in about 10–15% of cases and is seen in nonserous histologic subtypes such as mucinous and clear cell carcinomas [1].

The traditional definition of platinum resistance as reported in the previous GCIG Ovarian Cancer Consensus Conference (OCCC) refers to a disease which relapses within six months after finishing treatment with platinum. However, this definition has been challenged during the sixth OCCC which discouraged the use of platinum-free interval as the only criterion to define eligibility to clinical trial for patients with recurrent ovarian cancer [2].

Treatment is challenging, patients have to be informed that management always is considered palliative instead of curative, and potential toxicities, side effects, and risks must be discussed. Progression-free survival (PFS) and overall survival (OS) may not be the best endpoints in this subset of patients, as Health Related Quality of Life (HRQOL) and Patient Reported Outcomes (PROs) may be more adequate metrics in these cases with expected survival of less than 12 months. The choice of drug must be individualized to the patient and must be based on previous treatments, toxicity, drug availability, cost, physician experience, and patient preferences [3].

Several strategies are currently being investigated in an effort to improve outcome, including improvement of drug delivery by developing antibody-drug conjugates (ADCs) targeting several receptors, re-sensitizing the tumor by inhibiting DNA methylation, modulating cell-cycle using specific checkpoint kinase inhibitors, improving immune response by modulating tumor microenvironment, and optimizing the time for surgery, which as a sole therapy could be very important in removing as much tumor as possible in order to reduce the clonal diversity limiting the potential for sub-clonal populations to progress and become resistant.

The use of single-agent chemotherapy is considered standard of care in those patients that can be allocated to the definition of platinum-resistant. Four drugs are mainly used with similar response rates: pegylated liposomal doxorubicin (PLD), paclitaxel, gemcitabine, and topotecan. There is no preferred drug as first-line or subsequent therapy. The Cochrane consortium included 1323 cases of platinum-resistant EOC in a systematic review and concluded that topotecan, paclitaxel, and PLD have similar efficacy but with different adverse effects. Treatment response rates range from 15–20%, PFS is less than four months, and OS ranges between nine and 12 months [2].

Docetaxel and oral etoposide are other options that can be used as monotherapy. Currently, the evidence of an objective benefit in platinum-resistant patients remains weak, with response rates of 10–15% and PFS of three to four months.

Paclitaxel is one of the most commonly used cytotoxic agents. Its regimen was recently modified because the weekly administration showed response rates of 13–50% and caused less neurotoxicity, as compared with its every-three-week administration. Therefore, it has become the control arm of several randomized trials in patients with platinum-resistant EOC [4].

In a phase III multicenter trial, Ferrandina et al. compared gemcitabine versus PLD treatment, considering time to progression as the primary endpoint. No significant differences were found between the two treatments. Another phase III trial of gemcitabine compared with PLD was conducted by Mutch et al., recruiting patients experiencing recurrence within six months. The primary endpoint was progression-free interval. No differences were found either, with a similar OS in both groups.

Etirinotecan is a polymer conjugate of irinotecan with a longer half-life and fewer cholinergic effects. The findings of phase II trials have shown response rates of up to 15.4% in patients with platinum-resistant EOC. This drug has also shown a PFS of 4.4 months and OS of 10 months.

Bevacizumab was approved by the FDA for patients with platinum-resistant EOC in 2014; its benefits have been demonstrated in several studies with objective response rates of up to 20%. Candidate patients for bevacizumab are those who have received less than two regimens, have not previously taken bevacizumab, and have no history of bowel obstruction within six months. However, the most prominent activity is seen when bevacizumab is combined with chemotherapy.

Poly ADP-ribose polymerase (PARP) inhibitors are among the novel effective agents in the treatment of ovarian cancer. Olaparib, niraparib, and rucaparib are FDA approved as therapy for platinum-resistant disease with BRCA mutation after three lines of treatment. An objective response of 33% and an average response duration of 28 weeks were found in a phase II trial involving 24 patients with platinum-resistant disease and BRCA mutation. The QUADRA trial administered niraparib to BRCA mutation carriers with platinum-resistant EOC. This trial showed a response rate of 34% and an average response duration of 7.9 months [3].

ARIEL 4 is a randomized study of rucaparib versus standard chemotherapy as second-line treatment in patients with BRCA-mutated ovarian cancer. This study, which also included platinum-resistant patients, demonstrated an improved PFS compared to standard of care chemotherapy [5].

Endocrine therapy with tamoxifen versus chemotherapy in 138 platinum-resistant patients revealed a PFS of 8.3 and 12.7 weeks respectively. In asymptomatic women with elevated CA 125 levels, letrozole showed response rates >50% in tumor markers and radiological response rates of 9% [5].

Conclusion

In conclusion, platinum-resistant ovarian cancer is a complex and aggressive entity with very limited treatment options, and is a prolific area of research in order to counteract the different and multifactorial mechanisms of resistance. Cancer genome analysis has yielded promising results that will lead to personalized and targeted treatments according to specific genotypes. Monotherapy remains standard of care and must be carefully discussed with patients in order to select the best option.

References

1. McMullen M, et al. New approaches for targeting platinum-resistant ovarian cancer. *Semin Cancer Biol* 2020;2020:S1044–579X (20)30186–3. https://doi.org/10.1016/j .semcancer.2020.08.013

2. Pujade-Lauraine E, et al. Management of platinum-resistant, relapsed epithelial ovarian cancer and new drug perspectives. *J Clin Oncol* 2019;37(27):2437–2448. https:// doi.org/10.1200/JCO.19.00194

3. Lee JM, et al. New strategies in ovarian cancer treatment. *Cancer* 2019;125(Suppl. 24):4623–4629. https://doi.org/10.1002/cncr.32544

4. Poveda AM, et al. Bevacizumab combined with weekly paclitaxel, pegylated liposomal doxorubicin, or topotecan in platinum-resistant recurrent ovarian cancer: analysis by chemotherapy cohort of the randomized phase III AURELIA trial. *J Clin Oncol* 2014;33:3836–3838.

5. Oronsky B, et al. A brief review of the management of platinum-resistant-platinum-refractory ovarian cancer. *Med Oncol* 2017;34(6):103. https://doi.org/10 .1007/s12032-017-0960-z

19B What is the Optimal Therapeutic Option for Platinum-resistant Recurrent Ovarian Cancer?
Other

Olivia Lara and Bhavana Pothuri

Debate

The management of patients with platinum-resistant recurrent epithelial ovarian cancer (EOC) poses a significant challenge. Traditionally treatment has involved the use of non-platinum chemotherapeutic agents, including PEGylated liposomal doxorubicin (PLD), topotecan, gemcitabine, and paclitaxel, used as monotherapy with response rates of 10–15%, progression-free survival (PFS) of three to four months and overall survival (OS) of approximately 12 months [1]. These agents have had limited efficacy and failed to demonstrate a meaningful OS benefit at the risk of chemotherapy toxicity. Through advancements in integrated genomic analysis, an increased understanding of the underlying molecular characteristics of EOC has led to the development of various molecularly targeted strategies designed to advance the field beyond single agent chemotherapy.

Bevacizumab, a recombinant humanized monoclonal antibody that targets vascular endothelial growth factor, has single agent activity in EOC both as monotherapy and when combined with chemotherapy. The AURELIA (Avastin Use in Platinum-Resistant Epithelial OC) phase III study evaluated single agent chemotherapy with or without bevacizumab in patients with platinum-resistant disease and noted a near doubling of the PFS (3.4 vs. 6.7 months; hazard ratio (HR)=0.48; 95% confidence interval (CI): 0.38–0.60, p<0.001) with the addition of bevacizumab. Median overall survival increased by three months but was not statistically significant (13.3 vs. 16.6 months; HR=0.85, 95% CI: 0.66–1.08, p<0.174) [2]. This led to the FDA approval of bevacizumab for use with chemotherapy in patients with platinum-resistant EOC. This has spurred the integration of molecularly targeted agents in the management of EOC and utilization of bevacizumab has become a standard of care in the treatment of platinum-resistant ovarian cancer.

Inhibitors of poly (ADP-ribose) polymerase (PARP) have shown evidence of their efficacy in platinum-resistant patients as well. In a phase II study, which included 193 germline BRCA 1/2 mutation (gBRCAm) carriers with both platinum-sensitive and platinum-resistant EOC, the tumor response was 31% (95% CI: 24.6–38.1) and stable disease was seen in 40% of patients (95% CI: 33.4–47.7) [3]. Additionally in a phase Ib study of olaparib, RECIST responses were confirmed in eight (33.5%) of 24 platinum-resistant patients [4]. This has led to the FDA approval of olaparib as monotherapy for gBRCAm-related ovarian cancer after three or more prior regimens. Study 10 and the ARIEL 2 trial investigated rucaparib in 106 gBRCAm and tumor BRCA mutated (tBRCAm) patients who progressed on two prior therapies. Investigator-assessed objective response rate (ORR) was 66% (52/79; 95% CI: 54–76) in platinum-sensitive patients and 25% (5/20; 95% CI: 9–49) in platinum-resistant patients. This led to the FDA approval of rucaparib for treatment regardless of platinum sensitivity in gBRCAm and tBRCAm patients after two prior lines of therapy. In the phase II Quadra trial of single-agent niraparib the ORR of gBRCAm patients who had previously received three or more lines of therapy was 33% for platinum-resistant disease (n=21) and 19% for platinum-refractory disease (n=16) [5]. In a phase II trial investigating alterative combinations, olaparib was combined with cediranib in gBRCAm patients. The ORR in platinum-resistant patients was 20% (95% CI: 11–38%) with seven confirmed PRs. Median duration of response was six months and disease control rate (DCR) 43% in platinum-resistant patients [6]. Confirmatory studies of the combination olaparib and cediranib is currently under investigation in the NRG GY005 phase II/III trial that recently completed accrual (Clinicaltrials.gov identifier: NCT02502266).

Immunotherapy has shown some antitumor activity in platinum-resistant patients; the response rate with avelumab was 9.6% (12/125) and 9% (11/97) with pembrolizumab [7,8]. The TOPACIO/KEYNOTE-162 phase I and II trial evaluated pembrolizumab and niraparib in platinum-resistant ovarian carcinoma irrespective of BRCA mutation status. In the integrated phase I and II studies in ovarian carcinoma, ORR was 18% (95% CI: 11–29%), with a disease control rate of 65% (95% CI: 54–74%). This included three (5%) with complete response, eight (13%) with partial response, 28 (47%) with stable disease, and 20 (33%) with progressive disease [9]. In the phase II trial of Nivolumab and Ipilimumab in recurrent or persistent ovarian cancer, platinum-resistant patients represented 62% of patients and saw a favorable response to combination therapy [10]. In a single arm, phase II study (ClinicalTrials.gov identifier: NCT02440425) the combination of pembrolizumab and weekly paclitaxel has reported a preliminary response rate of 51% [11]. Results of a phase II trial evaluating pembrolizumab in combination with bevacizumab and oral metronomic cyclophosphamide showed an ORR of 37.5% which included platinum-sensitive and platinum-resistant patients who received a median number of five prior lines of chemotherapy (SGO Annual Conference 2019, Abstract LBA4). Immunotherapy in platinum-resistant disease has yielded promising yet mixed results. Further combinations including PLD and Atezolizumab are being studied in the ongoing phase II/III NRG GY009 study.

Finally, the use of novel therapeutics including antibody drug conjugates (ADC) have shown clinical activity in platinum-resistant disease. In an ongoing phase I study, ADC XMT-1536 demonstrated clinical responses and stable disease in platinum-resistant patients. Of the 20 patients evaluated, two (10%) confirmed complete response and five (25%) achieved partial responses for an objective response rate of 35% after treatment with XMT-1536. Additionally eight (40%) of 20 patients achieved stable disease [12]. Additional phase II trials are currently underway to determine the role of XMT-1536 in platinum-resistant ovarian cancer. Mirvetuximab soravtansine is another ADC composed of a humanized alpha-folate receptor (FRα)–binding monoclonal antibody with DM4, a potent antimitotic agent. In 46 patients in the phase I expansion cohort with platinum-resistant disease and FRα-positive tumors and up to five prior lines of systemic therapy, the ORR was 26% and the median PFS was 4.8 months [13]. A phase III trial, Mirasol is currently ongoing to confirm these findings. Other agents including ofranergene obadeno-vec (VB-111), a targeted anti-cancer gene therapy, in combination with weekly paclitaxel have shown interim favorable CA-125 tumor responses with an OS of 498 days compared to 172.5 days in the platinum-resistant group in phase III OVAL trial [14].

Conclusion

While the use of non-platinum single agent chemotherapy was once a standard of care for patients with platinum-resistant EOC, the use of molecular targeted therapies has changed the standard of care to include bevacizumab in these difficult-to-treat patients. PARPi are effective in treating gBRCAm and tBRCAm patients with recurrent platinum-resistant disease, and immunotherapy combinations as well as ADCs are being actively investigated to determine if they can play a critical role in the treatment of platinum-resistant ovarian cancer. Additional efforts are needed to understand the genomic events driving resistant EOC to provide continued rational development of new therapies in ovarian cancer.

References

1. Davis A, et al. "Platinum resistant" ovarian cancer: what is it, who to treat and how to measure benefit? *Gynecol Oncol* 2014;133: 624–631.

2. Pujade-Lauraine E, et al. Bevacizumab combined with chemotherapy for platinum-resistant recurrent ovarian cancer: the AURELIA open-label randomized phase III trial. *J Clin Oncol* 2014;32(13):1302–1308. https://doi.org/10.1200/JCO.2013.51.4489.

3. Kaufman B, et al. Olaparib monotherapy in patients with advanced cancer and a germline BRCA1/2 mutation. *J Clin Oncol* 2015;33:244–250.

4. Fong PC, et al. Inhibition of poly (ADP-ribose) polymerase in tumors from BRCA mutation carriers. *N Engl J Med* 2009;361:123–134.

5. Moore KN, et al. QUADRA: a phase 2, open-label, single-arm study to evaluate niraparib in patients (pts) with relapsed ovarian cancer (ROC) who have received ≥3 prior chemotherapy regimens. *J Clin Oncol* 2018;36:5514.

6. Liu JF, et al. A phase 2 biomarker trial of combination cediranib and olaparib in relapsed platinum (plat) sensitive and plat resistant ovarian cancer (ovca). *J Clin Oncol* 2018;36:5519.

7. Disis ML, et al. Efficacy and safety of avelumab for patients with recurrent or refractory ovarian cancer: phase 1b results from the JAVELIN solid tumor trial. *JAMA Oncol* 2019;5:393–401.

8. Matulonis UA, et al. Antitumor activity and safety of pembrolizumab in patients with advanced recurrent ovarian cancer: interim results from the phase 2 KEYNOTE-100 study. *J Clin Oncol* 2018;36:5511.

9. Konstantinopoulos PA, et al. Single-arm phases 1 and 2 trial of niraparib in combination with pembrolizumab in patients with recurrent platinum-resistant ovarian carcinoma. *JAMA Oncol* 2019;5:1141–1149.

10. Zamarin D, et al. Randomized phase ii trial of nivolumab versus nivolumab and ipilimumab for recurrent or persistent ovarian cancer: an NRG oncology study. *J Clin Oncol* 2020;38:1814–1823.

11. Wenham RM, et al. Phase II trial of dose dense (weekly) paclitaxel with pembrolizumab (MK-3475) in platinum-resistant recurrent ovarian cancer. 2016;34: TPS5612-TPS.

12. Richardson DL, et al. Phase I expansion study of XMT-1536, a novel NaPi2b-targeting antibody-drug conjugate (ADC): preliminary efficacy, safety, and biomarker results in patients with previously treated metastatic ovarian cancer (OC) or non-small cell lung cancer (NSCLC). *J Clin Oncol* 2020;38:3549.

13. Moore KN, et al. Safety and activity of mirvetuximab soravtansine (IMGN853), a folate receptor alpha-targeting antibody-drug conjugate, in platinum-resistant ovarian, fallopian tube, or primary peritoneal cancer: a phase i expansion study. *J Clin Oncol* 2017;35:1112–1118.

14. Arend RC, et al. Clinical trial in progress: pivotal study of VB-111 combined with paclitaxel versus paclitaxel for treatment of platinum-resistant ovarian cancer (OVAL, VB-111-701/GOG-3018). *J Clin Oncol* 2020;38:TPS6097-TPS.

20A
Should Patients with Platinum-sensitive Recurrent Ovarian Cancer Undergo Secondary Cytoreduction prior to Receiving Platinum-containing Second-line Chemotherapy?

Yes

Sarah Ehmann, Andreas du Bois, and Mareike Bommert

Debate

Cytoreductive surgery is an important part in the treatment of ovarian cancer, in the primary setting as well as in recurrence. One of the key prognostic factors which can be influenced in ovarian cancer patient management is the surgical cytoreductive outcome, but the ability to achieve complete resection and the right patient selection are of utmost importance to prevent surgical morbidity and mortality.

The Arbeitsgemeinschaft Gynäkologische Onkologie (AGO) published the Descriptive Evaluation of perioperative Selection KriTeria for OPerability in recurrent OVARian cancer (DESKTOP OVAR) series. The DESKTOP I trial created a predictive score for resectability taking into account three factors: no residual disease after primary debulking surgery, good performance status (PS), and ascites less than 500 mL in preoperative imaging. Localization of recurrent disease and therapy-free interval did not show any impact for complete resection in multivariate analysis [1]. The AGO score was successfully validated in the DESKTOP II trial and showed in the subgroup of AGO score positive patients with first recurrence a positive prediction regarding complete resectability in 76%. Surgery in AGO score negative patients might also be an option, but it is an individual decision and this endpoint was not addressed in the DESKTOP II trial. If complete resection was achieved even in AGO score negative patients, the progression-free survival (PFS) was comparable to AGO score positive patients [2]. MSKCC (Chi et al.) published selection criteria for offering secondary cytoreductive surgery which included disease-free interval, the number of recurrence sites, and the presence of peritoneal carcinomatosis. Bristow et al. showed in a meta-analysis that each 10% increase of complete resection rate in recurrent ovarian cancer resulted in an overall survival benefit of three months.

Worldwide, three prospective randomized multicenter trials in platinum-sensitive recurrent ovarian cancer were conducted to compare secondary cytoreductive surgery followed by platinum-based chemotherapy versus chemotherapy alone. The SOC-1 trial opened in 2013, included 357 patients and its primary endpoint was PFS and overall survival (OS). The iModel was used for patient selection and prediction of resection: it includes stage, residual disease after primary surgery, progression-free interval (PFI), PS, CA125, ascites at recurrence. The interim analysis showed a PFS benefit of 5.5 months (17.4 vs. 11.9) favoring surgery with a complete resection rate was 76.7%. OS data are not mature yet [3].

The GOG 213 trial started in 2007 and 485 patients participated. Two primary analyses were defined: chemotherapy with bevacizumab followed by bevacizumab maintenance therapy versus chemotherapy alone and on secondary surgery versus no surgery if the patient was also eligible for surgery. Its primary endpoint was OS. Focusing on the surgical part of this trial the patients were deemed by the investigator to be amenable to complete resection. Complete resection was reached in 63%. The median OS was 50.6 months in the surgical group versus 64.7 months in the no surgery group without reaching statistical significance (HR=1.29, 95% CI: 0.97–1.72, p=0.08) [4].

The DESKTOP III trial started in 2009 and had a standardized patient selection process based on the AGO score as well as a careful selection of the participating centers. It was a superiority trial with 407 patients and OS was the primary endpoint. Complete resection in secondary cytoreduction was achieved in 75%. Median OS was 53.7 months with and 46.0 months without surgery (HR=0.76, 95% CI: 0.59–0.97, p=0.03). Analyzing and comparing only patients with complete resection and patients without surgery an OS benefit of even 14.5 months was found (60.7 vs. 46.2 months), patients with surgery and incomplete resection did even worse with an OS of 28.8 months [5].

Conclusion

In conclusion, the extraordinary OS benefit of more than 14 months in the DESKTOP III trial was highest and exclusively seen in the cohort with complete resection, indicating the importance of the right patient selection as well as the right selection of the center, with an experienced team and interprofessional/interdisciplinary cooperation, to provide the best treatment results for our patients. Therefore, an assessment of all patients with recurrent ovarian cancer and a platinum-free interval of more than six months regarding their eligibility for secondary cytoreduction should be performed. Tools such as AGO score, imaging, patient, and tumor characteristics may be helpful for the identification of the right cohort. The remaining 25% of patients with incomplete resection due to tumor spread or other reasons should be evaluated for early initiation of platinum-based chemotherapy.

References

1. Harter P, et al. Surgery in recurrent ovarian cancer: the Arbeitsgemeinschaft Gynaekologische Onkologie (AGO) DESKTOP OVAR Trial. *Ann Surg Oncol* 2006;13:1702–1710. https://doi.org/10.1245/s10434-006-9058-0

2. Harter P, et al. Prospective validation study of a predictive score for operability of recurrent ovarian cancer: the Multicenter Intergroup Study DESKTOP II. A Project of the AGO Kommission OVAR, AGO Study Group, NOGGO, AGO-Austria, and MITO. *Int J Gynecol Cancer* 2011;21:289–295. https://doi.org/10.1097/IGC.0b013e31820aaafd

3. Zang R, et al. A randomized phase III trial of secondary cytoreductive surgery in later recurrent ovarian cancer: SOC1/SGOG-OV2. *J Clin Oncol* 2020;38:6001–

6001. https://doi.org/10.1200/JCO
.2020.38.15_suppl.6001

4. Coleman RL, et al. Secondary surgical
cytoreduction for recurrent ovarian cancer.
N Engl J Med 2019;381:1929–1939. https://d
oi.org/10.1056/NEJMoa1902626

5. Du Bois A, et al. Randomized phase III study to
evaluate the impact of secondary cytoreductive
surgery in recurrent ovarian cancer: final
analysis of AGO DESKTOP III/ENGOT-ov20.
J Clin Oncol 2020;38:6000. https://doi.org/10
.1200/JCO.2020.38.15_suppl.6000

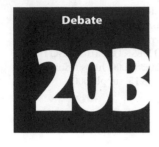

Should All Patients with Platinum-sensitive Recurrent Ovarian Cancer be Considered for Secondary Cytoreduction prior to Receiving Second-line Platinum Chemotherapy?

No

Anca Chelariu-Raicu and Robert L. Coleman

Debate

Ardent support of secondary cytoreductive surgery as a strategy in the treatment paradigm for patients with recurrent ovarian cancer has been levied for decades, largely by analogy to primary cytoreduction [1]. The primary rationale follows that removal of as much tumor as possible augments the effectiveness of subsequent chemotherapy and may enhance a more favorable tumor microenvironment for natural immune surveillance. However, the merit of this, as with any intervention, should be addressed in randomized clinical trials, if possible, to control bias, and compared to appropriate reference treatment assessing clinically relevant endpoints. This "tried and true" approach has been the foundation upon which current treatment standards have been defined. In the setting of recurrent ovarian cancer, a prolific expansion in efficacious therapies has been witnessed, challenging clinical trial endpoints, such as overall survival (OS), which may not be reached years after an index intervention [2].

When discussing role of surgery in recurrent ovarian cancer management, there are four key elements that establish the framework for debate: (1) most appropriate clinical setting; (2) patient candidacy/goal of surgery; (3) adjuvant therapy; (4) outcomes and endpoints. Our contention in this debate is that while seemingly discordant results have been presented among the three active clinical trials, the role of secondary cytoreduction is not clearly defined, particularly in the setting of highly effective adjuvant treatment, increasingly annotated by tumor genomic information [3–5].

Clinical Setting

We propose three subgroups of patients that are clinically relevant to the recurrent setting of ovarian cancer: patients without front-line maintenance, patients who progressed after front-line maintenance therapy with bevacizumab, and those who have progressed following poly (ADP-Ribose) polymerase (PARP) inhibitor therapy with or without combination bevacizumab. Herein, several key factors can be used to create an algorithm for an individual patient to evaluate potential response to systemic therapy: histologic type, platinum-free interval, molecular signature, pre-existing toxicities, and the impact of treatment on quality of life. In contrast, when considering a surgical approach, it is important to consider criteria such as chance to achieve complete gross resection, volume of disease, extensive platinum-free interval presence of ascites, and good performance status.

Goal of Surgery

In regards to surgical selection criteria, GOG-213 selected patients who were eligible for platinum-based therapy and deemed as reasonable candidates for surgery, including no extra-abdominal organ disease, ascites, and carcinomatosis. The pre-randomization stated objective for consideration of study participation was complete gross resection (CGR). However, DESKTOP III and SOC-1 trial used structured algorithms to provide guidance, though with the same goal, complete gross resection. Therefore, given the discrepant positive progression-free survival (PFS) results of these two trials relative to GOG-213, one may call into question the lack of more specific selection criteria for patient selection in GOG-213. However, it is important to note that the rate of CGR was numerically and statistically similar across all three studies (67–76.7%). The parity of these CGR rates minimizes one key variance often cited as a reason for the discordant observations seen in the three trials. It must not be discounted that individualization of clinical trial participation existed in each of these trials as patients matching eligibility criteria were not "required" to participate and may not have been enrolled due to one or both patient and investigator assessment factors, such as patient acceptance, medical safety of surgery, neoadjuvant chemotherapy in the first-line, and low likelihood of CGR based on disease distribution. Highlighting this point, in the SOC-1 trial, patients not meeting the iMODEL score were allowed to undergo additional evaluation with PET-CT where two physicians could override the criteria to enroll the subject, reaching 11% of patients who were enrolled by physician-directed individualization. In addition, while not stated in DESKTOP-III, 42% of patients meeting AGO surgical criteria in DESKTOP-II, did not undergo surgery, suggesting further patient individualization. Thus, championing discrepancy in trial results as a matter specific selection algorithm alone would appear to be misguided.

Adjuvant Therapy

All three trials were conducted during a time when treatment for platinum-sensitive recurrent ovarian cancer was changing, offering a greater variety of options, including concomitant and maintenance therapy; options that at the least have demonstrated better PFS, and in one, overall survival (OS). In contrast to GOG-213, which was designed to first address the impact of bevacizumab added to paclitaxel and carboplatin followed by maintenance bevacizumab until progression on OS, few patients enrolled in DESKTOP III or SOC-1 received any kind of maintenance therapy. This is critically important since the surgical effect might have been diluted by adjuvant therapy, particularly where maintenance was administered until disease progression. In a setting where prespecified and homogeneous chemotherapy is administered equally among the randomization cohorts, the effect of surgery on PFS is easier to determine. However, even in the absence of bevacizumab, platinum-based chemotherapy regimens have not demonstrated equipoise in formal phase III investigation. Similarly, several trials investigating the efficacy of PARP inhibition, for relapsed disease after complete or partial clinical response to platinum, demonstrated substantial improvements in PFS, independent of secondary cytoreduction [6–8]. Further, lack of a defined and balanced recurrence regimen strategy and the long anticipated post-progression survivorship in this disease setting differentially challenges any clear assessment of surgical treatment effect on OS. Despite this, the SOLO2 trial, which investigated the role of maintenance olaparib in unselected women with *BRCA*-mutated tumors is the first trial to report an improvement in median OS of 12.9 months [9]. Importantly, almost a third of patients treated with olaparib survived more than five years.

Outcomes and Endpoints

Interestingly, the median PFS, OS, and three-year OS rate among the surgical arms in the three trials are remarkably similar, highlighting some parity of prognostic factors. Moreover, the morphology of the Kaplan-Meier survival curves, which are at least 80% mature in GOG-213 and DESKTOP-III, are strikingly similar, demonstrating consistent time-dependent event rates. What is clear from evaluation of these three trials is that variance exists in the nonsurgical arms, with similarity observed in DESKTOP-III and SOC1, and discrepancy in GOG-213. With respect to PFS, this might be anticipated based on prior results of platinum-sensitive recurrence trials using bevacizumab, concomitantly and in maintenance, and may suggest a differentially more important role for adjuvant therapy (vs. surgical resection) in this population.

Conclusion

Taken together, each of the above-mentioned studies consists of an individual strength: the value of maintenance therapy in GOG-213 and structured surgical algorithms applied for patient selection in DESKTOP-III and SOC1. Although a trial investigating the role of secondary cytoreduction enrolling patients after both rigorous selection criteria for surgery and with an optimal (and biomarker directed) adjuvant therapy strategy would offer more clarity to the question, the likelihood such a trial could be completed is low. Further, the pace of drug discovery is swift and will continue to challenge treatment sequencing as newer therapies with incremental benefit will be adopted. Nevertheless, we strongly contend that continued investigation into innate and adapted tumor biology has the highest probability to identify patient cohorts where a multimodality approach would optimize patient survivorship. Until this time, the indication for secondary cytoreduction should be carefully considered.

References

1. Bristow RE, et al. Cytoreductive surgery for recurrent ovarian cancer: a meta-analysis. *Gynecol Oncol* 2009;112(1):265–274.

2. Insitute NC. Cancer Stat Facts: Ovarian Cancer. 2020.

3. Coleman RL, et al. Secondary surgical cytoreduction for recurrent ovarian cancer. *N Engl J Med* 2019;381(20):1929–1939.

4. duBois A, et al. Randomized phase III study to evaluate the impact of secondary cytoreductive surgery in recurrent ovarian cancer: final analysis of AGO DESKTOP III/ENGOT-ov20. *J Clin Oncol* (online) 2020;38. https://doi.org/10.1200/JCO.2017.35.15_SUPPL.5501

5. Zang R, et al. A randomized phase III trial of secondary cytoreductive surgery in later recurrent ovarian cancer: SOC1/SGOG-OV2. *J Clin Oncol* 2020 (online). https://doi.org/10.1200/jco.2020.38.15_suppl.6001

6. Coleman RL, et al. Rucaparib maintenance treatment for recurrent ovarian carcinoma after response to platinum therapy (ARIEL3): a randomised, double-blind, placebo-controlled, phase 3 trial. *Lancet* 2017;390(10106):1949–1961.

7. Mirza MR, et al. Niraparib maintenance therapy in platinum-sensitive, recurrent ovarian cancer. *N Engl J Med* 2016;375 (22):2154–2164.

8. Pujade-Lauraine E, et al. Olaparib tablets as maintenance therapy in patients with platinum-sensitive, relapsed ovarian cancer and a BRCA1/2 mutation (SOLO2/ENGOT-Ov21): a double-blind, randomised, placebo-controlled, phase 3 trial. *Lancet Oncol* 2017;18(9):1274–1284.

9. Poveda A, et al. Final overall survival (OS) results from SOLO2/ENGOT-ov21: a phase III trial assessing maintenance olaparib in patients (pts) with platinum-sensitive, relapsed ovarian cancer and a BRCA mutation. *J Clin Oncol* (online) 2020;38. https://doi.org/10.1200/jco.2020.38.15_suppl.6002

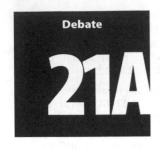

Should Tertiary Debulking for Patients with Recurrent Ovarian Cancer be Performed?

Yes

Karin K. Shih

Debate

The role of surgical cytoreduction in the management of primary ovarian cancer is well established. Unfortunately, the majority of patients develop recurrent disease. In the recurrent setting, the clinical benefit of surgical cytoreduction is debatable. The goal of treatment of recurrent ovarian cancer is to prolong remission, improve quality of life, and improve survival.

Recent results from randomized clinical trials evaluating the efficacy of surgical cytoreduction in the recurrent setting include results from the DESKTOP III trial [1]. In this prospective randomized trial, patients with platinum-sensitive recurrent ovarian cancer randomized to the surgery and chemotherapy arm had improved overall and progression-free survival compared with patients randomized to chemotherapy alone. Residual disease was a significant factor with patients who underwent complete gross resection [1] achieving a median overall survival of 61.9 months versus 28.8 months for patients who had residual disease after surgery versus 46 months for patients who received chemotherapy alone [1].

In contrast, results from the Gynecologic Oncology Group (GOG) 213 revealed no improvement in outcome with secondary cytoreductive surgery as compared with chemotherapy alone [2]. There are significant differences in these two trials which may explain the discordant findings. First, there was a substantial use of bevacizumab in GOG 213. Second, the resectability of disease was determined by surgeons which may confound results in each treatment arm. Moreover, the patient selection criteria in the DESKTOP III trial were stricter, with patients undergoing R0 resection at primary surgery.

In patients who achieve remission after treatment for recurrent ovarian cancer, relapse is common. In the tertiary recurrent setting, there are no randomized clinical trials to evaluate the survival benefit with surgical cytoreduction. Retrospective data suggests improved survival with appropriate patient selection (Table 21A.1). In a retrospective study of 77 patients, complete gross resection at tertiary cytoreductive surgery was significantly associated with disease-specific survival [3]. The median disease-specific survival of patients who underwent complete gross resection was 60.4 months compared with 27.9 months for patients with residual disease ≤ 0.5 cm and 13.6 months for patients with residual disease > 0.5 cm. Factors that portend a favorable tumor biology such as a longer treatment-free interval, platinum sensitivity, and single site of disease were associated with complete gross resection at time of tertiary surgical cytoreduction. A larger multicenter retrospective study at 14 centers evaluated 406 patients who underwent tertiary surgical cytoreduction [4]. The

Table 21A.1

	N	Treatment-free interval	Extent of disease at tertiary cytoreductive surgery	No gross residual disease	Overall survival and residual disease
Shih et al. 2010	77 patients	Median 17 months	62.3% single site	72.7%	60.4 months (no gross residual) 27.9 months (residual ≤ 0.5 cm) 13.6 months (residual > 0.5 cm)
Fotopolou et al. 2013	406 patients	Median 18 months	72.9% confined to pelvis	54.4%	49 months (no gross residual) 12 months (any residual disease)
Falcone et al. 2017	103 patients	All patients ≥ 6 months 63.1% (6–12 months) 36.9% (≥ 12 months)	43.7% single site	68.9%	43 months (no gross residual) 33 months (any residual disease)

median time from first to second relapse was 18 months and median overall survival was 26 months. Patients with no gross residual disease at tertiary surgical cytoreduction had a median overall survival of 49 months versus 12 months for patients with any tumor residual. More recently, a retrospective analysis of 103 patients enrolled at MITO affiliate centers included 103 patients who underwent tertiary surgical cytoreduction. The median overall survival for the entire cohort was 39.5 months [5]. However, patients who had no gross residual disease at tertiary surgical cytoreduction had median overall survival of 43 months, which was significantly higher than patients with any residual disease (33 months). Factors predictive of complete surgical cytoreduction included single site of disease as well as good performance status (ECOG = 0).

Patient selection is critical in evaluating the benefit of tertiary surgical cytoreduction. Factors that suggest favorable tumor biology include longer treatment-free interval, platinum sensitivity, single site of disease, and no residual disease at secondary surgical cytoreduction. As evident in the results from the DESKTOP III trial, stringent patient selection criteria are necessary to identify patients who will benefit from surgical cytoreduction in the recurrent setting.

Conclusion

There is a role for surgical cytoreduction in the setting of tertiary recurrent ovarian cancer. With appropriate patient selection, there may be a survival benefit with complete gross resection and surgical cytoreduction should be considered.

References

1. Dubois A, et al. Randomized phase III study to evaluate the impact of secondary cytoreductive surgery in recurrent ovarian cancer: final analysis of AGO DESKTOP III/ENGOT-ov20.*J Clinical Oncol* 2020;38:6000.

2. Coleman R, et al. Secondary surgical cytoreduction for recurrent ovarian cancer. *N Engl J Med* 2019;381:1929–1939.

3. Shih K, et al. Tertiary cytoreduction in patients in recurrent epithelial ovarian, fallopian tube, or primary peritoneal cancer: an updated series.*Gynecol Oncol* 2010;117:330–335.

4. Fotopoulou C, et al. Value of tertiary cytoreductive surgery in epithelial ovarian cancer: an international multicenter evaluation.*Ann Surg Oncol* 2013;20:1348–1354.

5. Falcone F, et al. Tertiary cytoreductive surgery in recurrent epithelial ovarian cancer: a multicenter MITO retrospective study.*Gynecol Oncol* 2017;147:66–72.

21B Should Tertiary Debulking be Performed for Patients with Recurrent Ovarian Cancer?

No

Antonio González-Martín

Debate

Surgery is considered a cornerstone in the treatment of advanced ovarian cancer. The absence of macroscopic residual tumor at the end of surgery is associated with a better outcome in primary debulking surgery and secondary cytoreduction for patients with a first relapse. Despite the absence of randomized clinical trials in the front-line setting, nobody questions the value of surgery in the initial management of primary advanced ovarian cancer due to extensive data showing a clear benefit in overall survival of complete cytoreduction after primary debulking surgery and interval debulking surgery. In the first relapse, three randomized clinical trials have produced apparently contradictory results. It is important to mention (for the best understanding of the question that we are dealing with), that only the studies including clearly defined selection criteria for cytoreduction, AGO-OVAR DESKTOP-III and SOC1, have produced a positive result in terms of progression-free survival. In addition, the AGO-OVAR study has also shown a benefit in overall survival.

The main weakness and argument against tertiary debulking surgery is the absence of good clinical evidence from randomized clinical trials, as we have for secondary cytoreduction, and even the lack of prospective series. To this author's knowledge, all the evidence that we have is from retrospective studies of highly specialized centers with high volume activity and, expectedly, highly influenced by selection bias, choosing probably patients with more "favorable" disease defined by longer disease-free interval, complete cytoreduction in prior secondary surgery and fewer locations of disease [1–4].

Unsurprisingly, the largest retrospective studies published have consistently shown that the achievement of complete cytoreduction in tertiary surgery is associated with a significantly longer overall survival than if any residual tumor is left [1,3,4]. So, the first question that the reader may raise is: do we have standardized criteria for selecting patients more likely to achieve complete cytoreduction with no gross residual at tertiary surgery? The answer is, unfortunately, not.

Many factors have been identified as predictors of complete cytoreduction at tertiary surgery in the multivariate analysis of retrospective studies. Fotopoulos et al. found platinum resistance, presence of positive lymph node at tertiary surgery, the persistence of tumor residuals at secondary surgery, tumor involvement of middle and upper abdomen, and presence of peritoneal carcinomatosis as significant risk factors for incomplete tumor resection

Table 21B.1 Retrospective studies of tertiary surgery with more than 100 patients

	Fotopoulos[1] (Multicenter)	Falcone[3] (MITO)	Manning-Geist[4] (MSKCC)
Date of publication	2013	2017	2021
Number of patients	406	103	114
Platinum-sensitive	38.2%	100%	88.6%
No gross residual at secondary surgery	38%	80.6%	67.6%
Peritoneal carcinomatosis	51.9%	56.3%*	55.3%*
Isolated recurrence at surgery	NA	43.7%	44.7%
CGR rate	54.1%	68.9%	89.5%

Abbreviations: CGR = complete gross resection; NA = not available; * = multiple tumor sites.

in a multicenter retrospective study with 406 patients. On the other hand, Falcone et al. have shown in a MITO retrospective study that the presence of a single lesion and a good performance status (ECOG 0) were the only independent predictors of complete surgical cytoreduction.

Interestingly, as summarized in Table 21B.1, the rate of complete cytoreduction of the three largest retrospective studies with more than 100 patients have shown a consecutive higher proportion of complete gross resection with best results in the most recently published, that could be explained for a better patient selection with a higher proportion of potentially good predictive factors for complete cytoreduction. In addition, we cannot rule out the influence of advances in surgery and radiographic imaging over time. In this regard, the retrospective series from Memorial Sloan Kettering by Manning-Geist et al. demonstrated the value of skilled radiology in accurately identifying patients likely to achieve a complete gross resection with high concordance between preoperative imaging and intraoperative findings (only 18.7% of patients with predicted single-site disease on imaging ultimately had three or more sites of disease).

As previously mentioned, the most potent factor that has been consistently identified as a predictive factor for survival was the absence of gross residual tumor after tertiary surgery. But we must also consider that tertiary surgery is not free of complications, with a reported rate of severe complications and 30-day operative mortality ranging from 13–31.1%, and from 0–5.9%, respectively. For this reason, seeking a prospective predictive model for complete gross resection at tertiary surgery allowing for a better selection of patients, as we have for the secondary cytoreduction, should be a priority for the international Gynecologic Oncology community. In addition, the value of complementary systemic chemotherapy and maintenance therapy after tertiary surgery is not known and should be further explored, but data from the retrospective studies suggest that it should not be skipped.

Conclusion

In conclusion, this author defends a position against the indiscriminative use of tertiary surgery, without validated assessment criteria for patient selection and outside of specialized centers, but, as a clinician treating patients with recurrent disease, I recognize that tertiary surgery may be considered in selected patients with a single site of recurrence, and especially after a long treatment-free interval.

References

1. Fotopoulou C, et al. Value of tertiary cytoreductive surgery in epithelial ovarian cancer: an international multicenter evaluation. *Ann Surg Oncol* 2013;20:1348–1354.

2. Fanfani F, et al. Is there a role for tertiary (TCR) and quaternary (QCR) cytoreduction in recurrent ovarian cancer?*Anticancer Res* 2015;35:6951–6956.

3. Falcone F, et al. Tertiary cytoreductive surgery in recurrent epithelial ovarian cancer: a multicentre MITO retrospective study. *J Gynecol Oncol* 2017;147:66–72.

4. Manning-Geist BL, et al. Tertiary cytoreduction for recurrent ovarian carcinoma: an updated and expanded analysis. *J Gynecol Oncol* 2021;162:345–352.

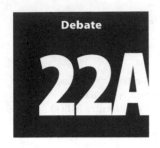

Is there a Role for Immunotherapy in Ovarian Cancer?

Yes

Claire F. Friedman

Debate

Epithelial ovarian carcinoma (EOC) remains a challenging malignancy to treat, with a five-year overall survival rate of approximately 50%. Unfortunately, despite front-line therapy including surgical resection and combination platinum-taxane chemotherapy, the vast majority of patients will recur and ultimately die from disease. Thus, there is a great unmet need for the development of novel complementary and augmentative therapeutic approaches. Translational studies would suggest that EOC is an excellent candidate for immuno-oncology (IO), given the high prevalence of tumor infiltrating lymphocytes at diagnosis and associated improved survival [1]. A number of IO approaches have been explored in EOC, with some promising data to date.

Checkpoint Inhibitors

Modest single agent activity has been seen for anti-PD-1 and anti-PD-L1 agents tested in patients with EOC (Table 22A.1) [2], with objective response rates (ORRs) ranging from 8–22%. The most promising data thus far has been seen in combination therapy. For example, in patients treated with the combination of ipilimumab plus nivolumab, the ORR was 33% in the nivolumab plus ipilimumab cohort, with a hazard of progression or death that was significantly lower in the combination group (hazard ratio (HR)=0.528; 95% CI: 0.339–0.821; two-sided p=.004) [3]. In addition to single-agent therapy checkpoint inhibitors (CPI), given preclinical data that demonstrate synergy with poly-ADP-ribose polymerase (PARP) inhibitors + anti-PD-1 combinations, there are several ongoing trials evaluating combination therapy. In the TOPACIO/KEYNOTE-162 study (ClinicalTrials.gov Identifier: NCT02657889), which enrolled patients with platinum-sensitive and resistant recurrent disease, the overall ORR was 25%; among the 11 patients with a BRCA mutation, the ORR was 45%. In contrast to these promising data, the JAVELIN Ovarian 100 study (ClinicalTrials.gov Identifier: NCT02718417), which studied the efficacy and safety of avelumab in combination with chemotherapy followed by maintenance avelumab in combination with talazoparib in patients with advanced EOC, failed to meet its primary endpoint of improved progression-free survival (PFS) and was discontinued early. Other studies have completed enrollment but have not reported on data, including the ATHENA study, which is assessing maintenance rucaparib plus nivolumab in EOC.

Lastly, there has also been interest in combining PD-1/PD-L1 blockade with anti-angiogenesis drugs. Unfortunately, the addition of atezolizumab to a backbone of

Table 22A.1 Clinical trials of checkpoint blockade in epithelial ovarian cancer

Study name	Drug	Patient population	ORR	Median PFS
PCD4989 g	Atezolizumab	Incurable or metastatic EOC (n=12)	22.2%	2.9 months (95% CI: 1.3, 5.5)
JAVELIN	Avelumab	Recurrent or refractory EOC (n=125)	9.6%	2.6 months (95% CI: 1.4–2.8)
KEYNOTE-028	Pembrolizumab	PD-L1-positive advanced metastatic EOC (n=26)	11.5%	1.9 months (95% CI: 1.8–3.5)
KEYNOTE-100	Pembrolizumab	Cohort A received one to three prior lines of treatment with a platinum-free interval (PFI) or treatment-free interval (TFI) between three and 12 months; cohort B received four to six prior lines with a PFI/TFI of ≥3 months	8%	2.1 months (95% CI: 2.1–2.2 cohort A, 2.1–2.6 cohort B)
	Nivolumab	Advanced or relapsed, platinum-resistant EOC (n=20)	15%	3.5 months (95% CI: 1.7–3.9)
NCT01611558	Ipilimumab	Recurrent platinum-sensitive EOC	10.3%	NA
NRG GY003	Nivolumab vs. ipilimumab plus nivolumab	EOC, one to three prior lines of therapy, PFI <12 months (n=100)	Nivolumab 12.2%, combination arm 31.4%	2.0 and 3.9 months, respectively

chemotherapy plus bevacizumab (ClinicalTrials.gov Identifier: NCT03038100) failed to significantly prolong PFS in patients with newly diagnosed EOC. More promisingly, in the phase II LEAP-005 basket study (ClinicalTrials.gov Identifier: NCT03797326), pembrolizumab plus the anti-angiogenic multikinase inhibitor lenvatinib demonstrated an ORR of 32.3% (95% CI: 16.7–51.4) in fourth line EOC. Median PFS for the ovarian cancer cohort was 4.4 months and the estimated six-month PFS was 47.1%.

Beyond Immune Checkpoint Inhibitors : T Cell-based Therapy

Adoptive cellular transfer (ACT) is the infusion of lymphocytes either derived from autologous tumor tissue or engineered to target tumor-specific antigens after activation and expansion ex vivo. A patient's T cells can either be engineered with a T-cell receptor (TCR) or an artificial chimeric antigen receptor (CAR) recognizing the respective antigen. Accordingly, binding of the TCR to a peptide antigen presented by the major histocompatibility complex (MHC) initiates signaling through the TCR/CD3 complex that is enhanced by costimulatory receptor signaling. A CAR uses the same CD3/costimulatory signaling pathway, however, binds the antigen independently of the MHC. A more recent strategy utilizes CAR T cells for tumor targeting that are additionally engineered with cytokines that are released upon CAR engagement, also known as a TRUCK (T-cells Redirected for Universal Cytokine-Mediated Killing) [4].

The repertoire of potential targets for ACT in ovarian cancer has grown exponentially, with potential targets including MUC16, mesothelin, and folate receptor. Clinical trials to date have primarily been designed to establish the safety of this approach, with some early signals of efficacy, including an ovarian cancer patient who achieved a partial response when treated with gavocabtagene autoleucel, a TCR directed against mesothelin (ClinicalTrials. gov Identifier: NCT03907852). There are multiple ongoing studies evaluating ACT in EOC with the hope that this may be an effective IO strategy moving forward.

Biomarkers

Pd-L1

KEYNOTE 100 was the largest study to attempt to prospectively define a PD-L1 expression cut point that would predict ORR to pembrolizumab among patients with recurrent EOC. The cut points were set as a combined positive score (CPS) of < 1, CPS ≥ 1, or CPS > 10. Among patients with from one to three prior lines of therapy, the ORR for each cut point was 4.1% (95% CI: 0.9–11.5), 5.7% (95% CI: 1.9–12.8), and 10% (95% CI: 2.8–23.7), respectively. Among patients with four to six prior lines of therapy, the ORR was 8.8% (95% CI: 1.9–23.7), 10% (95% CI: 3.3–21.8), and 18.2% (95% CI: 5.2–40.3), respectively [2]. This study suggested that defining a cut point of CPS > 10 may enrich for responders to CPI in EOC, but was not a perfect biomarker capable of discriminating responders from non-responders. The use of PD-L1 IHC as a biomarker is made more complicated by the fact that there may be significant differences in PD-L1 expression between primary tumor and peritoneal metastases [5].

Histologic Subtype

Several clinical trials have revealed increased sensitivity of ovarian clear cell carcinoma (OCCC) to CPI. In a phase II trial of nivolumab, two out of 20 cases of platinum-resistant ovarian cancer with a complete response (CR) were OCCC. In the KEYNOTE 100 study, 19 patients were OCCC. The ORR was 15.8% (95% CI: 3.4–39.6%) in OCCC, compared to 8.5% (95% CI: 5.5–12.4%) in the more common high-grade serous histology. Finally, in GY003, patients with OCCC (n=12) had improved odds of response (OR=5.21, 95% CI: 1.37–19.77) compared with the other histologic subtypes. These observations, although anecdotal and with limited numbers, suggest increased sensitivity of OCCC to CPI [1].

Future Directions

While the data for single agent CPI in EOC are disappointing, early data from combination studies and novel IO approaches such as ACT demonstrate the promise that these strategies have in EOC. While there have not been FDA approvals of IO to date in this disease type, and further work is needed to identify appropriate biomarkers to enrich the population of EOC patients most likely to respond to this approach, there will be a future role for immunotherapy in this disease.

References

1. Le Saux O, et al. *Challenges for immunotherapy for the treatment of platinum-resistant ovarian cancer.* Seminars in Cancer Biology 2020.

2. Borella F, et al. Immune checkpoint inhibitors in epithelial ovarian cancer: an overview on efficacy and future perspectives. *Diagnostics (Basel)* 2020;10(3):E146.

3. Zamarin D, et al. Randomized phase II trial of nivolumab versus nivolumab and ipilimumab for recurrent or persistent ovarian cancer: an NRG oncology study. *J Clin Oncol* 2020;38:1814–1823.

4. Chmielewski M, et al. TRUCKS, the fourth-generation CAR T cells: current developments and clinical translation. *Adv Cell Gene Ther* 2020;3:e84

5. Parvathareddy SK, et al. Differential expression of PD-L1 between primary and metastatic epithelial ovarian cancer and its clinico-pathological correlation. *Sci Rep* 2021;11:3750.

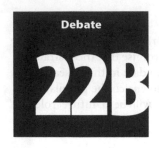

Debate

Is there a Role for Immunotherapy in Ovarian Cancer?
Not Yet

Tiffany Y. Sia and Dmitriy Zamarin

Debate

Immune checkpoint inhibitors (ICIs) have attracted attention recently and have received fast-track approvals from the Food and Drug Administration (FDA) in multiple cancer types, including cervical cancer and endometrial cancer. Normally, the expression of immune checkpoint receptors such as programmed death 1 (PD-1) and cytotoxic T lymphocyte-associated antigen 4 (CTLA-4) on T cells provides negative feedback mechanisms to prevent autoimmunity. Multiple cancers, including epithelial ovarian cancer (EOC), exploit these mechanisms to inhibit T cell activation, allowing them to escape immune detection. ICIs block immune checkpoint receptors, allowing for unchecked activation of cancer-targeted T cells leading to tumor cell destruction. Despite the success in various other cancer types, there are no approved immune therapies for ovarian cancer, as response of EOC to ICIs thus far have been modest.

For example, in KEYNOTE 100, an early phase II study of pembrolizumab (anti-PD-1 antibody) monotherapy in 376 patients with recurrent EOC, the ORR was 8% with a disease control rate of 37% [1]. This study also assessed expression of PD-L1 as a potential biomarker and demonstrated that PD-L1 expression by combined positive score (CPS) $\geq$ 10 was predictive of ORR, with ORR of 16.7% and 18.2% for CPS $\geq$ 10 in less and more heavily pretreated patients, respectively [1].

After moderate success with single agent ICIs, combination strategies to target different parts of the immune-suppressive pathways have been explored. In a phase II randomized trial of nivolumab with or without ipilimumab (anti-CTLA-4 antibody) in patients with persistent or recurrent EOC, objective response rates were 12% and 33% for the nivolumab and nivolumab plus ipilimumab groups, respectively [2]. Progression-free survival (PFS) was 2.0 months and 3.9 months, respectively, demonstrating that though ORR was increased, response to ICI had limited duration. Interestingly, there was a suggestion that patients with clear cell carcinoma were more likely to respond to the combination, though the numbers were small. Expression of PD-L1 was not found to be predictive of response in either cohort.

A number of studies have also explored chemotherapy in combination with ICIs in EOC. The recently published JAVELIN Ovarian 200 phase III trial compared avelumab (anti-PD-L1 antibody) monotherapy, avelumab in combination with pegylated liposomal doxorubicin (PLD), and PLD alone in 566 women with platinum-resistant or platinum refractory EOC. Chemotherapies used in platinum-resistant EOC, including PLD, had previously been shown to prime the immune system by enhancing antigen presentation, and were thought to be able to enhance the efficacy of immune checkpoint blockade (ICB). Unfortunately, the trial results did not show a benefit for either single-agent immunotherapy or for chemoimmunotherapy for patients with platinum-resistant EOC compared to single agent PLD, with an ORR of 4% for avelumab, 13% for avelumab with PLD, and 4% for PLD alone [3]. There was no improvement in either PFS or overall survival (OS) with avelumab alone or in avelumab plus PLD compared to single agent PLD. In a small subset of patients with tumors expressing both CD8 and PD-L1 that was not defined a priori, combination of avelumab and PLD therapy seemed to result in greater benefit than with monotherapy; however, the results were underpowered for this subgroup analysis [3].

Most recently, the IMagyn500 study was conducted to evaluate the efficacy and safety of ICI in combination with standard of care platinum-based chemotherapy and anti-VEGF therapy in EOC. Over the course of two years, 1301 patients with previously untreated stage III or IV EOC were randomized to atezolizumab (anti-PD-L1 antibody) plus bevacizumab plus chemotherapy versus placebo plus bevacizumab and chemotherapy. Although OS data for this trial are not yet mature, the trial showed no significant PFS improvement with ICB plus bevacizumab plus chemotherapy compared to bevacizumab and chemotherapy alone in the entire cohort and within the PD-L1 positive subgroup [4]. ORR were 93% in the atezolizumab group versus 89% in the placebo group in this previously untreated patient population.

Similarly, in the JAVELIN Ovarian 100 phase 3 trial, 998 patients with advanced treatment-naïve EOC were randomized to receive standard front-line platinum-based chemotherapy followed by avelumab maintenance, chemotherapy plus avelumab followed by avelumab maintenance, or chemotherapy followed by observation [5]. The trial was halted early as prespecified PFS futility boundaries were crossed, and PD-L1 status was not predictive of benefit [5].

Conclusion

Overall, the studies above highlight that ICIs either alone or in combination with chemotherapy to date have failed to demonstrate substantial clinical benefit in the majority of patients with EOC. Thus, we argue that outside of a clinical trial there is no clear evidence to support the routine usage of ICIs either alone or in combination with chemotherapy in EOC, even in a heavily pretreated platinum-resistant setting. We do note, however, that a minority of patients with EOC appear to derive durable clinical benefit and that there are some indicators or possibly increased responsiveness in some histologic subtypes such as clear cell carcinoma [1,2,6]. With identification of biomarkers predictive of response to ICIs in EOC, we remain hopeful that these drugs may play a role in therapy of some patients, although the biomarkers that have been predictive of response to ICIs in other cancer types (e.g., high tumor mutational burden, PD-L1 expression, homologous recombination deficiency) to date have not been found to be useful in EOC [2,5].

Lastly, our advances in understanding of EOC biology and immunology make room for further development of approaches aiming to address the resistance to ICIs. These include combinations of ICIs with additional chemotherapy regimens such as metronomic cyclophosphamide, anti-angiogenesis drugs, folate receptor antibodies, and PARP inhibitors. No less exciting are other novel immunotherapeutic strategies for EOC targeting, including bispecific antibodies, antibody-drug conjugates, cytokines, and adoptive cell therapies.

While many of these are still in the early stages of testing, we remain optimistic that immunotherapy will eventually find its way into the treatment armamentarium of gynecologic oncologists for most if not all ovarian cancers.

References

1. Matulonis UA, et al. Antitumor activity and safety of pembrolizumab in patients with advanced recurrent ovarian cancer: results from the phase II KEYNOTE-100 study. *Ann Oncol* 2019;30(7):1080–1087.

2. Zamarin D, et al. Randomized phase II trial of nivolumab versus nivolumab and ipilimumab for recurrent or persistent ovarian cancer: an NRG oncology study. *J Clin Oncol* 2020;38(16):1814–1823.

3. Pujade-Lauraine E, et al. Avelumab alone or in combination with chemotherapy versus chemotherapy alone in platinum-resistant or platinum-refractory ovarian cancer (JAVELIN Ovarian 200): an open-label, three-arm, randomised, phase 3 study. *Lancet Oncol* 2021;22 (7):1034–1046.

4. Moore KN, et al. Atezolizumab, bevacizumab, and chemotherapy for newly diagnosed stage III or IV ovarian cancer: placebo-controlled randomized phase III trial (IMagyn050/GOG 3015/ ENGOT-OV39). *J Clin Oncol* 2021;39 (17):1842–1855.

5. Monk BJ, et al. Chemotherapy with or without avelumab followed by avelumab maintenance versus chemotherapy alone in patients with previously untreated epithelial ovarian cancer (JAVELIN Ovarian 100): an open-label, randomised, phase 3 trial. *Lancet Oncol* 2021;22(9):1275–1289.

6. Hamanishi J, et al. Safety and antitumor activity of anti-PD-1 antibody, nivolumab, in patients with platinum-resistant ovarian cancer. *J Clin Oncol* 2015;33(34):4015–4022.

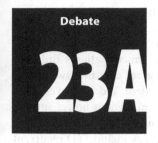

Debate

What is the Best Management Option for Malignant Bowel Obstruction?
Surgery

Joanie M. Hope and Jill S. Whyte

Debate

Malignant bowel obstruction (MBO) is one of the toughest clinical challenges in gyneco-logic oncology. Often the heralding sign of the "beginning of the end," together doctor and patient must decide whether to undergo palliative surgery motivated by the driving hope for more quality time. There is minimal debate that conservative options including bowel rest, nasogastric tube decompression, analgesics, and anti-secretory/motility agents should be exhausted prior to considering surgery. The controversy arises when medical management fails and the choice comes to accepting imminent death or attempting surgery to relieve obstruction, restore oral nutrition, allow potential for further cancer directed therapy, and achieve quality time.

Unfortunately, there are few rigorous clinical trials to guide management. Two Cochrane reviews addressing the role of palliative surgery in MBO in gynecologic cancers found only low-quality evidence comparing surgical and medical management and came to no definitive conclusions [1,2]. Ample data establish that palliative bowel surgery is ridden with complications and bad outcomes. Postoperative 30-day mortality after palliative bowel surgery is reported at 4–40% and rates of significant perioperative morbidity such as postoperative pain, bowel leaks, abscess, and sepsis are high, ranging from 5–86% [2]. Patients may end up in worse condition than had they not undergone surgery. Nevertheless, palliative bowel surgery remains the only approach offering the possibility of quality time in the face of recurrent malignant obstruction.

When conservative measures fail, a careful assessment of the potential role of surgery should be performed. The decision to proceed with surgery is highly individualized and must take into account location and cause of obstruction, performance status, prognosis, and goals for care. The best surgical candidates are obstructed in a single location, naive to prior bowel obstruction surgery, have few prior surgeries, chemotherapeutic options remaining, and minimal if any ascites or carcinomatosis [2]. Unfortunately, women pre-senting with MBO as a consequence of gynecologic cancer frequently do not meet these criteria.

Laparotomy may be offered to patients deemed good surgical candidates with a site of obstruction amenable to intervention. Both wisdom and technical prowess are critical for best outcomes as malignant bowel surgeries are among the hardest embarked upon by patient and gynecologic oncologist. The surgeon must be adept in adhesiolysis, bowel resections, bypass, diversions, and stoma formation, all in the setting of carcinomatosis;

as well as be able to problem solve and make intra-operative choices from the bird's eye perspective of where the patient is in her overall cancer journey.

The choice to proceed with surgery requires exceptional doctor–patient communication. Hope for more time is a tremendous influencer for terminal cancer patients and their families. It is incumbent upon gynecologic oncologists to take great care in how hope is proffered when discussing whether to undergo surgery. The patient and her loved ones cannot possibly foresee how significant the complications from malignant bowel surgery can be. Risks and alternatives must be vividly explained. Although every case should be approached individually, evidence based reasons to withhold surgery include: (1) recurrent obstruction treated with recent surgery; (2) multiple sites of obstruction; (3) inability to survive and heal from surgery; (4) rapidly growing disease likely to re-obstruct prior to completion of healing; (5) lack of any viable treatment options in the setting of rapidly growing disease; and (6) inability to consent and fully understand risk [1,2]. Additionally, the presence of ascites, malnutrition (albumin < 3.5), and poor performance status (ECOG 2–4) are associated with high rates of perioperative morbidity and mortality [1].

That said, with a carefully selected patient and a highly skilled surgical team, good outcomes are achievable in MBO surgery. A 2014 *JAMA* systematic review of 2347 articles reported that surgery palliated obstructive symptoms in 32–100% of patients with resumption of diet in 45–75% of cases [3]. While quality of life data and randomized controlled studies are sorely missing, there are multiple case reports and retrospective data of patients who achieve years of quality time following malignant obstruction surgery. We eagerly await the results of a randomized controlled study comparing surgery to medical therapy for MBO [4].

Moving forward, recurrent gynecologic cancer is becoming ever more approachable as a treatable chronic disease as the dualistic curative/terminal treatment paradigm is abandoned. Targeted biologic therapies, genetically driven personalized medicine, and immunotherapies are among the drugs revolutionizing cancer care. Many of these novel therapeutics are oral agents, making a functional GI tract even more critical. This onslaught of novel cancer therapy gives traction to the idea that if quality of life can be prolonged, science may indeed deliver new treatment hope in the metric of months if not years.

Conclusion

In closing, the best management option for MBO refractory to conservative measures is surgery, because surgery is the only way to offer real potential for quality, time, and ongoing treatment. Unfortunately, not all patients with malignant obstructions can be treated with surgery. In this very challenging conundrum, the rate-limiting step must be patient and not surgeon factors. The complex skill set needed for malignant bowel surgery and the willingness to operate when appropriate are essential components to state of the art gynecologic cancer care. In an era where aggressive debulking surgery gives way to a growing number of efficacious therapeutics, training future gynecologic oncologists in MBO surgical technique becomes paramount, especially as the indication for MBO surgery may increasingly become to offer meaningful life-prolonging therapy.

References

1. Cousins SE, et al. Surgery for the resolution of symptoms in malignant bowel obstruction in advanced gynaecological and gastrointestinal cancer. *Cochrane Database Syst Rev* 2016;1: CD002764.

2. Kucukmetin A, et al. Palliative surgery versus medical management for bowel obstruction in ovarian cancer. *Cochrane Database Syst Rev* 2010;7:CD007792.

3. Paul Olson T, et al. Palliative surgery for malignant bowel obstruction from carcinomatosis: a systematic review. *JAMA Surg* 2014;149(4):383–392.

4. SWOG S1316. Surgery or non-surgical management in treating patients with intra-abdominal cancer and bowel obstruction, ClinicalTrials.gov Identifier: NCT02270450.

What is the Best Management Option for Malignant Bowel Obstruction?

Percutaneous Endoscopic Gastrostomy

Claire V. Hoppenot and S. Diane Yamada

Debate

A malignant bowel obstruction (MBO) in the setting of recurrent or progressive gynecologic cancer is a terminal diagnosis. It is caused by progression of disease leading to carcinomatosis or widespread cancer involving the bowel. Median survival after diagnosis ranges from 76 to 141 days [1–3]. Half of patients will never recover from an initial diagnosis of MBO; of those who do, two thirds will have a recurrence of MBO symptoms [1].

In addition to a dismal prognosis, MBO is associated with pain and nausea, worsening nutrition, and difficulty tolerating additional treatments [1]. Utilizing qualitative interviews of 14 women with MBO (Hoppenot et al., personal communication) our group found that, in addition to survival, women with MBO prioritized symptom control, good communication with their physician, support at home, and ability to receive future treatments. Along similar lines, Lee et al. studied cohorts of gynecologic cancer patients with MBO before and after initiating a program of supported self-management that involved close telephonic and in-person follow-up from an interdisciplinary team [1]. Women after program initiation were less likely to undergo surgery (11% vs. 21%), but more frequently received chemotherapy (83% vs. 56%), which mirrors patient-identified goals from our qualitative study [1]. Patients were also less likely to have an Intensive Care Unit (ICU) admission and spent less time admitted to the hospital [1]. Despite these less "aggressive" measures, survival was longer in the intervention group by about five months.

Most importantly, a qualitative analysis of women who participated in the supported self-management program suggests that participants were most grateful for assistance with the medical and psychological effects of an MBO diagnosis [4]. In particular, they appreciated the access to health professionals to answer questions and slowly developed a better understanding of the implications of MBO as a terminal diagnosis [4].

The fact is that MBO secondary to recurrent gynecologic cancer is most commonly due to the presence of widespread disease. On pre-operative imaging of patients with recurrent gynecologic cancer, at least one third who underwent surgery for MBO had carcinomatosis and ascites [3]. While surgery can mitigate obstructive symptoms, it cannot address the carcinomatosis or ascites, leaving the patient at high risk of recurrent obstruction. Additionally, despite aggressive interventions, surgical patients survive only a few months longer than those who do not undergo surgery [2,3]. In the context of a terminal, incurable state, a focus on quality of life, not a few months length of life, may provide more benefit for patients. Quality of life from the patient's perspective is hard to measure, but surrogates such as ICU care in the last days of life (24% for surgical patients vs. 12% for gastrostomy tube (GT) patients, $p<0.05$) and death occurring in an acute care hospital (25% vs. 13%, respectively) suggest that GT are associated with less suffering than surgery at the end of life [2].

Gastrostomy tubes can control symptoms in medically refractory MBO to improve quality of life. These tubes, placed endoscopically or by interventional radiology, allow for venting of stomach contents to alleviate pain and nausea. A prospective study of GT for MBO showed relief of symptoms in 77% of patients [5]. Median survival after GT placement was about eight weeks and all deaths were due to disease progression [5]. Eighty-one percent were discharged home [5]. Complications were mild, including peristomal infections (14%) and intermittent catheter obstruction (8.4%) [5]. Rates of subsequent chemotherapy administration have ranged in the literature from 10–30%. In terms of quality of life measures following GT, only 25 of 142 patients had follow-up scores calculated; 16 (64%) had an improvement in overall quality of life, two (8%) had stable measures, and seven (28%) had nonsignificant worsening [5]. GT are safe, effective for symptom relief, and well tolerated.

In terms of future treatments, it is also unclear whether surgery increases chance of receiving further treatments, which patients valued, based on qualitative study. Although patients selected for surgery had a longer survival after their first MBO, our retrospective study of ovarian and uterine cancer patients showed similar rates of receiving chemotherapy after either surgery or GT (about 50%) [3].

Additionally, frequent admissions for MBO incur substantial costs. Lee et al. estimated the median cost for each admission to be over $8,000 in Canadian dollars [1]. In our retrospective study of ovarian and uterine cancer patients, 54% of ovarian cancer patients and 34% of uterine cancer patients were readmitted for MBO after a first admission [3]. Additional costs accrue from the higher level of care typically needed by surgical patients at the end of life [2]. A SEER-Medicaid retrospective study showed that GTs were associated with fewer readmissions compared to surgery (15% vs. 25%, $p<0.05$) and less need for ICU care (12% vs. 24%, $p<0.05$) [2].

In addition to incurred costs, offering surgery can send mixed messages and detract from patients' need for palliative care support. In our retrospective study, surgical patients were much less likely to have a palliative care consultation at the time of MBO (11% vs. 34% in nonsurgical patients), despite a median survival of less than six months and a planned palliative surgery [3]. In a large database study, palliative care referrals were again lower for surgical patients (2% vs. 8% for GT patients) [2]. Even within a program of supported self-management, patients sustained some uncertainty about prognosis after MBO [4]. It takes counseling and time for patients to comprehend the poor prognosis associated with MBO, and a focus on controlling symptoms and providing emotional and physical support stands to benefit patients the most during this transition.

Conclusion

In the setting of MBO in recurrent and progressive gynecologic cancer, management should focus on comfort care. For MBO symptoms refractory to medications, GTs are a safe and effective option. Offering surgery provides limited benefit and can send mixed messages about goals and options after a MBO diagnosis. A focus on symptom control with a GT and close emotional and medical supportive care can help achieve measures that are important to patients without compromising quality of life at the end of life.

References

1. Lee YC, et al. Optimizing care of malignant bowel obstruction in patients with advanced gynecologic cancer. *J Oncol Pract* 2019;15 (12):e1066–1071.

2. Lilley EJ, et al. Survival, healthcare utilization and end-of-life care in older adults with malignancy-associated malignant bowel obstruction; comparative study of surgery, venting gastrostomy, or medical management. *Ann Surg* 2018;267 (4):692–699.

3. Hoppenot C, et al. Malignant bowel obstruction due to ovarian or uterine cancer: are there differences in outcome? *Gynecol Oncol* 2019;154(1):177–182.

4. Cusimano MC, et al. Supported self-management as a model for end-of-life care in the setting of malignant bowel obstruction: a qualitative study. *Gynecol Oncol* 2020;157(3):745–753.

5. Zucchi E, et al. Decompressive percutaneous endoscopic gastrostomy in advanced cancer patients with small-bowel obstruction is feasible and effective: a large prospective study. *Support Care Cancer* 2016;24:2877–2882.

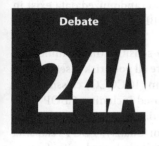

Debate

What is the Optimal Chemotherapy Regimen for Ovarian Germ-cell Tumors?
Bleomycin, Etoposide, and Cisplatinum (BEP)

Michael J. Seckl

Debate

Germ cell tumors predominantly arise in the gonads of children and young adults and are important to recognize as they are exquisitely sensitive to chemotherapy and highly curable. The behavior of the disease is likely different in pre-pubertal compared to post-pubertal cases. Malignant ovarian germ cell tumors (MOGCTs) are very rare, with an incidence between 1 in 250,000–500,000 women, and so studies to identify prognostic factors and optimal treatments have been hampered by small numbers of cases [1]. In contrast, testicular germ cell tumors (TGCTs) affect about 1:250 men and are the commonest cancer in this age group [1]. Consequently, most of the treatment discoveries have been made in the male disease where there have been sufficient cases to undertake larger and often randomized controlled trials [2]. Some historical perspective is helpful to understand how we have arrived at our current treatment paradigms in men before considering the female disease.

Prior to the discovery of cisplatin in the mid-1970s, most patients with advanced gonadal germ cell tumors that had spread beyond the affected primary site could not be saved. Indeed, although a number of agents had some activity including the vinca alkaloids, methotrexate, and bleomycin, the best hope for cure was in early stage (stage 1) surgically resected disease. However, matters dramatically changed when Einhorn and Donohue developed a regimen comprising bleomycin, etoposide, and cisplatin (BEP) which was less toxic than their prior regimen of cisplatin, vinblastine, and bleomycin (PVB). Subsequently, five-day BEP (etoposide 100 mg/m^2 and cisplatin 20 mg/m^2 days 1–5 with bleomycin 30,000 IU days 1, 8, and 15 repeated every three weeks) has proven in multiple randomized trials to be superior or at least not worse than more toxic alternative regimens [2]. Much work has since focused on how to reduce toxicities which can be life-threatening through, for example, the elimination of bleomycin or replacement of cisplatin with carboplatin in seminomas (the male equivalent of dysgerminomas in women). This is because bleomycin can cause pulmonary fibrosis and cisplatin (but much less so carboplatin) can trigger severe nephrotoxicity, peripheral neuropathy, hearing impairment, small vessel damage linked to high blood pressure, cardiac and cerebrovascular events. Helpfully, in seminomas, randomized data have shown that omission of bleomycin from BEP does not impair survival outcomes. Attention then switched to substituting cisplatin with carboplatin and currently investigators are considering whether platinum and etoposide could be replaced altogether with AUC 10 carboplatin alone. However, no randomized data exist in patients with seminoma to prove this to be equivalent to either BEP or platinum etoposide combinations [2].

For nonseminomatous TGCTs which are slightly less chemo-sensitive than seminomas, there is recognition that four cycles of BEP is not sufficient to cure all poor risk cases defined using The International Germ Cell Cancer Collaboration Group (IGCCCG) classification system. Whilst several alternative approaches have been proposed including CBOP-BEP, TIP, T-BEP, and high-dose chemotherapy, no randomized trial data exist that conclusively indicate these therapies are superior to four cycles of BEP [2]. Fortunately, TGCT relapsing after BEP chemotherapy can in 50–60% of cases be successfully salvaged with further intensive chemotherapy and/or surgery [2].

In MOGCTs, nonrandomized small phase II studies demonstrated that BEP is clearly active for both dysgerminomatous and nondysgerminomatous disease [1,3]. Arguments still continue regarding the need for adjuvant BEP in stage IA/B or some IC MOGCTs [1,3]. However, a key question for the present debate is whether we can mirror what was learnt in TGCTs by, for example, eliminating bleomycin for dysgerminomas or identifying poor risk MOGCTs needing more intensified therapies? In considering these issues it is essential to determine whether MOGCTs truly behave in a clinically and biologically identical fashion to testicular disease. An indication that this might not be the case came from reports showing that MOGCT relapsing after initial chemotherapy had dramatically lower salvage rates of around 30% [4] unlike the 50–60% seen in the testicular equivalent [2]. Moreover, data are emerging on how the distinct hormonal environment and genetic imprinting might influence the molecular pathogenesis and behavior of female versus male germ cell tumors [1,5]. At the very least, the clinical data suggest that in MOGCTs it is essential to optimize initial chemotherapy to maximize chances of long-term cure. Thus, attempts to reduce BEP-induced treatment toxicity by, for example, omitting bleomycin or switching cisplatin to carboplatin needs to be done with extreme caution. Indeed, there is a strong argument that treatment should be intensified in those women with advanced MOGCT who are more likely to relapse. So, can these individuals be identified? Efforts have been made to adapt the male IGCCCG system but currently, because of small MOGCT case numbers and inadequate power, there is no consensus apart from possibly stage IV disease where five-year survival may be between 60–75% [1]. However, this is not sufficient to enable accurate discrimination of patients for more intensified therapies.

Conclusion

In the future, our understanding of MOGCTs may be improved through centralization of care so that larger numbers of cases can be collected and managed in a uniform manner and/ or be available for clinical trials. Currently though, in the absence of data to indicate that any other chemotherapy is superior to three to four cycles of BEP, most investigators will continue to recognize this as the standard of care for virtually all women with MOGCTs of stage Ic or more.

References

1. Veneris JT, et al. Contemporary management of ovarian germ cell tumors and remaining controversies. *Gynecol Oncol* 2020;158:467–475.

2. Alsdorf W, et al. Current pharmacotherapy for testicular germ cell cancer. *Expert Opin Pharmacother* 2019;20:837–850.

3. Gershenson DM, et al. Management of rare ovarian cancer histologies. *J Clin Oncol* 2019;37:2406–2415.

4. Reddy Ammakkanavar N, et al. High-dose chemotherapy for recurrent ovarian germ cell tumors. *J Clin Oncol* 2015;33:226–227.

5. Oosterhuis JW, et al. Human germ cell tumours from a developmental perspective. *Nat Rev Cancer* 2019;19:522–537.

What is the Optimal Chemotherapy Regimen for Ovarian Germ-cell Tumors?
Other

Michael L. Friedlander

Debate

The notion that bleomycin, etoposide, and cisplatin (BEP) is the optimal chemotherapy regimen for all ovarian germ cell tumors (OGCTs) is flawed as there are a number of equally effective and potentially less toxic treatment regimens. The reductionist approach to prescribe BEP to all patients with OGCTs is based on strong opinion rather than strong evidence supported by well-designed randomized controlled trials in OGCTs. Indeed, there are no randomized trials to guide the choice of chemotherapy regimens in women with OGCTs and treatment guidelines have been extrapolated from clinical trials of males with germ cell tumors [1]. OGCTs are rare in adults, but more commonly diagnosed in young children and adolescents. OGCTs are highly curable and the focus over recent years has been on minimizing toxicity of treatment and in particular the delayed effects. In this regard, the pediatric trial groups are way ahead of gynecological/medical oncologists managing adult patients with OGCTs [2]. However, before discussing a risk-stratified approach to treatment of patients with OGCTs it is worthwhile to briefly review the landmark randomized trials in testicular germ cell tumors as well as the few phase 2 trials in OGCTs that have provided the evidence used to support treatment recommendations.

The major breakthrough in the management of germ cell tumors was the introduction of cisplatin in the 1970s and the highly effective, albeit toxic regimen of PVB (cisplatin, vinblastine, and bleomycin) reported by Einhorn and Donohue which was a transformational moment in oncology [1]. PVB was soon supplanted by BEP after Williams et al. reported equivalent efficacy, but with less toxicity than PVB in males with testicular cancer in 1987, and it became the standard of care [1]. It was also highly effective in OGCTs, with cures reported in over 95% of patients with stage 1 OGCTs and 75–80% of patients with stage 3 or 4 disease [2,3]. The success of BEP was widely heralded for good reason and it was rapidly integrated into practice. The acute toxicities were soon appreciated, but it took longer to learn of the late effects of BEP which now assume high importance given that the majority of patients with OGCTs are likely cured. The long-term side effects include secondary malignancies, cardiovascular disease, hypertension, Raynaud's phenomenon, pulmonary toxicity, nephrotoxicity, neurotoxicity, deafness, decreased fertility, and psychosocial problems amongst others [1–5].

In view of the early as well as late adverse effects, there have been attempts to avoid immediate treatment of patients with stage 1 OGCTs and rather than offer adjuvant BEP to all patients, which is all too common, an alternative strategy is close surveillance and treatment only for relapse [4].This does not impact on overall survival and has been standard of care for stage 1 testicular germ cell tumors for many years, as well as for pediatric and young adolescent patients with OGCTs. There has been much effort in de-escalating treatment, particularly in patients with advanced stage dysgerminomas. The Gynecologic Oncology Group (GOG) were prescient when they designed a phase 2 trial (GOG-116) which investigated carboplatin 400 mg/m^2 and etoposide 120 mg/m^2 days 1–3 every four weeks in 39 patients with stages 1b–3 dysgerminoma [3,5].No patients relapsed despite the very modest dose of carboplatin and three days of etoposide every four weeks for three cycles only. Unfortunately, the trial, reported in 2004, was closed early after the results of two trials in males with nonseminomatous testicular cancer reported inferior outcomes with carboplatin compared to cisplatin. However, the doses of carboplatin were low, with an AUC 5 in one trial and 500 mg/m^2 in the other and they did not include seminomas. Seminomas and dysgerminomas are very different to other germ cell tumors with very high response to carboplatin. Shah et al. reported the results of pooled data from six trials in the Malignant Germ Cell Tumor International Consortium (MaGIC) which included 126 patients with advanced stage (stages 1c–4) dysgerminomas who were treated with either carboplatin- or cisplatin-based chemotherapy [4]. Survival outcomes were equivalent with a 96% five-year survival in both groups. More recently, a study of single agent carboplatin at an AUC of 10 every three weeks for three to four cycles was reported to be highly effective in males with good prognosis metastatic seminomas with a three-year overall survival of 96% and three-year progression-free survival of 93.2%. A somewhat different approach in de-escalation of chemotherapy in seminomas was taken in the SEMITEP study, where the investigators used FDG PET scans to risk-stratify patients with metastatic seminoma after two cycles of treatment – 72% had a negative PET scan after two cycles of cisplatin and etoposide and ceased treatment and the 28% of patients who still had a positive PET-CT received an additional two cycles of EP. The three-year PFS in the de-escalated arm was 90% and the three-year overall survival was 100%.

Conclusion

Although BEP is an option for patients with nondysgerminomatous germ cell tumors, it is not the only option and again a risk stratification is important. The risk of recurrence as well as risk of acute/late toxicities should be considered as they impact on the selection of chemo-therapy regimen. Unfortunately, we still do not have an optimal risk classification for OGCTs unlike the IGCCC classification used to stratify patients with testicular cancers [4]. We need more than FIGO stage to make rational decisions regarding treatment regimens, particularly for patients with nondysgerminomas, rather than prescribe BEP for all regardless of risk. Treatment options include four cycles of etoposide and cisplatin instead of BEP x 3, in patients who are likely to have a good prognosis which is equivalent to BEP in males with good risk metastatic nonseminomatous germ cell tumors and avoids the toxicity of bleomycin [1]. An equally effective alternative is to substitute ifosfamide for bleomycin and to use three cycles only. While over 90% of males with good risk metastatic disease are cured, the outcomes are not as good for patients who fall into the intermediate or high-risk groups and who are treated with BEP, and more effective regimens are being investigated [1].Although relatively few patients with OGCTs fall into this category, their treatment should be discussed with a team experienced with the management of high-risk germ cell tumors as they may be suitable for clinical trials [4]. In conclusion, optimal management of patients with OGCTs requires a lot more thought than simply prescribing BEP to all.

References

1. Hanna N, et al. Testicular cancer: a reflection on 50 years of discovery. *J Clin Oncol* 2014;32(28):3085–3092

2. Newton C, et al. A multicentre retrospective cohort study of ovarian germ cell tumours: evidence for chemotherapy de-escalation and alignment of paediatric and adult practice. *Eur J Cancer* 2019;113:19–27.

3. Gershenson DM, et al. Conundrums in the management of malignant ovarian germ cell tumors: toward lessening acute morbidity and late effects of treatment. *Gynecol Oncol* 2016; 143(2):428–432.

4. Ray-Coquard I, et al. ESMO Guidelines Committee. Non-epithelial ovarian cancer: ESMO Clinical Practice Guidelines for diagnosis, treatment and follow-up. *Ann Oncol* 2018;29(Suppl. 4):iv1–iv18

5. Veneris JT, et al. Contemporary management of ovarian germ cell tumors and remaining controversies. *Gynecol Oncol* 2020;158(2):467–475.

25A

What is the Optimal Adjuvant Chemotherapy Regimen for Primary Granulosa Cell Tumor?

Bleomycin, Etoposide, and Cisplatinum (BEP)

Olivia Le Saux, Hélène Vanacker, and Isabelle Ray-Coquard

Debate

Adult granulosa cell tumors (AGCTs) are the most common type (85%) of granulosa cell tumors (GCTs) accounting for about 2–5% of ovarian neoplasms. AGCTs are found mainly in peri- and post-menopausal women, whereas juvenile granulosa cell tumors, which have different tumor biology, usually develop in adolescents and young females. The majority of GCT patients are diagnosed at an early stage and the disease is typically indolent. Surgical management is the cornerstone of both initial and recurrent disease treatment for AGCTs. The FIGO stage and age are the most often reported risk factors for recurrence. Consequently, for patients with stage IC and higher disease, some clinical guidelines recommend adjuvant chemotherapy, although the approach to such patients is controversial, and observation is also an acceptable strategy for completely resected and well-staged disease [1]. Indeed, although adjuvant chemotherapy has been associated with longer progression-free survival (PFS) among those with advanced GCT, there is no evidence supporting an overall survival (OS) benefit. As the benefit of postoperative treatment is unclear, practice is variable.

When chemotherapy is proposed, the most widely used platinum-based chemotherapy is the combination of bleomycin, platinum, and etoposide (BEP) due to the high response rate, reported by Gershenson et al. in 1996, of 83%, compared to 66% with platinum, vinblastine, and bleomycin (PVB), the historical regimen [2].

The positive arguments in favor are:

- **Bleomycin and etoposide are efficient drugs**. The benefit of bleomycin was highlighted in the study by Zambetti et al., which implemented PVB as a historical regimen of GCT [3]. In this study, PVB reported higher response rates (66%) compared to other platinum combination regimens without bleomycin (cisplatinum plus doxorubicin, or plus hexamethylmelamine, or plus doxorubicin and cyclophosphamide). Moreover, BEP showed superiority compared to EP in testicular germ cell tumors. The benefit of etoposide was emphasized by Gershenson et al. who reported a higher response rate with BEP versus PVB (83% vs. 66%). The added value of etoposide compared to vinblastine was confirmed in an earlier study published in the *New England Journal of Medicine* by

Williams et al. in 1987 in patients with testicular germ cell tumors which demonstrated reduced toxicity and equivalent efficacy.

- **To date, no trial has documented that carboplatin is equivalent to cisplatin in activity in GCT** [4]. In the retrospective series reported by Brown et al., taxanes were administered with a platinum agent, either carboplatin or cisplatin, and no comparison between the two agents was reported.

- **BEP is the regimen associated with the strongest level of evidence** (phase II study for BEP vs. retrospective study for platinum + paclitaxel, the most commonly used alternative). The GOG 115 trial was a single-arm phase II study to assess the efficacy and toxicity of the combination of BEP for incompletely resected stages II–IV or recurrent ovarian stromal malignancies [5]. Thirty-seven percent (14/38) of the patients undergoing second look laparotomy had negative findings (primary endpoint). The six complete responders were of long median duration (> 24 months). Myelotoxicity was tolerable. Based on the results of this trial, surgery followed by BEP has become the standard treatment option for patients with advanced ovarian GCT.

- **Comparison between BEP and taxanes platinum-based regimens did not totally conclude in favor of carboplatine + paclitaxel.** An indirect comparison via a retrospective review of all patients with sex cord stromal ovarian tumors seen at the M.D. Anderson from 1985 to 2002 demonstrated activity of both regimens. In this study, focusing on newly diagnosed disease, 11 patients received BEP (8/11 had residual disease after surgery) and eleven patients received a taxane +/- platinum agent (2/11 had residual disease). The authors reported a better (not statistically significant) ORR for BEP compared to taxanes +/- platinum agents for patients with measurable recurrent disease (ORR=71% vs. 37% respectively, p=0.677) [4]. There was also a trend towards increased median PFS for BEP versus taxanes +/- platinum agents for patients with recurrent disease (11.2 months vs. 7.2 months, p=0.312). These results should be considered even more attentively as the comparability of the two populations is to be confirmed (more residual disease, juvenile histology, and more advanced FIGO stage in the BEP regimen group). More recently, the randomized trial led by the Gynecologic Oncology Group and started in 2010 evaluating BEP versus paclitaxel plus carboplatin (PC) in this population of patients failed to demonstrate a benefit in favor of the PC regimen. This trial (NCT01042522) was closed early for futility of PC (Brown et al., *IGCS*, 2020). Median age was 48 years, 87% had GCT, the futility analysis was supported by 21 and 16 PFS events on the PC and BEP arms respectively, with an estimated HR=1.12 [95% CI: 0.58–2.16] in favor of BEP. PC patients had fewer grade ≥3 adverse events (PC 77% vs. BEP 90%). Differences included infections (0 vs. 10%), and low neutrophil count (65% vs. 84%). One death not otherwise specified occurred on PC regimen.

- **In terms of feasibility, short duration of therapy of three cycles for BEP versus six cycles for CP should be considered** when comparing the two regimens as it can be more convenient for patients.

- Trials analyzing BEP in GCT revealed significant bleomycin-related toxicity, including deaths from bleomycin-related pulmonary fibrosis. Etoposide can also result in the subsequent development of secondary malignancies. Nevertheless, **none of the trials reported on quality of life, and toxicity and adverse-event data were incompletely reported, limiting the interpretation.**

Table 25A.1 BEP regimen's activity in this patient population

Study	N of GCT patients	Study design	Population	ORR %	PFS (mo) median (95% CI)	Overall survival (mo) median (95% CI)
Gershenson (1996) [2]	6	Prospective	IA, IIC, IIIC, or recurrent	83.3	14 (NA)	28 (NA)
GOG-115 (1999) [5]	48	Phase II	Stage II, III, IV	40	66 (13, NR)	NR (47, NR)
Brown (2005) [4]	20	Retrospective	Newly diagnosed	71	46 (NA)	97 (NA)
Pautier (2008) [6]	20	Prospective	Advanced ovarian granulosa cell tumors: initial metastatic (n=5) or recurrent (n=15)	90	25 (NA)	46 (NA)
Ray-Coquard (2010) [7]	44	Prospective	Newly diagnosed and first relapse	84 in first line 50 at first relapse	65 (60–68)	NR
GOG-264 (2020) [8]	55	Randomized phase II	Newly diagnosed, stage IIA–IVB, ≤8 weeks after surgery	NA	19.7 (10.4–52.7)	NA

Abbreviations: NA = not available; NE = not reached.

Conclusion

To conclude, for younger, fit patients, and more specifically juvenile histology, we typically recommend using BEP as there is no reliable evidence for the superiority of PC, while we prefer PC for patients >50 years old, due to toxicity concerns.

References

1. ESMO. Non-epithelial ovarian cancer: ESMO Clinical Practice Guidelines for diagnosis, treatment and follow-up. *Ann Oncol* 2018;29:iv1–iv18.

2. Gershenson DM, et al. Treatment of poor-prognosis sex cord-stromal tumors of the ovary with the combination of bleomycin, etoposide, and cisplatin. *Obstet Gynecol* 1996;87:527–531.

3. Zambetti M, et al. cis-platinum/vinblastine/ bleomycin combination chemotherapy in advanced or recurrent granulosa cell tumors of the ovary. *Gynecol Oncol* 1990;36 (3):317–320.

4. Brown J, et al. The activity of taxanes compared with bleomycin, etoposide, and cisplatin in the treatment of sex cord-stromal ovarian tumors. *Gynecol Oncol* 2005;97:489–496.

5. Homesley HD, et al. Bleomycin, etoposide, and cisplatin combination therapy of ovarian granulosa cell tumors and other stromal malignancies: a gynecologic oncology group study. *Gynecol Oncol* 1999;72:131–137.

6. Pautier P, et al. Combination of bleomycin, etoposide, and cisplatin for the treatment of advanced ovarian granulosa cell tumors. *Int J Gynecol Cancer Off J Int Gynecol Cancer Soc* 2008;18:446–452.

7. Ray-Coquard I, et al. Management of rare ovarian cancers: the experience of the French website «Observatory for rare malignant tumours of the ovaries» by the GINECO group: Interim analysis of the first 100 patients. *Gynecol Oncol* 2010;119:53–59.

8. Brown J, et al. 125 Results of a randomized phase II trial of paclitaxel and carboplatin versus bleomycin, etoposide and cisplatin for newly diagnosed and recurrent chemonaive stromal ovarian tumors. *Int J Gynecol Cancer* 2020;30:A56.

25B What is the Optimal Adjuvant Chemotherapy Regimen for Primary Granulosa Cell Tumor?
Carboplatin/Paclitaxel

Dib Sassine and Chrissy Liu

Debate

Patients with early-stage granulosa cell tumors (IA or IB) may be treated with surgical therapy alone and expect an excellent prognosis. Patients with stage IC or greater disease, recurrent granulosa cell tumors, and sub-optimally reduced disease may benefit from adjuvant chemotherapy [1]. The type of adjuvant chemotherapy has been controversial and varies based on clinical guidelines. The National Comprehensive Cancer Network (NCCN) guidelines recommend platinum-based chemotherapy and endorses paclitaxel and carboplatin (PC), etoposide and cisplatin, or bleomycin, etoposide, cisplatin (BEP) [2]. In this debate the authors support the use of paclitaxel plus carboplatin based on (1) BEP lacks durable activity, (2) PC demonstrates favorable outcomes in a retrospective analysis, (3) PC has a better safety profile compared to BEP, (4) the dosing regimen for PC is more convenient, and (5) there is insufficient data comparing PC to BEP.

Granulosa cell tumors (GCTs) represent up to 90% of malignant sex-cord stromal tumors of the ovary. Usually, they are unilateral, large, and are prone to rupture that can cause hemoperitoneum in about 10% of cases. They are divided into adult and juvenile type, with the adult type being predominant [3]. While complete gross resection is the cornerstone treatment of most GCT, adjuvant chemotherapy is suggested by certain specialists in advanced cases (stage IC and above) as well as in the recurrent setting.

Bleomycin, Etoposide, and Cisplatin Has Not Demonstrated Durable Remission in Patients

In 1999, the Gynecologic Oncology Group (GOG) investigated BEP in patients with incompletely resected stage II–IV or recurrent sex cord stromal tumor (SCSTs), and found that 37% (14/38) of patients who underwent second-look laparotomy had negative findings [4]. Six complete responders had a 24.4 month median duration of response (DoR) [4]. However, only one of seven patients with advanced disease experienced a durable remission [4]. Despite being a single arm, small study, and requiring a dose reduction of bleomycin due to two fatalities, the authors concluded that the modified BEP regimen is tolerable and active, which led to the commonly used treatment option for patients with advanced ovarian SCST. Gershenson and colleagues noted similar limitations in durable remission in a prior publication, where only one of seven patients with metastatic disease experienced a durable remission (14%) [5].

While the most common chemotherapy regimen is BEP, carboplatin and paclitaxel have shown to be effective. Brown et al. conducted a retrospective review of patients at MD Anderson Cancer Center: in the primary adjuvant setting, 89% of patients with GCT were disease free at completion of the treatment and almost 80% had durable remission, with a median PFS not reached at 51 months. In the setting of measurable recurrent disease, the response rate was 42% with a median follow-up of 100 months [6]. This study suggested that a platinum and taxane combination is active in GCT [6].

Paclitaxel and Carboplatin Has a More Favorable Side-effect Profile than Bleomycin, Etoposide, and Cisplatin

Brown and colleagues showed that patients on PC had fewer grade 3 or higher adverse events than BEP (77% vs. 90%) [7]. Specifically, PC is associated with lower rates of infection (0% vs. 10%), neutropenia (65% vs. 84%), and leukopenia (22% vs. 40%) when compared to BEP [7]. In the trials conducted by Gershenson et al. and Homesley et al., two patients developed pulmonary toxicity and two patients died as a result of bleomycin-related pulmonary fibrosis, respectively [4,5]. Etoposide has been linked to the development of subsequent secondary malignancies [6]. Although modifying doses and monitoring hematologic and pulmonary function can lower the morbidity associated with BEP, there is still potential for serious adverse effects. We think such toxicities should not be considered acceptable in this relatively young population, especially in the setting of nondurable remission with BEP. On the other hand, toxic effects in patients treated with PC for newly diagnosed or recurrent disease included febrile neutropenia, anemia, thrombocytopenia, and hypersensitivity, which are "largely acceptable" and treatable adverse events [6].

The dosing schedule for PC is more convenient. Paclitaxel 175 mg/m^2 and carboplatin AUC=6 IV are given once every three weeks for a total of six cycles. The BEP regimen requires multiple infusions five days a week: bleomycin 20 units/m^2 IV push on day 1, etoposide 75 mg/m^2 IV on days 1–5, and cisplatin 20 mg/m^2 IV on days 1–5 every three weeks for a total of three or four cycles. The burden from daily infusions, travel to the infusion center, and treatment-related toxicity can negatively impact a patient's quality of life.

Conclusion

To date, there has been no successful head-to-head comparison between PC and BEP. Brown and colleagues initiated a noninferiority trial evaluating BEP versus PC in newly diagnosed advanced or recurrent chemotherapy-naïve SCST. This study was discontinued at the interim futility analysis, as PC failed to improve PFS [7].

Because adult type GCTs are typically indolent and recur late, follow-up periods are long, and analyzing overall survival of any adjuvant therapy is difficult in the setting of GCT. Although there is a paucity of data, good response rates have been reported in paclitaxel and carboplatin. One ongoing clinical trial is evaluating the use of PC versus BEP in SCST surgery (NCT02429700) and is still recruiting, with PFS being the primary outcome. Hopefully this study will potentiate the evidence for the use of PC in patients with GCT.

References

1. DiSaia PJ, et al. *Clinical Gynecologic Oncology* (9th edn.). London: Elsevier, 2018.

2. Network NCC. NCCN Guidelines Version 1.2022 Ovarian Cancer. Published 2022.

3. Young RH. Ovarian sex cord-stromal tumours and their mimics. *Pathology* 2018;50(1):5–15.

4. Homesley HD, et al. Bleomycin, etoposide, and cisplatin combination therapy of ovarian granulosa cell tumors and other stromal malignancies: a gynecologic oncology group study. *Gynecol Oncol* 1999;72(2):131–137.

5. Gershenson DM, et al. Treatment of poor-prognosis sex cord-stromal tumors of the ovary with the combination of bleomycin, etoposide, and cisplatin. *Obstet Gynecol* 1996;87(4):527–531.

6. Brown J, et al. The activity of taxanes in the treatment of sex cord-stromal ovarian tumors. *J Clin Oncol* 2004;22 (17):3517–3523.

7. Brown JMA, et al. 125 Results of a randomized phase II trial of paclitaxel and carboplatin versus bleomycin, etoposide and cisplatin for newly diagnosed and recurrent chemonaive stromal ovarian tumors. *Int J Gynecol Cancer* 2020;30:A56.

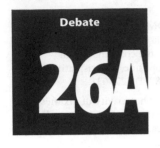

What is the Best Management Strategy for a Recurrent Granulosa Cell Tumor?

Surgery

Alice Bergamini, Luca Bocciolone, and Gioriga Mangili

Debate

Among patients diagnosed with stage I granulosa cell tumors (GCTs) of the ovary, 25% will experience recurrent disease, after a median of four to six years from initial diagnosis [1]. GCTs are rare tumors and have a slow, indolent course, with recurrences registered even after several decades from initial diagnosis [2].

Due to the rarity of this tumor type and the low number of events, data deriving from randomized trials are lacking. For these reasons, strong evidence regarding the optimal treatment of GCT recurrence is limited and mainly derives from small size retrospective series.

The most recent NCCN clinical guidelines indicate either surgery, radiotherapy, hormonal therapy, or chemotherapy as possible options for the treatment of recurrent disease. Conversely, ESMO Clinical Practice Guidelines consider surgery as the most effective treatment for recurrent ovarian GCTs.

Several factors support surgery as the best therapeutic option for these patients, with chemotherapy to be reserved in case of recurrent unresectable disease or when optimal cytoreduction is not feasible.

Residual disease at primary surgery is known to be a prognostic factor for survival [3], but also suboptimal cytoreduction at secondary debulking surgery is associated with a decreased overall survival (OS). In a retrospective study of the MITO group, five-year OS decreased from 87.4% in the case of no residual disease to 55.6% in the case of suboptimal cytoreduction [4].

Hölscher et al. in 2009 made a comparison on the outcomes of GCT treatment before and after 1988 and found a significant improvement in five-year and ten-years OS, from 55.8% to 89.1% and 42.8% to 85.2% respectively [5]. They concluded that these results could be related to the continued advances made in the surgical field towards optimal tumor resection with no residual disease.

Recurrences in GCTs are typically multifocal, similar to epithelial ovarian cancer. In a retrospective study from Fotopolou et al., including 45 patients with relapsed GCT, 38.5% had tumor on the pelvic side wall, 30.8% had bowel involvement, 5% showed tumor on the liver, while 15.4% had tumor on the diaphragm, 15.4% on the abdominal wall, and 11.5% on the omentum. Only 7.7% had mesenteric involvement [6]. Despite this pattern at relapse, higher rates of optimal tumor cytoreduction have been reported when compared to epithelial ovarian cancer, as high as 85% [7,8]. Notably, most of the recurrences are asymptomatic and incidentally diagnosed during follow-up [9]. These cases are therefore generally associated with absence of large amounts of ascites, better performance status and higher tolerance to complex surgical procedures compared to patients with epithelial ovarian cancer.

Achieving optimal cytoreduction requires a complex multidisciplinary surgical approach, often with extensive peritonectomy, bowel resections, splenectomy or liver resections, and pancreatectomy [6]. Surgical complexity should be balanced in relation to patient's performance status.

Lymphadenectomy is not considered a standard procedure during primary surgery for GCT, as lymph node metastases occur in only 4.5–5.5% of cases [6,7]. Abu Rustum et al. reported that up to 15% of patients with first recurrence had positive retroperitoneal lymph nodes [8]. Thus, status of the retroperitoneum should be assessed during second cytoreductive surgery, and bulky nodes should be removed.

The slow growth and indolent course of GCT supports surgery compared to chemotherapy for the treatment of recurrent disease that is considered poorly chemoresponsive. From available retrospective data, chemotherapy administered after optimal secondary surgery for recurrence does not seem to improve survival [4], but evidence is still controversial.

In the retrospective experience deriving from MITO-9, 33% of patients with recurrent GCT who had received surgery only as salvage treatment versus 37.5% of those treated with surgery plus chemotherapy developed a second recurrence.

A recent retrospective study by Zhao et al. evaluated the outcome of 40 patients with recurrent GCT. Three were treated with surgery alone, 31 with surgery plus chemotherapy, and six by chemotherapy alone. Multivariate analysis showed that the administration of chemotherapy following surgery and residual tumor at second cytoreductive surgery are the only independent risk factors for PFS [10].

Conclusion

From the abovementioned evidence, we can conclude that surgery should be the primary approach for patients with recurrent GCTs, with the aim of achieving optimal cytoreduction. Chemotherapy should be reserved in cases with suboptimal cytoreduction or unresectable disease.

References

1. Thrall MM et al. Patterns of spread and recurrence of sex cord-stromal tumors of the ovary. *Gynecol Oncol* 2001;122:242–245.

2. Hines JF, et al. Recurrent granulosa cell tumor of the ovary 37 years after initial diagnosis: a case report and review of the literature. *Gynecol Oncol* 1996;60 (3):484–488.

3. Sun HD, et al. A long-term follow-up study of 176 cases with adult type ovarian granulosa cell tumors. *Gynecol Oncol* 2012;124(2):244–249.

4. Mangili G, et al.Recurrent granulosa cell tumors (GCTs) of the ovary: a MITO-9 retrospective study. *Gynecol Oncol* 2013;130 (1):38–42.

5. Hölscher G, et al. Improvement of survival in sex cord stromal tumors – an observational study with more than 25 years follow-up. *Acta Obstet Gynecol Scand* 2009;88:440e8.

6. Fotopolou C, et al. Adult granulosa cell tumors of the ovary: tumor dissemination pattern at primary and recurrent situation,

surgical outcome. *Gynecol Oncol* 2010;119:285–290.

7. Lee YK, et al. Characteristics of recurrence in adult-type granulosa cell tumos. *Int J Gynecol Cancer* 2008;18:642–647.

8. Abu-Rustum NR, et al. Retroperitoneal nodal metastasis in primary and recurrent granulosa cell tumors of the ovary. *Gynecol Oncol* 2006;103:31.

9. Wang PH, et al. Outcome of patients with recurrent adult-type granulosa cell tumors – a Taiwanese Gynecologic Oncology Group study. *Taiwan J Obstet Gynecol* 2015;54(3):253–259.

10. Zhao D, et al. Characteristics and treatment results of recurrence in adult-type granulosa cell tumor of ovary. *J Ovarian Res* 2020;13(1):19.

26B What is the Best Management Strategy for Recurrent Granulosa Cell Tumor?
Chemotherapy

Amanika Kumar and Simrit Warring

Debate

When considering the best management of recurrent granulosa cell tumors (rGCTs), surgery is certainly an essential part of treatment for patients due to the indolent nature of this disease. However, given the long survivals and multiple recurrences many patients will experience, chemotherapy is an important component of overall treatment. Systemic therapy can increase the interval of time between surgeries, thereby potentially improving overall survival (OS) and treatment-related morbidity and mortality.

Despite the rarity of disease and limited available data, there are several studies to suggest efficacious chemotherapy regimens in rGCTs. The recommended first-line chemotherapy regimen has changed from VAC (vincristine, Adriamycin, and cyclophosphamide) to BEP (bleomycin, etoposide, and cisplatin) and more recently to carboplatin and paclitaxel; hormonal agents have also been used effectively in rGCTs and immunotherapeutic targets are of interest for future clinical trials.

Multiple small cohort studies have shown the efficacy of BEP in GCTs. In 1996, Gershenson et al. studied BEP in nine patients with sex cord stromal tumors (SCSTs). The studies showed a median progression-free survival (PFS) of 14 months and OS of 28 months [1], with 83% of patients demonstrating some response. Then Gynecologic Oncology Group (GOG) 115 was reported in which 51.2% (n=41) patients with recurrent disease and receiving BEP had a median PFS of 66 months [2]. Other follow-up cohort studies show similar efficacy with median PFS of 25–66 months and OS of 28–97 months [1–4], suggesting BEP to be an active chemotherapy regimen for advanced primary and recurrent SCSTs (Table 26B.1).

More recently, taxane and platinum therapies have shown activity in GCTs with less toxicity than BEP therapy. In the GOG187 phase II trial, 31 patients with recurrent SCSTs received single-agent paclitaxel resulting in a 3.2% complete response and 25.8% partial response with a median PFS of 10 months and OS of 73.6 months [5]. Ray-Coquard et al. completed the first randomized control trial of SCSTs and found that 71% of patients were progression-free at 6 months after treatment with weekly single-agent paclitaxel treatment further validating taxane therapy as an option for treatment for SCSTs [6]. Brown et al. compared BEP to taxane-based chemotherapies and showed that taxanes, alone or in combination with platinum, are not inferior to BEP treatment in 30 patients with recurrent measurable disease with median PFS of 7 months, median OS of 49 months, 7% complete response, 30% partial response, 20% stable disease, and 40% progressed disease [3]. This

Table 26B.1 Systemic treatment of granulosa cell tumors

Therapy
BEP [1–4]
Taxane +/– platinum [3,5]
Bevacizumab [7]
Hormonal treatment [8]

suggests that taxane-based therapy is an effective and a less toxic approach for treatment of SCSTs. GOG264 is an ongoing multi-institutional cooperative trial that randomizes newly diagnosed patients with advanced stage SCSTs and chemo-naive patients with recurrent SCSTs to either carboplatin/paclitaxel or BEP treatment.

Bevacizumab has also shown efficacy in GCT treatment. In a GOG phase II trial, 36 women with recurrent SCST (88.9% GCT) were given bevacizumab treatment with a 16.7% partial response, 77.8% stable disease, 5.6% progressive disease, and median PFS of 9.3 months [7]. A more recent study compared the addition of bevacizumab to single-agent paclitaxel and demonstrated no additional benefit in the rate of PFS at 6 months (72% vs. 71%) [6].

Given these tumors express steroid hormone receptors, equally relevant with regards to nonsurgical systemic treatment is the use of hormone therapy (HT), such as steroidal progestins, selective estrogen receptor modulators, gonadotropin-releasing hormone agonists, and aromatase inhibitors. In 31 patients who had all previously been treated with surgery, a systematic review assessed the effectiveness of HT in GCT, which included letrozole, tamoxifen, anastrozole, megestrol acetate, ganirelix, goserelin, medroxyprogesterone acetate, and diethylstilbestrol. The findings revealed there was a 25.8% complete response, 45.2% partial response, median PFS of 18 months (range 0–60 months), 12.9% with stable disease, and 16.1% with progressive disease [8]. Additional hormonal therapies and agents targeted to the estrogen pathway are an area of future research, including ribociclib, palbociclin, and fulvestrant. Immunohistochemistry has been utilized to investigate potential biomarkers to inform clinical trials in GCT. In 2019, Mills et al. argued against a significant role for immunotherapy in the absence of additional stimulation to make targets further immunogenic, though they did suggest that many GCTs were potential candidates for anti-androgen therapy [9]. There is currently an open label phase II clinical trial utilizing enzalutamide for metastatic or advanced nonresectable GCT underway. In 2020, Pierini et al. published findings on Forkhead Box L2 (FOXL2), a protein expressed by GCTs, showing promise as an immunologic therapeutic target [10]. A combination anti-PD-L1 with FoxL2-TT vaccine reduced tumor progression and improved survival in animal studies, suggesting potential long-term benefits and serving as a foundation for immunotherapy clinical trials.

Conclusion

While chemotherapy has not shown strong OS benefit, the extension of PFS is meaningful and can lead to longer intervals between surgery and perhaps an overall decrease in the total number of surgeries a patient has in their lifetime. The intraoperative and postoperative risks associated with multiple surgeries for recurrent GCTs are not insignificant and must be considered when choosing best management for recurrences. There is ongoing research to better understand the various systemic treatment approaches for GCTs including chemotherapeutic agents, bevacizumab, HT, and immunotherapy. Overall, a multimodal approach is essential for the effective treatment of recurrent GCTs with systemic chemotherapy being an important part of the treatment paradigm for this tumor.

References

1. Gershenson DM, et al. Treatment of poor-prognosis sex cord-stromal tumors of the ovary with the combination of bleomycin, etoposide, and cisplatin. *Obstet Gynecol* 1996;87(4):527–531.

2. Homesley HD, et al. Bleomycin, etoposide, and cisplatin combination therapy of ovarian granulosa cell tumors and other stromal malignancies: a Gynecologic Oncology Group study. *Gynecol Oncol* 1999;72(2):131–137.

3. Brown J, et al. The activity of taxanes compared with bleomycin, etoposide, and cisplatin in the treatment of sex cord-stromal ovarian tumors. *Gynecol Oncol* 2005;97(2):489–496.

4. Pautier P, et al. Combination of bleomycin, etoposide, and cisplatin for the treatment of advanced ovarian granulosa cell tumors. *Int J Gynecol Cancer* 2008;18(3):446–452.

5. Burton ER, et al. A phase II study of paclitaxel for the treatment of ovarian stromal tumors: an NRG Oncology/ Gynecologic Oncology Group study. *Gynecol Oncol* 2016;140(1):48–52.

6. Ray-Coquard I, et al. Effect of weekly paclitaxel with or without bevacizumab on progression-free rate among patients with relapsed ovarian sex cord-stromal tumors: the ALIENOR/ ENGOT-ov7 randomized clinical trial. *JAMA Oncol* 2020; 6(12):1923–1930.

7. Brown J, et al. Efficacy and safety of bevacizumab in recurrent sex cord-stromal ovarian tumors: results of a phase 2 trial of the Gynecologic Oncology Group. *Cancer* 2014;120 (3):344–351.

8. van Meurs HS, et al. Hormone therapy in ovarian granulosa cell tumors: a systematic review. *Gynecol Oncol* 2014;134 (1):196–205.

9. Mills AM, et al. Emerging biomarkers in ovarian granulosa cell tumors. *Int J Gynecol Cancer* 2019;29(3):560–565.

10. Pierini S, et al. Ovarian granulosa cell tumor characterization identifies FOXL2 as an immunotherapeutic target. *JCI Insight* 2020;5(16):e136773.

Is progression-free survival a rational surrogate endpoint in front-line ovarian cancer clinical trials?

Yes

Daniel Margul and Thomas J. Herzog

Debate

Progression-free survival (PFS) is not only a rational surrogate in front-line ovarian cancer, but is actually the preferred endpoint for the following reasons.

Front-line Ovarian Cancer Trials that Use Overall Survival as the Primary Endpoint Are Problematic Because of the Very Long Survival After Secondary Treatment for the First Recurrence/Progression

The number of approved agents for ovarian cancer has escalated rapidly, leading to numerous active options for post-progression therapy, thereby diluting the relationship between PFS and overall survival (OS). The result is that contemporary management of ovarian cancer produces a relatively long post-progression survival (PPS). The disease course includes undulating tumor burdens with multiple lines of interventions and therapies leading to an OS to PFS ratio ranging from 2.5–4.1.

Primary and Secondary Cross-over Treatments

Primary cross-over is when a patient in the control arm receives the experimental agent in a later line after coming off a trial for progression or toxicity. Novel treatments tested in a specific trial may lead to a substantial increase in PFS, but due to crossover in subsequent lines of therapy, no OS advantage is seen in the specific trial as the control group ends up benefiting from the experimental agent in later lines of treatment. This effect was observed in GOG 47 (doxorubicin/cyclophosphamide ± cisplatin) as patients randomized to doxorubicin/cyclophosphamide frequently received cisplatin upon progression, confounding the OS endpoint. Similarly, in GOG 132 (paclitaxel, cisplatin, or the combination of both agents) cisplatin along or in combination yielded superior PFS; however, OS was similar in all arms since the majority of patients in the single agent groups immediately received the other agent after completion of the protocol or prior to progression. Secondary cross-over occurs when a patient receives other active agents in later lines of treatment which may or may not have been given to patients in the experimental arm of a specific trial. This intervention also obscures the ability to demonstrate an OS effect.

Numbers Required for Enrollment Make Overall Survival Trials Impractical

Due to the aforementioned long PPS time, powering studies to detect a treatment effect for OS requires far greater sample sizes than for PFS. For example, if a novel treatment improves PFS from six to nine months, a typical study with 80% power would require 280 patients. If PPS is not affected, the same study at 80% power would require 2440 patients to preserve a statistically significant OS effect.

A Rapidly Evolving Clinical Landscape in the Era of Molecular Genomics Makes Prolonged Overall Survival Trials Clinically Irrelevant

Drug development in recent years has rapidly evolved with the elucidation of molecular and/or genetic etiologies of many cancers. Rapid discovery of actionable mutations is outpacing our capacity to contemporaneously evaluate these targets. Time from study conception to OS readout in front-line ovarian cancer often exceeds eight-plus years, thereby making trial conclusions clinically irrelevant as the discovery is so dated relative to the rapidly evolving standard of care if OS is the primary endpoint.

Progression-free Survival is a Valid Surrogate for Overall Survival when Assessed Properly

Overall survival is clearly objective, but the subjectivity of PFS can be minimized. To mitigate bias, clinical trials using PFS should blind the study treatments with placebo use and/or incorporation of blinded independent central review. Assessment time bias should be abrogated via assuring imaging and assessment visits are symmetrical in all study arms. With these measures, most criticisms of PFS as an effective primary endpoint lose credibility.

Recent approvals in front-line ovarian cancer by the United States Food and Drug Administration

	Frontline	Platinum Sensitive	Platinum Resistant	Clear Cell, Mucinous, LG-serous
OS	Approve	Approve	Approve	Approve
PFS (statistically significant) + other (QoL/PRO)	Approve	Approve	Consider	Consider
PFS (statistically significant) with clinically meaningful MOE	Consider	Consider	Consider	Consider
Objective Response Rate (with supportive duration of response)	No	No	Consider	Consider

Abbreviations: MOE = magnitude of effect, median difference between the experimental arm(s) relative to the control.

Regulatory Preference for Progression-free Survival

Virtually all recent approvals in front-line ovarian cancer by the US FDA have utilized PFS as the primary end-point. The agency has embraced PFS, and it has codified this position in workshop proceedings that describe the FDA position by line of therapy, as seen in Table 27A.1. Notably, the FDA does require data to assure no diminution in OS when using PFS.

References

1. Herzog TJ, et al. Ovarian cancer clinical trial endpoints: Society of Gynecologic Oncology White Paper. *Gynecol Oncol* 2014;132 (1):8–17.

2. Broglio KR, et al. Detecting an overall survival benefit that is derived from progression-free survival. *JNCI J Natl Cancer Inst* 2009;101(23):1642–1649.

3. Herzog TJ, et al. SGO guidance document for clinical trial designs in ovarian cancer: a changing paradigm. *Gynecol Oncol* 2014;135:3–7.

4. Herzog TJ, et al. FDA ovarian cancer clinical trial endpoints workshop: Society of Gynecologic Oncology White Paper. *Gynecol Oncol.* 2017;147(1):3–10.

27B Is progression-free survival a rational surrogate endpoint in front-line ovarian cancer clinical trials?

No

Eric Pujade-Lauraine, Benoit You, and Jean Sebastien Frenel

Debate

As specified by the fifth Ovarian Cancer Consensus Conference (OCCC) consensus statements [1], the endpoints in clinical trials need to demonstrate whether the treatment results in clinical benefit. The authors will discuss here whether progression-free survival (PFS) is a surrogate marker for patient clinical benefit in front-line ovarian cancer (OC) clinical trials.

Is the Progression-free Survival Criterion as Currently Assessed Clinically Relevant?

The answer is clearly No. Clinical trials define PFS as the time interval between the date of randomization (or first dose of protocol treatment) and disease progression (or death) according to the latest version of the RECIST definition. RECIST disease progression is assessed radiologically. The biomarker CA125 is only used to make the difference between complete and partial remission depending on whether CA125 level falls within normal range or not.

Though radiographs have the merit to be potentially checked by several different independent radiologists, it appears that the standard follow-up of ovarian cancer patients in routine practice does not include systematic radiological examinations in most countries. During surveillance after chemotherapy doctors indicate radiological examination mainly based on patient symptoms or CA125 level evolution.

The appearance of symptoms at relapse is the critical signal for indicating a new treatment. The main reason for waiting for the appearance of symptoms despite evidence of disease progression on CA125 levels or radiologic examinations is that the objective of treatment at relapse becomes palliative as the cure rate of patients with recurrent disease is very low. And even worse, treating the patient on the basis of earlier signals such as a CA125 level increase may be deleterious for the quality of life of patients, exposing them to an increased number of chemotherapy lines without prolonging their overall survival [2].

Based on the acknowledgement that RECIST progression may have no clinical impact on treatment decision, most recent trials including maintenance treatment allow the patient to pursue the treatment identically despite the observation of a RECIST radiologically proven disease progression.

To sum-up, the current PFS criterion is an artificial construction which is not based on routine practice patient follow-up nor on a clinically meaningful endpoint.

Is Progression-free Survival a Clinically Relevant Survival Landmark for Patients Treated in Front-line?

The answer is clearly No.

The main objective of new experimental OC treatments in front-line is to increase patient cure rate [1]. We have to recognize that overall survival (OS) superiority is difficult to demonstrate due to long post-progression survival and cross-over. In addition, OS is an endpoint which is more and more remote in advanced OC with the progress of first-line therapy. The recent result disclosure of the AGO-Ovar 17 trial which has the merit of a seven-year follow-up shows a median OS between 54 and 60 months of advanced stage patients treated with chemotherapy plus bevacizumab and this before the introduction of PARP inhibitors in first-line management [3].

Thus, the search for an OS surrogate marker appears justified. Does PFS fulfill the requirements for an OS surrogate marker? The recent GCIG meta-analysis from 11,029 patients included in randomized first-line trials concluded that the correlation between PFS and OS at the trial level was low, acknowledging the meta-analysis included very few positive trials in terms of survival gain, which limits the conclusions that we can draw from the outcomes [4]. In other words, demonstrating a reduction of PFS hazard ratio (HR) in advanced ovarian cancer does not guarantee that a reduction in OS HR or an increase in "cure rate" will be observed.

The recognition that PFS is such a poor surrogate marker of OS and a mediocre indicator of first-line treatment clinical benefit has led to the addition of several other criteria of efficacy in OC trials [1]. The authors will not outline here all the weaknesses of PFS2; time to first subsequent treatment (TFST) and time to second subsequent treatment (TSST), but thus far these metrics have added little to the interpretation of trial efficacy and they have not yet proven their ability to compensate for the shortcomings of PFS in reliably predicting clinical benefit.

Interestingly, some other surrogate markers have been proposed for patients in the neo-adjuvant setting. Lecuru et al. have suggested that the ultimate goal for these patients could be to combine RECIST response to chemotherapy at three cycles and complete resection at interval surgery. These two criteria have a loose correlation between them and their combination appears to be correlated to PFS and OS [5].

Is Prolonging the Time to Next Relapse (Progression-free Survival) a Clinically Sound Objective?

This is doubtful. The main reason leading to the belief that prolonging the time without relapse is beneficial for patients is based on the concept that rechallenging the patient with chemotherapy is the worst thing that can happen for them. While there is plenty of evidence that relapse is a particularly painful event, there are few prospective data evaluating the quality of life (QoL) change when the patient resumes chemotherapy at relapse. The question is particularly relevant when the patient is relapsing under a maintenance therapy which has its own toxicity and thus may itself induce some QoL deterioration which could be potentially worse or equal to that of chemotherapy.

To circumvent the inability of PFS superiority alone to adequately demonstrate clinical patient benefit, the fifth OCCC requires that PFS should be supported by additional endpoints such as relevant patient-reported outcomes (PROs) [1]. The issue is that "relevant PROs" tools correlated to patient well-being still need to be validated in OC. Recently, a simple assessment called "TWIST," time without symptoms or toxicity, has shown clinically meaningful promise as a PRO tool [6]. However, there is not yet a consensus on which symptoms and toxicity should be taken into account in the model and whether the symptoms described by the doctor (CTCAE v5.0) or by the patient (specific OC QoL questionnaires) should be assessed.

Conclusion

In conclusion, PFS is a second-best option as surrogate endpoint in front-line ovarian cancer clinical trials. PFS is a criterion which is not clinically relevant, PFS is not correlated with OS, and prolongation of PFS does not in itself mean a superior clinical benefit for the patient. To try to palliate its numerous weaknesses in evaluating efficacy in OC, PFS is currently surrounded by several additional criteria such as PFS2, TFST, TSST and assessment of PROs. There is one exception to this grim picture of the lack of utility for PFS: when the magnitude of PFS prolongation is clearly superior to the risks, such as with PARP inhibitors in OC with homologous recombination deficiency [7].

References

1. Bookman MA, et al. Fifth Ovarian Cancer Consensus Conference. Harmonising clinical trials within the Gynecologic Cancer InterGroup: consensus and unmet needs from the Fifth Ovarian Cancer Consensus Conference. *Ann Oncol* 2017;28(Suppl. 8): viii30–viii35.

2. Rustin GJ, et al. MRC OV05; EORTC 55955 investigators. Early versus delayed treatment of relapsed ovarian cancer (MRC OV05/ EORTC 55955): a randomised trial. *Lancet* 2010;376(9747):1155–1163.

3. Pfisterer J, et al. Optimal duration of bevacizumab combined with carboplatin and paclitaxel in patients with primary epithelial ovarian, fallopian tube or peritoneal cancer. *J Clin Oncol* 2021;39 (15):5501.

4. Paoletti X, et al.Gynecologic Cancer InterGroup (GCIG) Meta-analysis Committee. Assessment of progression-free survival as a surrogate end point of overall survival in first-line treatment of ovarian cancer: a systematic review and meta-analysis. *JAMA Netw Open* 2020;3(1): e1918939.

5. Lecuru F, et al. Surrogate endpoint of progression-free (PFS) and overall survival (OS) for advanced ovarian cancer (AOC) patients (pts) treated with neo-adjuvant chemotherapy (NACT): Results of the CHIVA randomized phase II GINECO study. *Ann Oncol* 2019;30 (Suppl. 5):3251.

6. Friedlander M, et al.Health-related quality of life and patient-centred outcomes with olaparib maintenance after chemotherapy in patients with platinum-sensitive, relapsed ovarian cancer and a BRCA1/2 mutation (SOLO2/ENGOT Ov-21): a placebo-controlled, phase 3 randomised trial. *Lancet Oncol* 2018;19(8):1126–1134.

7. Moore K, et al. Maintenance olaparib in patients with newly diagnosed advanced ovarian cancer. *N Engl J Med* 2018;379 (26):2495–2505.

Fertility-sparing Surgery in Early-stage Endometrial Cancer is Safe and Does not Compromise Oncological Outcome

28A

Yes

Enes Taylan and Kutluk Oktay

Debate

Endometrial cancer is the most common gynecologic malignancy in the United States, and the standard-of-care for its treatment is total hysterectomy with bilateral salpingo-oophorectomy (TH-BSO). Although the majority of patients are typically diagnosed after menopause, up to 6.5% of cases are seen in reproductive-age women at 45 years old or younger who may wish to preserve their fertility. Moreover, the share of young women is expected to grow with the increasing incidence of obesity, metabolic syndrome, and nulliparity due to delayed childbirth, all of which are significant risk factors for endometrial cancer.

As a result, preserving fertility for a future chance of childbearing is increasingly becoming an essential component of care in women with endometrial cancer. Therefore, it is critical to provide timely fertility preservation counseling to reproductive-age women with early-stage endometrial cancer who have not yet completed childbearing [1,2].

Conservative Fertility Preserving Surgery

Endometrial cancer tends to have more favorable outcomes in young women than in older patients due to preponderance of well-differentiated (grade 1, endometrioid) endometrioid subtype tumors with limited myometrial invasion. These tumoral lesions are typically related to unopposed estrogen exposure of endometrium, and up to 55% will complete regress with systemic or localized progestin therapy. Several recent studies have shown that hysteroscopic resection of the localized endometrial tumor followed by levonorgestrel-releasing intrauterine device (LR-IUD) placement or systemic progestin therapy is another effective fertility-preserving strategy providing up to 88.9% complete response rate [1]. However, it should be noted that these treatment options should be considered in patients with stage 1A disease, and only after an accurate pathological diagnosis of endometrioid subtype is established. In addition, the risk of recurrence (5%) and potential future hysterectomy should be kept in mind.

Another fertility-sparing surgical approach for women with early-stage endometrial cancer is the preservation of ovaries at the time of hysterectomy. Recent studies have shown that preserving ovaries prevented menopause-associated morbidity and did not increase the risk of endometrial cancer recurrence [1]. These patients can then attempt having a child using in vitro fertilization (IVF) followed by embryo transfer to a gestational surrogate.

Aromatase Inhibitor Protocols to Stimulate Ovaries for Oocyte and Embryo Freezing

Over the past few decades, remarkable advances have been achieved in developing efficient and safer controlled ovarian hyperstimulation (COH) protocols for oocyte retrieval to cryopreserve oocytes or embryos in women with estrogen-sensitive cancer [2,3]. A major concern with COH in women with endometrial cancer is that elevated systemic estrogen levels can potentially worsen the prognosis. To overcome this, we developed an aromatase-inhibitor protocol where letrozole is combined with reduced doses of gonadotropin stimulation in assisted reproduction cycles. This protocol has been widely studied by the same team in women with breast cancer and it has been shown to provide success rates that equal or exceed the success rates with conventional protocols, without reducing the relapse-free survival. Using the same novel protocol in a small case series, we generated embryos in endometrial cancer patients who have had hysterectomy with ovarian preservation, and the transfer of these embryos to gestational surrogates resulted in live births without compromising oncological treatment [4].

In women who may need TH-BSO, but there is insufficient time to wait for next menses to start ovarian stimulation, we developed a "random start COH protocol" where the letrozole-FSH protocol can be started at any time during the menstrual cycle. This strategy provides successful retrieval of an adequate number of oocytes in less than two weeks without causing any significant delay in the cancer treatment [5]. Later studies showed that embryo quality is similar regardless when the ovarian stimulation is started during the ovarian cycle.

Ovarian Tissue Cryopreservation and Transplantation

For women with endometrial cancer without evidence of ovarian involvement and who do not have sufficient time for ovarian stimulation to cryopreserve oocytes or embryos, ovarian tissue cryopreservation (OTC) and subsequent autotransplantation can be offered as an alternative fertility-preserving surgery option. Quiescent primordial follicles, which are embedded in the ovarian cortex and constitute the ovarian reserve, can be efficiently cryopreserved without a need for ovarian stimulation or any regard to the day of menstrual cycle. Having developed and performed the first successful procedures in 1999, our team recently showed that auto-transplantation of frozen-thawed ovarian cortical tissues via orthotopic or heterotopic approaches could efficiently establish ovarian function in patients with various malignancies, including endometrial cancer, resulting in successful retrieval of oocytes, generation of embryos, and live births [1,3].

Conclusions

The foregoing indicates that there are numerous fertility preservation options that can preserve reproductive potential in young women with early-stage endometrial cancer. The current literature on conservative surgery for early-stage cancer provides a good safety profile, however, larger studies with longer follow-up durations are still needed to establish the safety of these strategies in oncological care. While the results obtained during the past two decades with cancer patients indicate that oocyte and embryo freezing with aromatase inhibitor protocols and ovarian tissue cryopreservation followed by auto-transplantation are safe, specific data for endometrial cancer patients is limited. While all patients should be counseled about the availability and success of fertility preservation approaches, the limitations of the available data should also be disclosed to them. Judging from the progress within the past two decades however, the potential for fertility preservation success looks promising for women with endometrial cancer.

References

1. Taylan E, et al. Fertility preservation in gynecologic cancers. *Gynecol Oncol* 2019;155:522–529.

2. Oktay K, et al. Fertility preservation in patients with cancer: ASCO clinical practice guideline update. *J Clin Oncol* 2018;36:1994–2001.

3. Oktay K, et al. Robot-assisted orthotopic and heterotopic ovarian tissue transplantation techniques: surgical advances since our first success in 2000. *Fertil Steril* 2019;111:604–606.

4. Azim A et al. Letrozole for ovulation induction and fertility preservation by embryo cryopreservation in young women with endometrial carcinoma. *Fertil Steril* 2007;88:657–664.

5. Sonmezer M, et al. Random-start controlled ovarian hyperstimulation for emergency fertility preservation in letrozole cycles. *Fertil Steril* 2011;95:2125. e9–2125.e11.

Fertility-sparing Treatment for Early-stage Endometrial Cancer is Safe and Does Not Compromise Oncological Outcome

No

Jessica E. Parker and David S. Miller

Debate

While the average age of patients diagnosed with endometrial cancer is 62 years old, around 4% of women are diagnosed under the age of 40. The gold standard treatment of endometrial cancer is total hysterectomy, bilateral salpingo-oophorectomy, and retroperitoneal lymph node assessment. This is, in many cases, curative but can be life-altering in women desiring fertility. Fertility-sparing options include progestin treatment with oral agents such as megestrol acetate, medroxyprogesterone, or a levonorgestrel-releasing intrauterine device. The National Comprehensive Cancer Network (NCCN) supports these options in well selected patients without any evidence of myometrial invasion who strongly desire fertility [1]. However, this is not based on randomized or prospective trials but rather retrospective data.

In one comprehensive review, a durable complete response to continuous progestin therapy was seen in only 50% of patients [2]. However, the rate of recurrence even after a complete response is relatively high at 35–40%. Most studies on response to progestin treatment include endometrial intraepithelial neoplasia/complex atypical hyperplasia (EIN/CAH) in their analysis as well, which is known to have a higher response rate and lower recurrence rate than endometrial cancer, even with the 40% risk of underlying endometrial cancer with an EIN/CAH preoperative diagnosis [1,2]. The impact of fertility-sparing treatment on actual survival in endometrial cancer is not well reported. In the most recent study and one of the largest published on this topic to date, younger age (<40 years) was associated with a worse progression-free survival (PFS) (HR=3.96, p<0.001) on multivariate analysis. This difference was no longer significant when patients who underwent fertility-sparing therapy were excluded from the analysis (HR=1.17, p=0.71), suggesting that the difference in PFS is directly attributed to fertility-sparing treatment. While overall survival was not impacted by age, the importance of time without progression of disease, and therefore off cancer treatment, has significant quality of life implications that should not be ignored [3]. The risks of continuous progestin therapy including venous thromboembolism, weight gain, headaches, sleep disorders, and mood and libido changes should also be carefully weighed when considering the medical implications as well as the quality of life of the patient.

If gynecologic oncologists are to pursue fertility-sparing treatment for our patients despite these risks and patients understand and accept them, we must consider the benefit that may be ascertained by forgoing standard of care surgery. Studies evaluating outcomes after progestin treatment for endometrial cancer or even EIN/CAH have revealed poor pregnancy outcomes, with pregnancy rates of only 35% and live birth rates of 28% after treatment. One recent study evaluated the addition of metformin to progestins in the fertility-sparing treatment of endometrial intraepithelial neoplasia and cancer. The live birth rate reported in this study was only 17%, and 81% of patients achieving live birth required the use of assisted reproductive technology. It is important to note that the live birth rate was even lower than the 22% risk of endometrial cancer recurrence. This was despite a complete response rate of 69% and an overall response rate of 79% [4]. Another study found an even lower rate of conception of 5% [3]. Therefore, pregnancy outcomes in this population are low.

Outside of continuous progestin therapy, another option for fertility-sparing management of endometrial cancer is hysterectomy with ovarian preservation. The NCCN suggests that ovarian preservation for premenopausal women with stage 1A or 1B endometrial cancer may be safe as it did not appear to increase cancer-specific mortality in one study with follow-up of 16 years [1]. However, this presents a potentially fatal risk of missing ovarian metastases or even synchronous ovarian primary cancer. One study of 102 patients under the age of 45 years undergoing hysterectomy for presumed early-stage endometrial cancer showed that 25% of these patients had a coexisting ovarian malignancy on final pathology. Of these patients, 58% had inner myometrial invasion and 69% had well-differentiated endometrial cancer. This suggests that the apparent low risk endometrial cancer does not preclude coexisting ovarian cancer diagnosis [5]. In another study, the rate of synchronous ovarian cancer was significantly higher in patients under the age of 40 compared with those between 41–60 years (9% vs. 1%, p<0.001). Similar to the prior study, the majority of endometrial cancers with synchronous ovarian cancer had <50% myometrial invasion (91%) and lacked lympho-vascular space invasion (82%). This presents a missed opportunity for the patient and her family to treat this cancer as well as consider genetic testing for familial syndromes associated with ovarian or endometrial cancer.

Conclusion

Based on the available evidence, one cannot definitively state that oncologic outcomes for patients undergoing fertility-sparing treatment for endometrial cancer are the same as for those patients undergoing standard of care surgical management. In fact, there appears to be a lower PFS in these patients with a relatively low durable response rate and high recurrence rate. Patients who decline the standard of care must be prepared to assume these risks with a small likelihood of taking home a child. Therefore, patients should be counselled in a frank and honest manner against fertility-sparing treatment in lieu of standard therapy in endometrial cancer.

References

1. National Comprehensive Cancer Network. Uterine Neoplasms (Version 2.2020). Available from: www.nccn.org/profes sionals/physician_gls/pdf/uterine.pdf [last accessed September 19, 2020].

2. Gunderson CC, et al. Oncologic and reproductive outcomes with progestin therapy in women with endometrial hyperplasia and grade 1 adenocarcinoma: a systematic review. *Gynecol Oncol* 2012;125:477–482.

3. Son J, et al. Endometrial cancer in young women: prognostic factors and treatment outcomes in women aged <40 years. *Int J Gynecol Cancer* 2020;30:631–639.

4. Acosta-Torres S, et al. The addition of metformin to progestin therapy in the fertility-sparing treatment of women with atypical hyperplasia/endometrial intraepithelial neoplasia or endometrial cancer: little impact on response and low live-birth rates. *Gynecol Oncol* 2020;157 (2):348–356.

5. Walsh C, et al. Coexisting ovarian malignancy in young women with endometrial cancer. *Obstet Gynecol* 2005;106(4):693.

29A

Sentinel Lymph Node Mapping Should be the Standard for Staging Patients with High-grade Endometrial Cancers
Yes

Patricia Rivera, Andrea Mariani, and Brooke A. Schlappe

Debate

High-grade endometrial cancers consist of FIGO grade 3 endometroid, clear cell, and papillary serous carcinomas and carcinosarcomas. These cancers are rare and given their propensity to metastasize carry a poor prognosis. Lymph node (LN) metastasis has been noted in up to 20–40% of patients with high-grade disease regardless of the depth of myometrial invasion and as such LN evaluation is recommended for surgical staging regardless of uterine factors. There is strong evidence that reveals LN evaluation via sentinel lymph node (SLN) mapping versus complete lymphadenectomy (LND) to be non-inferior in terms of detection of metastatic lymphatic disease and adverse outcomes. For this reason, as well as the increased potential for injury to surrounding structures, lymphedema, and lymphocyst formation with LND, SLN mapping should be the standard for staging patients with high-grade endometrial cancers and is acceptable per the standard guidelines [1].

Opponents to SLN assessment cite two primary concerns which may theoretically lead to worse oncologic outcomes with the use of this technique as compared to a full LND in high-grade disease: (1) Limited ability to accurately detect metastatic disease, and (2) Loss of the "therapeutic" removal of microscopic metastatic disease. The current available data do not support these concerns.

Several studies support adequate detection of metastatic disease using a SLN algorithm. In a prospective trial with evaluable high-risk disease, all patients underwent LN assessment using a SLN algorithm followed by complete LND. Using the SLN algorithm, the detection rate, sensitivity, false negative predictive value, and false negative rate were 89%, 95%, 1.4%, and 5%, respectively [2]. In the largest prospective trial in endometrial cancer SLN assessment, of which 28% of patients (n=101) had high-grade histologies, the sensitivity in detection of metastatic disease and negative predictive value of the SLN algorithm was 97.5% and 99.6%, respectively [3]. These data confirm results from multiple retrospective cohort studies and support the adequate detection of metastatic disease using the SLN algorithm in patients with high-grade endometrial cancers.

A recent retrospective cohort study evaluating the use of a SLN algorithm versus LND in serous and clear cell endometrial carcinoma demonstrated no difference in detection of advanced stage disease with the SLN algorithm despite the removal of more LNs in those who underwent a LND (median pelvic nodes removed 11 vs. 30 [p<0.001], median para-aortic LNs removed 4 vs. 17 [p<0.001]) [4]. These data are consistent with the results of other cohort studies comparing a SLN algorithm to LND in high-grade disease.

Several retrospective cohort studies demonstrate improved survival with increasing number of LNs removed, supporting the theory that LND is therapeutic. These studies, however, do not utilize a SLN algorithm which identifies metastatic disease with the removal of fewer LNs. The improved survival in these studies likely comes from the improved diagnosis of advanced stage disease, not the removal of microscopic nodal disease. This is confirmed in several studies comparing oncologic outcomes in high-grade endometrial cancer with the use of a SLN algorithm and a full LND. The previously mentioned retrospective multicenter study compared outcomes of SLN mapping (n=118) with LND (n=96) in patients with clear cell and serous endometrial carcinoma. There was no statistic-ally significant difference in overall survival (OS) nor recurrence-free survival (RFS) between the two cohorts [4]. Another multicenter study reviewed outcomes of SLN (n= 56) and LND (n=48) in patients with nonbulky stage IIIC endometrial cancer (46% were high risk, defined as high-grade endometrioid with deep invasion or nonendometrioid) there was no difference in OS between the SLN or LND cohorts [5]. Other single institution retrospective studies confirm similar oncologic outcomes when a SLN algorithm is used in high-grade endometrial cancer.

There does not appear to be an increased risk of nodal recurrences with the use of a SLN algorithm. In the previously mentioned retrospective multicenter study, there was no clear difference in the rates of nodal recurrence, though the numbers were too small for statistical analysis. In a subset with negative LNs, the SLN cohort did have an increased risk of progression (HR=3.12, 95% CI: 1.02, 9.57) but this was felt to be due to differences in surveillance techniques between the cohorts [4]. Multinu et al. found no statistically significant difference in the relative risks of any progression nor the risk of paraaortic progression when SLN was compared to the LND, with paraaortic recurrences occurring in 4/48 of the LND cohort and 6/56 of the SLN cohort. There was no statistically significant difference in lymphatic PFS in patients in the SLN cohort with 10 or fewer LNs removed versus more than 10 LNs [5]. These data do not support the theory that LND is therapeutic.

Conclusion

Use of a SLN algorithm has proven to be non-inferior to LND in staging high-grade endometrial cancer. With less morbidity and similar advanced stage detection rates, it should be the standard for staging patients with high-grade endometrial cancer.

References

1. Holloway RW, et al. Sentinel lymph node mapping and staging in endometrial cancer: a society of gynecologic oncology literature review with consensus recommendations, *Gynecol Oncol* 2017;146:405–415. https://doi .org/10.1016/j.ygyno.2017.05.027

2. Soliman PT, et al. A prospective validation study of sentinel lymph node mapping for high-risk endometrial cancer. *Gynecol Oncol* 2017;146:234–239. https://doi.org/10.1016/j .ygyno.2017.05.016

3. Rossi EC, et al. A comparison of sentinel lymph node biopsy to lymphadenectomy for endometrial cancer staging (FIRES trial): a multicentre, prospective cohort study, *Lancet Oncol* 2017;18:384–392. https://doi.org/10.1016/S1470-2045(17)30068-2

4. Schlappe BA, et al. Multicenter study comparing oncologic outcomes after lymph node assessment via a sentinel lymph node algorithm versus comprehensive pelvic and paraaortic lymphadenectomy in patients with serous and clear cell endometrial carcinoma, *Gynecol Oncol* 2020;156:62–69. https://doi.org/10.1016/j.ygyno.2019.11.002

5. Multinu F, et al. Role of lymphadenectomy in endometrial cancer with nonbulky lymph node metastasis: comparison of comprehensive surgical staging and sentinel lymph node algorithm. *Gynecol Oncol* 2019;155:177–185. https://doi.org/10.1016/j.ygyno.2019.09.011

Debate

29B

Sentinel Lymph Node Mapping Should be the Standard for Staging Patients with High-grade Endometrial Cancers

No

Camilla Yu, Payam Katebi Kashi, and Amanda N. Fader

Debate

There is rationale for sentinel lymph node biopsy (SLNB) in endometrial cancer. Randomized controlled trials (RCTs) have demonstrated that complete lymphadenectomy in women with primary low-grade endometrial cancer (LGEC) who are at low risk for metastatic disease increases perioperative morbidity without any clear influence on progression-free survival (PFS) or overall survival (OS). Unlike LGEC, those with high-grade endometrial cancer (HGEC) are at increased risk for pelvic and para-aortic lymph node metastases, with some studies citing up to 40% risk regardless of uterine factors. In order to accurately tailor adjuvant treatments for women affected by HGEC, comprehensive pelvic and para-aortic lymphadenectomy offers the most complete evaluation of the lymph node basin and in a large, retrospective study, may also improve survival outcomes independent of adjuvant therapy. Additionally, while limited prospective studies exist, there are currently no RCTs studying oncologic outcomes of SLNB in women with HGEC.

The high rate of lymphatic dissemination in high-grade cancers as well as the lack of data regarding long-term survival outcomes and therapeutic impact of SLNB versus complete lymphadenectomy raise concerns for under-treatment of women with HGEC staged with SLNB. Until these gaps are clarified, complete lymphadenectomy should remain the standard of care in the surgical staging of women with HGEC.

Background

Metastatic lymphatic disease is among the most important prognostic factors in endometrial cancer. Historically, endometrial cancer has been staged via comprehensive pelvic and aortic lymph node dissection. There are well defined risks to performing a comprehensive lymphadenectomy, including a low risk of intraoperative vascular and nerve-related injuries and a higher risk of lower extremity lymphedema. The use of SLNB in the staging of apparent uterine-confined endometrial cancer has gained tremendous ground in the last decade, with purported benefits such as a high sensitivity and low negative predictive value in the hands of experienced surgeons, decreased surgical time and morbidity, as well as a decreased risk of postoperative complications. However, many of the studies cited to support SLNB in this setting focus on women with LGEC who have an overall very low risk for nodal involvement and recurrence.

In contrast, HGEC, comprised of p53 aberrant tumors such as grade 3 endometrioid subtypes, serous, papillary, and clear cell carcinomas as well as uterine carcinosarcoma, carry an elevated risk for lymph node metastases (i.e., 20–40%), irrespective of uterine factors, due to their biological aggressiveness. Compared to LGEC, those with HGEC often require systemic adjuvant therapies and have a much worse prognosis. Additionally, among those patients with non-endometrioid histologies who have lymphatic spread, 70% were found to have para-aortic lymph node metastases [1]. Therefore, accurately identifying patients with HGEC who have metastatic lymphatic disease is paramount, as it impacts adjuvant therapy strategies and potential survival outcomes. The use of SNLB in the staging of HGEC remains controversial.

Sentinel Lymph Node Studies in Endometrial Cancer Largely Focus on Low-grade Endometrial Cancers

The vast majority of literature regarding SLNB in endometrial cancer is retrospective, and demonstrates the feasibility and relative accuracy of SLNB in the setting of LGEC [2,3]. One of the higher quality prospective studies, the multi-institutional FIRES trial, reported a 99.6% (95% CI: 97.9–100) sensitivity and 97.2% (95% CI: 85–100%) negative predictive value (NPV) in this technique. However, the study population was comprised primarily of women with LGEC; only 28% of study subjects had HGEC, and therefore, the study was underpowered to examine outcomes in this setting [4]. Since the publication of the FIRES trial, several other studies have attempted to clarify the role of sentinel lymph node mapping HGEC. While the sensitivities and mapping rates demonstrated in these studies are comparable to those found in studies including both high- and low-grade endometrial cancers, most studies contain small datasets with varying false negative rates, reaching as high as 22% as seen in one single institution study [5]. These false negative rates may be further underestimated given the low rate of para-aortic lymphadenectomies, and in particular those extending above the inferior mesenteric artery, performed in studies validating SLNB protocols in women with HGEC. The recently published SENTOR study, which included 156 patients, 80% of who had HGEC, is the first prospective trial that is adequately powered to evaluate the accuracy of SNLB in women with HGEC with sensitivity of 97.4% (95% CI: 93.6) and NPV of 99% (95% CI: 96–100%) [6]. However, the SENTOR study was not adequately powered to evaluate long-term survival outcomes, recurrence, and morbidity outcomes associated with SLNB alone. Given the high propensity for lymphatic spread of HGEC, the use of SLNB in lieu of comprehensive lymphadenectomy risks missing the presence of extra-uterine disease, potentially leading to under-staging and under-treatment of disease.

Absence of Survival Data in Existing Sentinel Lymph Node Endometrial Cancer Trials

In examining other solid tumor types, such as breast cancer and melanoma, SLNB has become the standard of care after rigorous validation of techniques and outcomes data through RCTs. A meta-analysis consisting of four RCTs in breast cancer patients demonstrated no long-term survival benefit to complete axillary node dissection compared to SLNB [7]. Similarly, the MSLT-1 study, a phase III trial studying patients undergoing wide local excision for melanoma, demonstrated improved disease-free survival outcomes at 10 years for patients treated with SLNB compared to just wide local excision alone [8].

To date, there are no RCTs evaluating survival outcomes of women with HGEC staged using SLNB alone compared to comprehensive lymphadenectomy (Table 29B.1) Although two RCTs have demonstrated no therapeutic benefit of comprehensive pelvic and aortic lymphadenectomy in women with endometrial cancer compared to hysterectomy alone, these trials largely included low-risk, LGEC patients, and were not powered to examine PFS and OS outcomes in women with HGEC. These two RCTs only examined the therapeutic effect of pelvic lymphadenectomy and no para-aortic lymphadenectomies were performed in either study. Furthermore, both RCTs utilized selective rather than systematic lympha-denectomy. The ASTEC trial in particular was limited, with ≤9 lymph nodes removed in 35% of patients and ≤4 lymph nodes removed in 12% of patients in the lymphadenectomy group. In both the ASTEC trial as well as the study by Benedetti-Panici et al., the rates of adjuvant therapy in both study arms were similar, with almost equal numbers of patients receiving adjuvant chemotherapy and/or radiation therapy, which further confound post-operative and survival outcomes.

In contrast, the Japanese SEPAL study demonstrated a significantly longer overall survival in a cohort of women with intermediate and high-risk endometrial cancer who underwent systematic pelvic and aortic lymph node dissection compared to those undergo-ing pelvic lymphadenectomy alone. On multivariate analysis, systematic lymphadenectomy remained independently associated with improved survival even after controlling for adju-vant chemotherapy. These data suggest that detecting positive lymph nodes may have led to chemotherapy administration; chemotherapy alone may not be sufficient to treat para-aortic disease [9,10].

Further evidence supporting a survival benefit of full lymphadenectomy is found in a recent abstract presented at the Society for Gynecologic Oncology meeting in 2019. Buskwofie et al. examined data from the National Cancer Database. This study identified 16,950 women diagnosed with type II uterine cancers between 2010–2015 and demon-strated para-aortic lymph node metastases in 39% of patients who also had known positive pelvic lymph nodes, and in 3% of patients without pelvic lymph node metastasis. This study concluded that women treated with para-aortic lymphadenectomy were 12% less likely to die from their disease (HR=0.88, 95% CI: 0.83–0.93) [11]. These data suggest that it is essential to validate the use of SLN biopsy in women with HGEC through large RCTs before considering a paradigm shift in the surgical staging of women with HGEC. Additionally, randomized data is needed on perioperative outcomes associated with SLN biopsy com-pared to comprehensive lymphadenectomy, especially pertaining to lymphedema. A National Cancer Institute-NRG Oncology study is planned.

Conclusion

While the data supporting the use of SLNB in HGEC is preliminarily promising, the question of clinical and survival benefit for patients remains. Ultimately, further investiga-tion, ideally in a randomized trial setting, is required before universal adoption of SLNB as a staging technique for women with HGEC. Until that time, if SLNB is to be employed, close adherence to the NCCN SLN algorithm, which endorses complete lymphadenectomy for an

Table 29B.1 Summary of studies examining sentinel lymph nodes in endometrial cancer

	Study designs	Patients with SLN (Total)	Tumor grade		Histologic subtypes		Statistical power to examine oncologic outcomes in HGEC?
			LGEC⊤ n(%)	HGECπ n(%)	Endometrioid EC n(%)	Non-Endometrioid EC n(%)	
Prospective studies							
Cusimano et al. (SENTOR) 2020 [6]	Prospective cohort	156	30 (19)	126 (81)	65 (42)	91 (58)	No
Soliman et al.	Prospective	101	44 (44)	57 (56)	44 (44)	57 (56)	No
Rossi et al. (FIRES) 2017 [4]	Prospective cohort	293	254 (87)	39 (13)	252 (86)	41 (14)	No
Retrospective studies							
Tanner et al. 2017 [5]	Retrospective	52	0	52 (100)	14 (27)	38 (73)	No
Eriksson et al. 2016 [2]	Retrospective	642	450 (70)	192 (30)	642 (100)	0 (0)	No
RCT							
No study	None	0	0	0	0	0	None

Key: ⊤ = low-grade endometrial cancer; π = high-grade endometrial cancer.

unmapped hemi-pelvis as well as removal of abnormal-appearing lymph nodes, is critical in order to minimize false negatives and potential poorer outcomes for women. If the recent findings of the randomized surgical LACC trial in cervical cancer have proven anything, it is that we should be cautious in our surgical approach to gynecologic cancer, not assume that retrospective or underpowered prospective data is accurate, and look before we take a surgical leap.

References

1. Mariani A, et al. Prospective assessment of lymphatic dissemination in endometrial cancer: a paradigm shift in surgical staging. *Gynecol Oncol* 2008;109(1):11–18.

2. Eriksson AGZ, et al. Comparison of a sentinel lymph node and a selective lymphadenectomy algorithm in patients with endometrioid endometrial carcinoma and limited myometrial invasion. *Gynecol Oncol* 2016;140(3):394–399.

3. Buda A, et al. Lymph node evaluation in high-risk early-stage endometrial cancer: a multi-institutional retrospective analysis comparing the sentinel lymph node (SLN) algorithm and SLN with selective lymphadenectomy. *Gynecol Oncol* 2018;150(2):261–266.

4. Rossi EC, et al. A comparison of sentinel lymph node biopsy to lymphadenectomy for endometrial cancer staging (FIRES trial): a multicentre, prospective, cohort study. *Lancet Oncol* 2017;18(3):384–392.

5. Tanner EJ, et al. The utility of sentinel lymph node mapping in high-grade endometrial cancer. *Int J Gynecol Cancer* 2017;27(7):1416–1421.

6. Cusimano MC, et al. Assessment of sentinel lymph node biopsy vs lymphadenectomy for intermediate- and high-grade endometrial cancer staging. *JAMA Surg* 2021; 156(2):157–164.

7. Petrelli F, et al. Axillary dissection compared to sentinel node biopsy for the treatment of pathologically node-negative breast cancer: a meta-analysis of four randomized trials with long-term follow up. *Oncol Rev* 2012;6(2):e20.

8. Morton DL, et al. Final trial report of sentinel-node biopsy versus nodal observation in melanoma. *New Engl J Med* 2014;370(7):599–609.

9. Todo Y, et al. Survival effect of para-aortic lymphadenectomy in endometrial cancer (SEPAL study): a retrospective cohort analysis. *Lancet* 2010;375:1165–1172.

10. Frost JA, et al. Lymphadenectomy for the management of endometrial cancer. *Cochrane Database Syst Rev* 2015;2015(9): CD007585.

11. Buskwofie A, et al. Role of paraaortic nodal evaluation in women with uterine cancer. *Gynecol Oncol* 2019;154:105–106.

Molecular Profiling Should be Done to Guide the Management of Endometrial Cancer?

30A

Yes

Karen Cadoo

Debate

Molecular profiling is emerging as a critical tool for accurate stratification and treatment planning in endometrial cancer (EC). Decision making and application of clinical trial data has been challenged by the heterogenic biology and outcomes in ECs. We rely on clinical variables to assess risk and determine optimal therapy, including patient age, tumor stage and grade, and myometrial, lymphovascular, and cervical stromal invasion. These variables provide imprecise estimates with the potential for both under and over treatment of patients. Critically, intra observer variability affects classification and therefore applicability of relevant data. It was shown, for example, that centralized pathology review in the PORTEC-3 study changed clinico-pathological data in 43% of patients [1].

With the integration of molecular data, we have the opportunity to be more precise for our patients. We have learned from The Cancer Genome Atlas (TCGA) that ECs fall into four distinct clusters or molecular subgroups [2]. Cluster one is defined by tumors with a *POLE* ultramutated phenotype. These tumors often have a grade 3 and histologically aggressive appearance but in fact have a good prognosis. Accurate classification and risk stratification of these tumors facilitates optimal management. We await further data; however, it may be possible to de-escalate adjuvant therapy that would have been prescribed based on clinical features in these cancers. In cluster two, tumors have mismatch repair (MMR) deficiency /microsatellite instability (MSI) and are frequently but not exclusively endometrioid cancers. Tumors are hypermutated, immunogenic, and responsive to immunotherapy. This applies currently in the advanced disease setting; ongoing clinical trials are exploring the role of immunotherapy in the adjuvant setting. Cluster three ECs are genomically relatively stable and MMR proficient, with a moderate number of mutations. This group does not have a surrogate marker for identification and were classified by TCGA as copy number low. This is considered a misleading term as they often harbour copy number alterations, leading to the proposed terminology of "no specific molecular profile/ no surrogate marker profile." It is likely that further work will better define this subgroup in the future. Cluster three tumors frequently have alterations in the *PTEN/ PIK3CA* pathway which have the potential to be therapeutically targetable. Cluster four is characterized by extensive copy number alterations, few DNA methylation changes, and frequent TP53 mutations. While these tumors are predominantly serous histologically, molecular data has shown that 25% of high-grade endometrioid tumours share these characteristics, again highlighting that defining these tumors by their molecular profile is vital. Traditionally, serous and clear cell EC have frequently been categorized together in clinical trials as high grade, with the implication that prognosis and the impact of the intervention is expected to be similar in both subtypes. However, clear cell cancers are distributed across the four TCGA clusters, again with potential prognostic significance [3]. In fact, all stages, grade, and histologic type of EC can be found across the TCGA subgroups. We need to integrate this histomolecular data to accurately identify what the tumor represents to avoid both under and over treatment in the adjuvant setting. While the TCGA methodology is not practical for routine use, more pragmatic approaches have been proposed using surrogate markers to identify molecular subgroups providing the option to integrate into routine clinical care [4].

With integration of this more accurate tumor classification we will learn how to better tailor therapy not just based on appropriate risk assessment but also predication of how a given intervention may affect different subtypes. The ongoing PORTEC-4 study, for example, is investigating the use of a molecular integrated risk profile to define appropriate adjuvant therapy (NCT03469674). In addition, we have novel clinical trial designs where eligibility for inclusion is molecularly rather than histology driven. This also provides the opportunity to run clinical trials in rarer cancers and rare subtypes of cancers, increasing the possibility for drug approvals and availability. Importantly, molecularly driven studies have already led to drug approval on the basis of a genomic biomarker with pembrolizumab being the first agnostic drug approval based on the genomic biomarker of MMR deficient/MSI high tumor rather than a histology or disease specific indication. For patients who have recurrent EC, molecular data and in particular, next generation sequencing, may identify potential targets for therapy. In a study of advanced EC patients undergoing next generation sequencing, 65% had a likely therapeutically actionable alteration. While patients who enrolled in a clinical trial and benefitted from targeted therapy represented just 10% of patients in this study, the proportion of EC patients who will benefit from this approach will become far higher as routine sequencing is integrated into care and more molecularly driven clinical trials become available.

Aside from the implications in terms of therapy planning in adjuvant and recurrent EC, routine molecular profiling provides opportunities for our patients and their family members for more accurate future cancer risk identification. Many women with EC are fortunately cured of their disease. Identification of MMR deficient/MSI high EC acts as a screening tool for Lynch syndrome. It is critical to identify women who have Lynch syndrome, providing an important opportunity for reduction of future cancer risks in both the patient and their family. It is also imperative to accurately classify the origin of MMR deficiency. Previously women with MMR deficient EC, in the absence of *MLH1* promoter hypermethylation or an identified germline mutation to explain the immunohistochemical loss, may have been considered to have occult Lynch syndrome. In these ECs with molecular testing double somatic MMR mutations may be identified, providing reassurance in these tumors that an occult germline mutation is unlikely. This avoids the emotional and financial toll of intensive cancer screening for a high penetrance cancer predisposition mutation if it is not required [5].

Conclusion

Molecular profiling of all EC enables accurate stratification of risk and optimized therapy planning and clinical trial enrollment. The identification of specific molecular subgroups has changed the understanding of EC biology and it is continuing to evolve. Molecular profiling is an essential tool for optimal patient care for all EC patients.

References

1. de Boer SM, et al; for PORTEC Study Group. Clinical consequences of upfront pathology review in the randomised PORTEC-3 trial for high-risk endometrial cancer. *Ann Oncol* 2018;29(2):424–430. https://doi.org/10.1093/annonc/mdx753

2. Cancer Genome Atlas Research Network, Kandoth C, et al. Integrated genomic characterization of endometrial carcinoma. *Nature* 2013;497(7447):67–73. https://doi.org/10.1038/nature12113. Erratum in: *Nature* 2013;500(7461):242.

3. DeLair DF, et al. The genetic landscape of endometrial clear cell carcinomas. *J Pathol* 2017;243(2):230–241. https://doi.org/10.1002/path.4947

4. Stelloo E, et al. Improved risk assessment by integrating molecular and clinicopathological factors in early-stage endometrial cancer: combined analysis of the PORTEC cohorts. *Clin Cancer Res* 2016;22(16):4215–4224. https://doi.org/10.1158/1078-0432.CCR-15-2878

5. Salvador MU, et al. Comprehensive paired tumor/germline testing for lynch syndrome: bringing resolution to the diagnostic process. *J Clin Oncol* 2019;37(8):647–657. https://doi.org/10.1200/JCO.18.00696

30B Molecular Profiling Should be Done to Guide the Management of Endometrial Cancer?

No

Michael Wilkinson, Paul Downey, and Donal J. Brennan

Debate

The treatment of endometrial carcinoma (EC) has been traditionally guided by microscopic features, but the concept of molecular subtyping of endometrial cancer is nothing new. In 1983, Bokhman proposed that endometrial cancers be divided into two pathogenic groups: type 1 endometrial tumors – low-grade, low-stage, good prognosis tumors classically associated with PTEN mutations and activation of the PI3-kinase pathway (typically endometrioid histology) – and type 2 endometrial tumors – high-grade, non-endometrioid poorer prognosis tumors associated with p53 and Her2 mutations (classically serous and clear cell histology) [1].

The more recent iteration of molecular profiling of endometrioid cancers (The Cancer Genome Atlas (TCGA) and subsequently the ProMisE and TransPORTEC) is an evolving piece of work (Figure 30B.1). Subtle differences have started to emerge between different iterations of the molecular classification which appears to be reproducible, simple to apply, and has clear prognostic implications. It has also recently been endorsed by the World Health Organization who simultaneously removed other pathologic variants (e.g., secretory, villoglandular, sertoliform, and microglandular from their classification of female genital tumors) [2].

Advances in molecular classification of endometrial cancer certainly have the potential to guide exciting developments in the twenty-first century, but whether the molecular stratification of endometrial cancer ultimately reduces mortality from endometrial cancer remains to be seen. Likewise, it is apparent that this is a dynamic area that may not yet have reached a conclusion, for example where will L1CAM and CTNNB1 mutations fit into this classification going forward? The pace of change in our evolving understanding of molecular profiling is rapid, and incorporating routine molecular profiling into the management of endometrial cancer may be premature at this point, particularly without universal access to this technology. The focus at this point should be on appropriately powered prospective randomized controlled trials (RCTs) designed to evaluate the utility of these molecular stratifications, with a particular emphasis on their predictive rather than their prognostic capacities. Currently the best data we have to support this approach

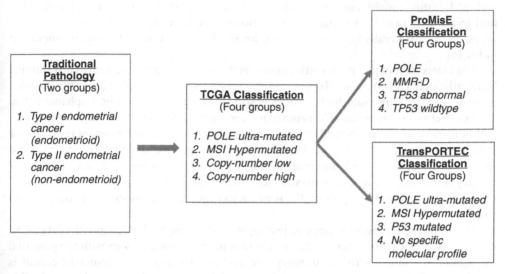

Figure 30B.1 The molecular classifications of endometrial cancer.
This figure shows the evolution of the classification of endometrial cancer from the original classification on the left of the figure to the newly adapted ProMisE and TransPORTEC classifications on the right.

is a post-hoc analysis of PORTEC3 and the only predictive signal suggests a benefit for chemoradiotherapy in the p53 mutated group – which can be identified using immuno-histochemistry [3].

As the clamour to introduce molecular subtyping increases, it is prudent to note that this will not obviate the need for histopathologic assessment of all endometrial tumors, which is required to establish the epithelial origin, out-rule a biphasic tumor, and attribute the appropriate histological subtype (endometrioid vs. non-endometrioid). Simultaneously, on the basis of hematoxylin and eosin (H&E) evaluation, this assessment can stratify tumors into those with a low risk of recurrence, identify low-grade tumors with intermediate recurrence risk (e.g., low-grade tumors with lympho-vascular space invasion (LVSI) and tumors with a microcystic elongated and fragmented pattern of invasion (MELF-like invasion)) and tumors that are potentially MMR deficient (endo-metrial cancers with tumor infiltrating lymphocytes, tumors arising in the lower uterine segment, and tumors with MELF-like invasion). An ad-hoc adoption of molecular subtyping for all endometrial cancers will not replace these important observations.

The molecular classification of endometrial cancer has its origins in large-scale next-generation sequencing – a technology that has promised a lot but delivered very little in day-to-day oncological care. While there may be a place for targeted molecular profiling, e.g., in the identification of less aggressive grade 3 ECs based on POLE mutation status tumors, access to POLE sequencing has proven to be difficult outside of a research setting, and numerous technical issues have been highlighted throughout the literature. Furthermore, it is becoming increasingly obvious that not all POLE mutations are equal. While some will argue that the identification of MMR-deficient endometrial cancer may identify women who could respond to immunotherapy, access to immunotherapy is restricted to high income countries. Until there is widespread access to molecular profiling, the use of immunohistochemistry for MMR profiling, ER and p53 status should remain standard practice. We should remind ourselves that multiple breast cancer molecular classifications have been developed over the last 15 years, all of which really have been focused on ER, PR, and Her2 status and proliferation index [4].

The assessment of any proliferative endometrial lesion will always require conventional histopathologic examination. Histomorphology using a simple H&E stain (with the addition of selected immunohistochemistry) is widely available and can be implemented in a cost-effective and reproducible manner in low- to middle-income settings. A low-tech pathologic assessment often yields the only information required for treatment purposes for the most common type of endometrial carcinomas – low grade endometrial cancer confined to the inner half of the endometrium without LVSI. These tumors are typically cured by surgery alone. Most of these patients will die of cardiovascular disease as a result of their comorbidities and additional prognostic or predictive molecular profiles are unlikely to add value.

The implementation of molecular testing should not be to the detriment of standard histomorphological assessment – this would be a major retrograde step with the potential for significant clinical error. Histomorphological classification of endometrial cancer is widely available worldwide and can be attained in a cost effective and reproducible manner. Molecular profiling is a highly specialized investigation requiring skilled interpretation, and adds considerable cost to cancer care. Its introduction to the management of endometrial cancer will further alienate cancer centers in developing countries and raise concerning ethical issues. While molecular profiling may have a role especially in identifying good prognosis POLE mutated cancers (which would otherwise have a potential for overtreatment) and in identifying an underlying familial cancer syndrome, this is not required for most endometrial cancers, and we should wait for the results of forthcoming RCTs. Until then, the focus should remain on improved training of gynecological pathologists worldwide to improve morphological assessment and provide appropriate immunohistochemistry assessment (IHC). Endometrial cancer affects women of all socioeconomic classes and cultures worldwide. A globally standardized means of classifying tumors is crucial for the delivery of equitable healthcare and research progression worldwide.

Conclusion

Ultimately, until results of PORTEC-4A [5] and other ongoing RCTs are available and demonstrate significant patient benefits in terms of improved overall survival or reduced treatment-related morbidity, we should temper our enthusiasm. We should learn from previous experience of over-enthusiastic adoption of new technologies which subsequently failed in phase 3 randomized trials – from minimally invasive surgery for early-stage cervical cancer to immunotherapy for ovarian cancer; gynecological oncology is littered with examples of overzealous early adoption of new techniques before evidence of benefit is available.

References

1. Bokhman JV. Two pathogenetic types of endometrial carcinoma. *Gynecol Oncol* 1983;15(1):10–17.

2. International Agency for Research on Cancer. *WHO Classification of Tumours. Female Genital Tumours* (5th edn.). 2020.

3. León-Castillo A, et al. Molecular classification of the PORTEC-3 trial for high-risk endometrial cancer: impact on prognosis and benefit from adjuvant therapy. *J Clin Oncol* 2020;38 (29):3388–3397.

4. Buus R, et al. Molecular drivers of oncotype DX, prosigna, endopredict, and the breast cancer index: a TransATAC study. *J Clin Oncol* 2020;2020:Jco2000853.

5. van den Heerik A, et al. PORTEC-4a: international randomized trial of molecular profile-based adjuvant treatment for women with high-intermediate risk endometrial cancer. *Int J Gynecol Cancer* 2020;30 (12):2002–2007.

What is the Best Adjuvant Therapy for Management of Stage III Endometrial Cancer?
Chemotherapy Alone

Daniela Matei

Debate

Regarded as a malignancy with high risk for local recurrence and highly responsive to radiation, locally advanced endometrial cancer was traditionally approached with surgery, followed by pelvic external beam radiotherapy (EBRT) aiming to sterilize potential residual malignant sites in the tumor and lymphatic draining bed. Many studies have demonstrated the efficacy of postoperative EBRT preventing pelvic and regional recurrences, however more than a third of women with stage III endometrial cancer treated with surgery and radiotherapy alone, experience failure at distant sites, ultimately succumbing to recurrent disease. The recognition of nodal metastasis as a harbinger of future systemic recurrence has brought interest to exploring chemotherapy as a treatment modality in this setting. The Gynecologic Oncology Group (GOG) trial GOG-122 randomized phase III trial comparing whole abdominal irradiation (WAI) to chemotherapy with doxorubicin and platinum showed that administration of systemic treatment improved the overall survival (OS) by 10% compared to radiotherapy. This study put for the first time the spotlight on chemotherapy as a potential primary treatment approach for locally advanced endometrial cancer [1]. However, 20% of patients treated with chemotherapy alone in this study experienced loco-regional failure, raising the question whether a combined modality approach could further improve outcomes for patients with stage III uterine cancer.

Several subsequent trials explored chemoradiation following surgery for this patient population. GOG-184 compared two chemotherapy regimens (double vs. triple agent combinations) together with volume directed EBRT and yielded a three-year progression-free survival exceeding 60% for both groups [2]. While hailed as a successful approach, toxicity was high in this study, with 20% of patients failing to complete the intended six cycles of chemotherapy. Approximately 80% of the intended dose of chemotherapy was given to those patients who completed chemo-radiotherapy. Grade 3 and 4 hematological toxicity occurred in more than half of treated patients, while grade 3–4 gastrointestinal adverse events were recorded in ~25% of women. Additionally, late grade 3 and 4 gastrointestinal toxicities were noted in 5% of patients treated on this study and worsening neurotoxicity scores were detectable after chemo-radiation, being more significant in women who received the platinum-containing regimen [2]. These observations underscore the high level of acute and late toxicity associated with the combined treatment strategy.

Taking a different perspective, adjuvant chemo-radiotherapy was compared to EBRT alone in patients with early-stage high risk and stage III endometrial cancer in PORTEC-3 trial. The combined regimen improved both OS and recurrence-free survival (RFS) over radiotherapy alone in the mixed high-risk patient population examined in this study, of which only half represented stage III endometrial cancer. This subgroup, at risk for both local and systemic failure, drove most of the benefit form the combined approach in this trial [3,4]. Despite these highly compelling results supporting use of a chemoradiation strategy, the question as to whether the combined modality approach adds anything to the benefits of systemic chemotherapy alone had not been addressed in either trial. Further, the results of the PORTEC-3 clearly demonstrated the advantages conferred by chemotherapy administration in patients with stage III endometrial cancer, but failed to dissect out whether EBRT provided any additional benefit in this setting.

To address this remaining question, GOG-258 compared chemoradiation with systemic chemotherapy alone in women with stage III/IVA endometrial cancer [5]. Although the combined approach significantly reduced the rate of loco-regional relapse, contrary to expectations, the study failed to demonstrate that the combination regimen was superior to chemotherapy alone in prolonging RFS. At five years, 58% of patients were alive free of disease recurrence on both arms of the study. The three-year RFS exceeded 60% for both strategies, being comparable to the outcomes observed in GOG-184 where all patients received chemo-radiotherapy, including a highly myelosuppressive three-drug regimen. The lack of difference in outcome between patients receiving systemic treatment only and multi-modality strategy was likely driven by an unexpected increase in rate of distant failure in the group of patients receiving chemoradiotherapy. Whether the increase in visceral metastases reflected the consequences of the inability to deliver full doses of chemotherapy to those patients allocated to the multi-modality treatment strategy or to the delay in initiating the systemic treatment remains controversial. Only 75% of patients allocated to the chemoradiation arm completed the intended four cycles of chemotherapy. Coupled with findings that patients receiving a combined therapeutic approach had an increased rate of constitutional, gastrointestinal, renal/genitourinary, and musculoskeletal toxicities, and reported worse quality of life scores, driven by more frequent gastrointestinal symptoms in the group allocated to additional EBRT, the findings of this trial support omitting radiotherapy for the treatment of women with endometrial cancer with nodal metastases.

Conclusion

It appears that for those patients whose tumors have escaped the containment of the uterus, the risk of distant failure by far outweighs the danger of local recurrence, being the dominant factor regulating survival. Addressing the risk of pelvic recurrence with EBRT shifts the attention away from the far higher threat of distant metastasis, diminishes tolerability and ability to deliver full doses of systemic treatment. With the cat out of the bag in stage III endometrial cancer, chemotherapy wins all.

References

1. Randall ME, et al. Randomized phase III trial of whole-abdominal irradiation versus doxorubicin and cisplatin chemotherapy in advanced endometrial carcinoma: a Gynecologic Oncology Group study. *J Clin Oncol* 2006;24:36–44.

2. Homesley HD, et al. A randomized phase III trial in advanced endometrial carcinoma of

surgery and volume directed radiation followed by cisplatin and doxorubicin with or without paclitaxel: a Gynecologic Oncology Group study. *Gynecol Oncol* 2009;112:543–552.

3. de Boer SM, et al. Adjuvant chemoradiotherapy versus radiotherapy alone for women with high-risk endometrial cancer (PORTEC-3): final results of an international, open-label, multicentre, randomised, phase 3 trial. *Lancet Oncol* 2018;19(3):295–309.

4. de Boer SM, et al. Adjuvant chemoradiotherapy versus radiotherapy alone in women with high-risk endometrial cancer (PORTEC-3): patterns of recurrence and post-hoc survival analysis of a randomised phase 3 trial. *Lancet Oncol* 2019;20:1273–1285.

5. Matei D, et al. Adjuvant chemotherapy plus radiation for locally advanced endometrial cancer. *N Engl J Med* 2019;380:2317–2326.

What is the Best Adjuvant Therapy for Management of Stage III Endometrial Cancer?

Combined Chemotherapy and Radiation Therapy

Stephanie M. de Boer and Catheryn M. Yashar

Debate

Stage III endometrial cancer (EC) comprises women with local and/or regional spread of the tumor: invasion of the tumor to the serosa and/or adnexae (IIIA), vaginal and/or parametrial involvement (IIIB) or metastases to pelvic and/or para-aortic lymph nodes (IIIC). Stage III is considered high-risk EC (HREC) and identifies women at increased risk of recurrence and EC-related death. Optimal adjuvant treatment has been studied for decades. To optimize both locoregional and distant control, concurrent chemoradiotherapy was investigated. Two randomized trials (both including stage III EC patients) were published in 2019; the Gynecologic Oncology Group (GOG)-258 trial and the Post-Operative Radiotherapy in Endometrial Carcinoma (PORTEC)-3 trial. In both trials chemoradiotherapy (CTRT) was investigated, compared with chemotherapy (CT) alone in the GOG-258 trial and radiotherapy (RT) alone in the PORTEC-3 trial.

In the PORTEC-3 trial, women with HREC were randomized to pelvic RT with or without concurrent and adjuvant chemotherapy (two cycles of cisplatin 50 mg/m² during radiotherapy, followed by four cycles of carboplatin AUC5 and paclitaxel 175 mg/m²). Of 660 eligible patients, 45% of women had stage III disease: 13% (n=83) stage IIIA, 6% (n=42) stage IIIB, and 26% (n=170) stage IIIC. Updated survival analysis with a median follow-up of 72 months showed a significant improvement of 5% in five-year overall survival (OS; 81% vs. 76%, HR=0.70) and 7% in five-year recurrence-free survival (RFS; 76% vs. 69%, HR=0.70) in favor of CTRT [1]. The benefit of chemotherapy was most pronounced for women with stage III and/or serous cancers. For women with stage III EC, a significant and clinically relevant benefit of 10% in OS (78% vs. 68%; HR=0.63) and 12.5% in RFS (71% vs. 58%; HR=0.61) was found in favor of CTRT compared to only 2% in OS and 4% in RFS for stages I–II EC. Both OS and RFS were significantly improved for serous cancers with CTRT as well; five-year OS was 71% (CTRT) versus 53% (RT; HR=0.48) and five-year RFS was 60% (CTRT) versus 48% (RT; HR=0.42). Notably, the addition of chemotherapy to RT demonstrated increased toxicity and lower quality of life during treatment and the first year thereafter. The persistence of sensory neuropathy among women treated with chemotherapy is the most clinically relevant and most bothersome long-term symptom, reported by 25% of women at two years after treatment [2].

The GOG-258 trial randomly assigned 813 women with stages III–IVA EC (97% stage III, 94% lymphadenectomy) to either pelvic RT with concurrent cisplatin and adjuvant carboplatin and paclitaxel (in the same schedule as used in the PORTEC-3 trial), or chemotherapy alone (six cycles of carboplatin and paclitaxel given every three weeks) [3]. With a median follow-up of 47 months overlapping RFS curves were reported (five-year RFS: 59% CTRT vs. 58% CT). Significantly more pelvic and para-aortic lymph node recurrences were reported in patients treated with chemotherapy alone: HR=0.43 (95% CI: 0.28–0.66). Women treated with CTRT had a trend for more distant recurrences as the first failure (HR=1.36, 95% CI: 1.00–1.86). It was not reported how many women with pelvic or para-aortic lymph node recurrences in the chemotherapy-alone arm had salvage radiotherapy. Grade 3, 4, or 5 acute adverse events were reported in 202 patients (58%) in the CTRT group and 227 patients (63%) in the chemotherapy-only group; A grade 4 or higher acute adverse event occurred in 48 patients (14%) in the chemoradiotherapy group and in 108 patients (30%) in the chemotherapy-only group.

Comparing the stage III subgroup of the PORTEC-3 and the GOG-258 trial (97% stage III), it is notable that the RT arm of the PORTEC-3 had a similar RFS (58%) compared with both treatment arms of the GOG-258 (59% and 58%), while the RFS was 71% in the CTRT arm of the PORTEC-3. In GOG-258, 73% of the trial participants were stage IIIC while in PORTEC-3 58% of the stage III women had stage IIIC, so it is difficult to directly compare these two groups.

These two randomized trials demonstrated that radiotherapy improved locoregional control, even after lymphadenectomy. The addition of chemotherapy improved both OS and RFS, especially for stage III and/or serous cancers: the question remains which patients derive the most benefit from chemotherapy. HREC stage III is a very heterogeneous group of tumors. Currently, decisions on adjuvant treatment are based on traditional histopathological factors. After the EC molecular classification was introduced by The Cancer Genome Atlas (TCGA), a transition towards molecular-based classification was initiated [4]. This molecular classification consists of four subclasses based on mutational burden and copy number alterations with clear prognostic impact; p53-mutant (p53abn), POLE ultra-mutated (POLEmut), mismatch-repair deficient (MMRd), or no specific molecular profile (NSMP).

The TransPORTEC consortium investigated the TCGA-defined prognostic molecular subgroups on 410 of 660 tumor tissues from patients enrolled in the PORTEC-3 trial [5]. The molecular classification had strong prognostic value with a five-year RFS of 98% for POLEmut (12% of cases), 72% for MMRd (33%), 74% for NSMP (32%) and 48% for p53abn (23%; p<0.001). Even among stage III patients, all four molecular subgroups were reported. Women with p53abn EC had a significant benefit from CTRT (22% five-year RFS and 23% five-year OS benefit), while POLEmut EC had excellent outcomes regardless of adjuvant treatment received (100% vs. 97%). For women with MMRd EC no benefit of CTRT was found (68% vs. 76%) and for women with NSMP EC a trend towards benefit from CTRT was observed (80% vs. 68%). These results suggest that molecular factors should direct adjuvant treatment in HREC.

Conclusion

In conclusion, radiotherapy for stage III EC significantly improved locoregional control and should therefore remain the backbone for management of stage III EC. The addition of chemotherapy is beneficial for a subgroup of patients but comes at the expense of increased adverse events and a (transient) impairment in quality of life. The EC molecular classification should be incorporated in the risk stratification of these patients to identify truly high-risk patients and those that derive the most benefit from chemotherapy. For others treatment de-escalation should be considered or specific, targeted treatments may be preferable.

References

1. de Boer SM, et al. Adjuvant chemoradiotherapy versus radiotherapy alone in women with high-risk endometrial cancer (PORTEC-3): patterns of recurrence and post-hoc survival analysis of a randomised phase 3 trial. *Lancet Oncol* 2019;20(9):1273–1285.

2. de Boer SM, et al. Toxicity and quality of life after adjuvant chemoradiotherapy versus radiotherapy alone for women with high-risk endometrial cancer (PORTEC-3): an open-label, multicentre, randomised, phase 3 trial. *Lancet Oncol* 2016;17(8):1114–1126.

3. Matei D, et al. Adjuvant chemotherapy plus radiation for locally advanced endometrial cancer. *N Engl J Med* 2019;380 (24):2317–2326.

4. Kandoth C, et al. Integrated genomic characterization of endometrial carcinoma. *Nature* 2013;497(7447):67–73.

5. León-Castillo A, et al. Molecular classification of the PORTEC-3 trial for high-risk endometrial cancer: impact on prognosis and benefit from adjuvant therapy. *J Clin Oncol* 2020;38 (29):3388–3397.

32A How Should Stage IA Serous Papillary Endometrial Cancer Confined to a Polyp or the Endometrial Lining be Managed?

Observation

Ryan M. Kahn and Ginger J. Gardner

Debate

Uterine papillary serous cancer (UPSC) accounts for only 10% of endometrial malignancies, however, attributes to over 50% of endometrial cancer deaths annually [1]. USPC is commonly more aggressive than the endometrioid subtype, with a higher propensity for lymphovascular invasion as well as intraperitoneal and intra-abdominal spread at time of diagnosis.

Despite the known increased aggressiveness and risk of relapse in USPC, a standardized treatment paradigm for early-stage disease confined to the endometrium remains lacking. There has been conflicting evidence on the benefit of adjuvant therapy in this population and debate as to whether these patients require adjuvant therapy at all. As of 2021, the National Comprehensive Cancer Network (NCCN) suggests observation, chemotherapy, or radiotherapy all as acceptable management options following surgical staging for stage IA USPC without myometrial invasion [2].

The appropriate surgical staging for USPC is critical. In addition to a total hysterectomy and removal of the bilateral adnexa, this specifically includes peritoneal evaluation with systematic intraoperative peritoneal survey, washings, omental tissue sampling, and nodal assessment. Even in the absence of myometrial invasion, previous studies have demonstrated UPSC rates of omental involvement up to 11% [3]. This highlights the necessity of optimal staging in this population, as omental involvement could drastically change both stage of disease and management.

In addition to guiding future adjuvant treatment decisions, studies have shown that adequate surgical staging in patients with USPC could also lead to improved outcomes. A 2016 retrospective review of 77 patients with stage IA USPC and clear cell endometrial cancer by Velker et al. reported over 90% of recurrences (11/12) within the study had occurred in patients that had either incomplete or suboptimal surgical staging [4]. When stratified by staging adequacy, the five-year recurrence-free survival (RFS) was 97% in the adequately staged cohort, compared with 68% in the suboptimally staged cohort (p=0.01).

The previously described study by Velker et al. represents one of the largest initial series of patients with stage IA UPSC who underwent observation as a primary treatment strategy. Among the 77 patients with stage 1A uterine cancer (70% with USPC), 27 patients underwent adjuvant therapy versus 50 patients who underwent observation with a median follow-up time of 34 months (range 1–108) [4]. Congruent with previous studies, myometrial involvement was an independent risk factor for increased recurrence rates with 22% (10/45) recurring among the myometrial invasion cohort versus 6% (2/32) recurring in patients without invasion.

The five-year RFS rates among the observation and adjuvant treatment groups were 84% and 63% respectively (p=0.27). Furthermore, when stratifying for those who underwent observation alone, crude rates of recurrence were 25% (6/24) in those with invasion versus 4% (1/26) in those without invasion. Ultimately, this led the authors to conclude that it is reasonable to favor observation in USPC in the absence of myometrial invasion [4]. It should be noted, there was a strong trend of increased recurrence rates in patients with myometrial invasion who underwent observation alone. Limitations in this study include the histologic heterogeneity with the combination of USPC with clear cell tumors.

Similar outcomes were reported in a 2013 Canadian population-based retrospective cohort study of 127 patients with stage I UPSC by van der Putten et al. [3]. Median follow-up time was 25 months (range 2–98 months). The five-year disease-free survival (DFS) rates were 80.7% for those with stage I USPC without myometrial invasion and 74.4% for stage I USPC with myometrial invasion. Among patients with stage IA disease with myometrial invasion, the recurrence rates were 3% (1/35) for those who received chemoradiotherapy (three cycles of adjuvant chemotherapy followed by radiation) versus 18% (4/21) for those who either received observation or radiotherapy alone [3].

However, when stratifying for those without myometrial invasion, recurrence rates were 10% (3/30) after observation versus 18% (2/11) after adjuvant treatment (p=0.60). Based on these results, the authors concluded that observation alone renders a favorable prognosis in patients with stage IA USPC without myometrial invasion and therefore do not routinely need to receive adjuvant therapy [3].

Expanding beyond using myometrial invasion as the sole determining factor for treatment decisions in stage IA disease, a 2020 retrospective National Cancer Database (NCDB) study by Mysona et al. developed a clinical scoring system to further classify stage IA USPC patients that may or may not benefit from adjuvant therapy [5]. This study included 1751 total patients with stage IA USPC; of which, 58% (1012/1751) received chemotherapy while 34% (587/1751) underwent observation. Using a machine learning, random survival forest algorithm, the authors developed a Cox regression model with risk factors including age, CDCC scoring (Charlsen/Deyo Comorbidity Index), nodal status, omentectomy, lymphovascular invasion, peritoneal cytology, and tumor size. Using a binned scoring system, they were able to categorize by low-risk, moderate-risk, and high-risk scores [5].

This random forest survival algorithm, which is publicly available online as a free-of-cost clinical calculator, projected an overall survival (OS) of 87% for patients with stage IA USPC receiving adjuvant chemotherapy versus 84% for those not receiving chemotherapy (p=0.29) [5]. This method identified roughly one-third of patients within the study's low-risk cohort who would not benefit from chemotherapy and would be able to avoid the associated risks and side effects of chemotherapy.

Conclusion

Ultimately, identifying the optimal treatment for women with stage IA UPSC without myometrial invasion after surgery is critical. Until further studies show a benefit, observation should be performed for patients with no evidence of myometrial invasion at this time. The previously described negative studies regarding stage IA USPC outcomes amongst small populations on retrospective reviews need to be considered carefully. Prospective randomized clinical trials are necessary to definitively show that observation can be equivalent to adjuvant therapy in patients without myometrial invasion. In specific UPSC populations, clinicians must balance the unproven benefit of adjuvant treatments with the possible toxicities and quality of life outcomes. Additional answers likely lie within an improved molecular understanding of this disease. Just as there is an established association with HER2 status and uterine serous carcinoma outcomes, further molecular classifications – such as *POLE* mutations, *p53* aberrancy, and copy-number repeats, among others – will likely shed light on future directions and individualized treatment strategies for this clinical conundrum.

References

1. del Carmen MG, et al. Uterine papillary serous cancer: a review of the literature. *Gynecol Oncol* 2012;127(3):651–661.

2. Abu-Rustum NR, et al. NCCN Guidelines® Insights: Uterine Neoplasms, Version 3.2021. *J Natl Compr Canc Netw* 2021;19(8):888–895.

3. van der Putten LJ, et al. Population-based treatment and outcomes of stage I uterine serous carcinoma. *Gynecol Oncol* 2014;132 (1):61–64.

4. Velker V, et al. Role of adjuvant therapy for stage ia serous and clear cell uterine cancer: is observation a valid strategy? *Int J Gynecol Cancer* 2016;26 (3):491–496.

5. Mysona DP, et al. Clinical calculator predictive of chemotherapy benefit in stage 1A uterine papillary serous cancers. *Gynecol Oncol* 2020;156 (1):77–84.

How Should Stage IA Serous Papillary Endometrial Cancer Confined to a Polyp or the Endometrial Lining be Managed?

Adjuvant Chemotherapy

Alessia Aloisi, Federica Tomao, and Eleonora Zaccarelli

Debate

Uterine serous carcinoma is a rare, aggressive, high-risk histological subtype of endometrial cancer. Although it represents less than 10% of all endometrial cancers, it accounts for more than 50% of relapses and deaths attributed to endometrial carcinoma. This is most likely due to a higher incidence of extrauterine disease at presentation, to higher rates of recurrence, and a higher tendency for distant metastases compared to other histological subtypes.

A Gynecologic Cancer InterGroup review suggests that more than 50% of patients affected by serous endometrial cancer is diagnosed at early stage (International Federation of Gynecology and Obstetrics, FIGO, stage I); however, the overall survival (OS) rates (range 65–85%) reported for these patients are much lower compared to the most common endometrioid early-stage subtypes (>90%) [1].

The increased risk of recurrence, especially with distant metastasis, and the lower OS warrant a consideration of adjuvant therapy even for patients with an early-stage disease.

Data from international literature, investigating the role of adjuvant chemotherapy in a stage IA polyp-confined serous endometrial cancer, are inconsistent due to its rarity and to the lack of prospective trials (most of the data are from retrospective studies and involve small numbers of patients). Particularly, heterogeneous adjuvant treatment regimens (radiotherapy, chemotherapy, combination of radiotherapy and chemotherapy) were investigated with mixed high-risk histologies and stages.

In this regard, there is no international consensus on what is the optimal adjuvant treatment for stage IA serous endometrial cancer without myometrial invasion.

According to the European Society of Gynecologic Oncology (ESGO) and the National Comprehensive Cancer Network (NCCN) Guidelines, 2020, patients can be treated either with observation, vaginal brachytherapy or adjuvant chemotherapy (platinum/taxane combination) with or without vaginal brachytherapy.

The largest single-center retrospective study conducted by Viswanathan et al. suggested a survival benefit for the combination of chemotherapy and radiotherapy in uterine serous cancer [2]. However, a subgroup analysis of the NSGO9501/EORTC 55991 and MaNGO-ILIADE III trials did not show a survival benefit for patients with early stage serous or clear-cell tumors [3].

To date, the largest cohort of patients ever evaluated that reviewed 1709 patients with stage I uterine serous carcinoma with no myometrial invasion selected from the National Cancer Database, showed that adjuvant chemotherapy (with or without radiotherapy) is significantly associated with a survival benefit (five-year OS 81.9% vs. 91.3%) [4]. However, some considerations should be taken into account, such as absence of a central pathology review, lack of information about residual tumor on the hysterectomy specimen or about cause of death, and absence of data on the surgical staging for which staging misclassifications cannot be excluded.

According to a review of the literature [5], seven studies that included an overall cohort of 160 patients reported oncologic outcomes on FIGO stage IA, polyp limited, serous endometrial cancer. Only three of the studies required complete surgical staging in their inclusion criteria. Among 160 patients, 13 women experienced a relapse, with a majority of them recurring with extrapelvic metastases. Of these, seven were sent for observation, while the remaining six were submitted to an adjuvant treatment (one patient underwent brachy-therapy, one patient was submitted to EBRT, two to adjuvant chemotherapy + EBRT, and two to adjuvant chemotherapy + vaginal brachytherapy). Overall, among 13 patients who relapsed, only four had received chemotherapy as adjuvant treatment, though the statistical significance of this association, due to the small number of cases analyzed, is aleatory.

Another multi-institutional retrospective review of data by Mahdi et al. examined the impact of adjuvant therapy and pelvic radiation on pattern of recurrence and oncologic outcomes in stage IA noninvasive uterine papillary serous carcinoma [6]. In this paper, adjuvant therapy was associated with greater survival only in patients who did not undergo complete surgical staging.

Finally, data from the Cancer Genome Atlas (TCGA) network have shown that endometrial cancer can be divided into four clinically significant molecular subtypes with differing clinical prognoses: POLE ultramutated, microsatellite instability hypermutated (MSI-H), copy number low, and copy number high. Patients with POLE-mutated tumors usually have an excellent prognosis while those with copy-number-high tumors have poor oncologic outcomes. The MSI-H and copy-number-low groups, instead, usually have intermediate, stage-dependent prognoses.

Copy-number-high tumors, which are characterized by TP53 mutations, comprise some high-grade endometrioid adenocarcinomas, some clear cell carcinomas, and all serous cancers, confirming its bad prognosis [5]. Because of this new scenario, the current knowledge about the indication regarding adjuvant treatment of endometrial cancer, especially in nonendometrioid histotypes, might be completely changed in the near future.

Conclusion

In conclusion, the utility of adjuvant treatment in stage IA serous papillary endometrial cancer confined to a polyp or the endometrial lining remains controversial and a clinical dilemma. Observation has been reported as sufficient in most cases, even if adjuvant therapy could be considered in nonstaged patients, when complete surgical staging is not feasible, in case of risk factors such as positive peritoneal citology or large residual tumor on the hysterectomy specimen or within clinical trials. Future prospective clinical trials, including the constantly evolving molecular categorization, are needed to explore more effective treatment strategies for this unique patient population.

References

1. Boruta DM, et al. Management of women with uterine papillary serous cancer: a Society of Gynecologic Oncology (SGO) review. *Gynecol Oncol* 2009;115:142–153.

2. Viswanathan AN, et al. The importance of chemotherapy and radiation in uterine papillary serous carcinoma. *Gynecol Oncol* 2011;123:542–547.

3. Hogberg T, et al. Sequential adjuvant chemotherapy and radiotherapy in endometrial cancer – results from two randomised studies. *Eur J Cancer* 2010;46:2422–2431.

4. Nasioudis D, et al. Adjuvant treatment for patients with FIGO stage I uterine serous carcinoma confined to the endometrium. *Int J Gynecol Cancer* 2020;30(8):1089–1094.

5. Welp A, et al. Distant recurrence in a patient with polyp-confined stage IA serous endometrial carcinoma treated with adjuvant chemotherapy: a case report and review of literature. *Gynecol Oncol Rep* 2019;31:100512.

6. Mahdi H, et al. Adjuvant vaginal brachytherapy decreases the risk of vaginal recurrence in patients with stage I non-invasive uterine papillary serous carcinoma. A multi-institutional study. *Gynecol Oncol* 2015;136(3):529–533.

Debate

33A

What is the Optimal Sequence of Therapy for Patients with Stage IIIC Endometrial Carcinoma Treated with Multimodal Therapy?
Sandwich Therapy

Lauren Thomaier Bollinger and Melissa A. Geller

Debate

For surgically staged stage III endometrial cancer, National Comprehensive Cancer Network (NCCN) guidelines recommend systemic therapy ± external beam radiotherapy ± brachytherapy. Recent prospective data suggest that treatment with pelvic radiation prior to chemotherapy (CT) is not associated with a survival benefit compared to CT alone. A subset analysis of PORTEC-3 did however demonstrate that patients with Stage III disease treated with chemotherapy and radiation experienced longer five-year progression-free survival at 69% versus 58% (p=0.03) [1]. The optimal sequencing of chemotherapy and radiation remains a source of debate. "Sandwich" therapy consists of radiation therapy (whole pelvis ± para-aortic ± brachytherapy) sandwiched between six total cycles of chemotherapy (typically, carboplatin and paclitaxel). The "sandwich" modality evolved as a solution to reduce distant recurrence and minimize locoregional recurrence while limiting toxicity in order to achieve optimal therapeutic dosing of both radiation and chemotherapy. Multicenter and single institution comparative retrospective studies have shown the superiority of sandwich therapy compared to sequential therapy (adjuvant chemotherapy followed by radiation or radiation followed by chemotherapy) for patients with stage III disease (Table 33A.1).

Multiple retrospective analyses show improved outcomes with "sandwiching" radiation between chemotherapy. In a multicenter retrospective analysis of 265 patients with optimally resected Stage IIIC recurrent endometrial cancer, 61 patients (23%) received "sandwich" adjuvant therapy. Combination adjuvant therapy resulted in a significantly lower risk of death and progression compared to chemotherapy alone. Patients treated with the "sandwich" method had a significantly superior overall survival (OS) compared to those treated with either radiation followed by chemotherapy or chemotherapy followed by radiation (p=0.04). Ninety-eight percent of patients treated with "sandwich" therapy were alive at three years versus 90% and 82% of patients treated with sequential therapy [2].

There is also prospective evidence supporting "sandwich" therapy's tolerability and efficacy. We performed a prospective, single-arm phase II trial of 42 patients with Stage III, IV and recurrent endometrial cancer who received three cycles of docetaxel (75 mg/m^2) and carboplatin (AUC 6) on an every 21-day schedule followed by involved field irradiation

Table 33A.1 Studies supporting the use of "sandwich" therapy for stage III endometrial cancer

Author	PMID	Year	Design	N % stage IIIC	Findings
Secord et al. (USA) [2]	23085460	2013	Retrospective, multicenter **Combo CT+RT:61%** (n=161*) - **Sandwich:** 38% (n=61) CT followed by RT and then CT - **Sequential:** 16% (n=26) RT followed by CT; 43% (n=68) CT followed by RT - **Concurrent:** 2% (n=3) RT and CT; 1% (n=2) RT and CT followed by CT **RT alone:** 17% (n=45) **CT alone:** 17% (n=46)	265 100%	**Sandwich:** superior three-year OS (98%) compared to RT+CT (90%) or CT+RT (82%) **RFS CT alone vs. combo CT+RT:** HR=2.2 (95% CI: 1.2–4.2; p=0.02) **OS CT alone vs. combo CT+RT:** HR=4 (95% CI: 1.6–10, p=0.004)
Geller et al. (USA) [3]	21239048	2011	Prospective, single institution **Sandwich:** three cycles of docetaxel (75 mg/m²) and carboplatin (AUC 6) on a q21 day schedule followed by involved field irradiation (45 Gy) ± brachytherapy and three additional cycles of docetaxel and carboplatin	42 51%	**KM estimates OS** at one, three, and five years: 95% (95% CI: 82–99%), 90% (95% CI: 75–96%), 71% (95% CI: 45–86%) **KM estimates PFS** at one, three, and five years: 87% (95% CI: 72–94%), 71% (95% CI: 51–83%), 64% (95% CI: 42–80%)
Glasgow et al. (USA) [4]	27408749	2016	Long-term follow-up data of phase II trial **Sandwich:** docetaxel (75 mg/m²) and carboplatin (AUC = 6) every three	41 51%	**OS five years** 70% (95% CI: 53–82%) **PFS five years** 66% (95% CI: 48–78%)

Table 33A.1 (cont.)

Author	PMID	Year	Design	N % stage IIIC	Findings
			weeks for three cycles before and after RT		OS and PFS estimates remain high and in-field recurrences low
Frimer et al. (USA) [5]	30371562	2018	Prospective, single institution stages I, II, III, or IV uterine serous carcinoma, completely resected **Sandwich:** CT (paclitaxel (175 mg/m^2) and carboplatin (AUC 6–7.5) every three weeks for three cycles) followed by RT to 45 Gy (EBRT +/- HDR brachytherapy) followed by three additional cycles of CT (carboplatin AUC 5–6)	132 18%	**Stage III disease OS probability** at two, five years: 74%, 44% OS far higher survival than what has been reported in single-modality trials 81% completed six cycles of CT and RT Grades 3 and 4 hematologic toxicities: 22% and 14% of cycles, respectively Grades 3 and 4 nonhematologic toxicities: 6.9% of cycles

Abbreviations: AUC = area under curve; CT = chemotherapy; HDR = high-dose radiation; KM = Kaplan-Meier; OS = overall survival; PFS = progression-free survival; RFS = recurrence-free survival; RT = radiotherapy.
* = mode of sequencing was unknown in one patient.

(45 Gy) ± brachytherapy followed by three additional cycles of docetaxel and carboplatin. Just over half of these patients had stage IIIC disease and included unfavorable histologies. Kaplan-Meier (KM) estimates at one, three, and five years for OS were 95% (95% CI: 82–99%), 90% (95% CI: 75–96%), and 71% (95% CI: 45–86%) [3]. "Sandwich" therapy was well-tolerated with only 14 (34%) and 16 (39%) patients exhibiting grade 3 and 4 hematologic toxicities, respectively; lower than the toxicity reported in the chemoradiation arm of PORTEC-3 [1]. In follow-up of our study after a median of five years, 15 of 41 patients (37%) had died. The KM estimate for OS remained high at five years (70% (95% CI: 53–82%)) with an estimated median OS of 8.2 years. There were no further pelvic recurrences and only one distant recurrence in the cohort [4]. Frimer and colleagues similarly reported acceptable toxicity, high survival (74% at two years) and high therapy completion rate (81%) in a prospective study of patients with uterine serous carcinoma treated with "sandwich" adjuvant therapy [5].

Conclusion

Despite mounting evidence to support its use, no prospective randomized trial has included a treatment arm in which CT is given *before* radiotherapy or sequenced in a "sandwich" fashion to maximize local and systemic control. Such a trial is necessary to determine the most effective adjuvant treatment for patients with stage IIIC endometrial cancer.

References

1. de Boer SM, et al. Adjuvant chemoradiotherapy versus radiotherapy alone for women with high-risk endometrial cancer (PORTEC-3): final results of an international, open-label, multicentre, randomised, phase 3 trial. *Lancet Oncol* 2018;19(3):295–309.

2. Secord AA, et al. A multicenter evaluation of adjuvant therapy in women with optimally resected stage IIIC endometrial cancer. *Gynecol Oncol* 2013;128(1):65–70.

3. Geller MA, et al. A phase II trial of carboplatin and docetaxel followed by radiotherapy given in a "sandwich" method for stage III, IV, and recurrent endometrial cancer. *Gynecol Oncol* 2011;121(1):112–117.

4. Glasgow M, et al. Long-term follow-up of a phase II trial of multimodal therapy given in a "sandwich" method for stage III, IV, and recurrent endometrial cancer. *Gynecol Oncol Res Pract* 2016;3:6.

5. Frimer M, et al. Adjuvant pelvic radiation "sandwiched" between paclitaxel/carboplatin chemotherapy in women with completely resected uterine serous carcinoma: long-term follow-up of a prospective phase 2 trial. *Int J Gynecol Cancer* 2018;28(9):1781–1788.

33B

What is the Optimal Sequence of Therapy for Patients with Stage IIIC Endometrial Carcinoma Treated with Multimodal Therapy?

Sequential

Nasuh Utku Dogan and Selen Dogan

Debate

Introduction

Endometrial cancer (EC) is the most common genital tumor in the developed world and in the majority of cases, EC is diagnosed in early stage. Five to ten percent of EC patients present at advanced stage with a poor prognosis. Surgery is the cornerstone of treatment and curative in early stage; but in locally advanced stage, adjuvant treatment is required to decrease risk of recurrence. Five-year survival rate is 96% in early disease while this decreases to 67% in localized disease and falls to 17% in metastatic phase. There is no optimal treatment for women diagnosed with stage III–IV EC. In the Gynecology Oncology Group (GOG)-122 the superiority of chemotherapy over whole abdomen radiation was demonstrated. Studies thereafter showed that combination of chemotherapy and radiation improved survival compared to monotherapy either with chemotherapy or radiation. Systemic treatment by means of chemotherapy improves overall survival in stage III disease but is not good enough to prevent in particular pelvic recurrence, which can be seen in 18–40% of cases. On the contrary, when external beam radiotherapy is given as a sole treatment, there is a high rate of distant metastasis. Although the effect of combination treatment proves to be effective, the optimal sequence of treatment is not clear. One approach is the sandwich method (three cycles of chemotherapy followed by radiation and then three more cycles of chemotherapy). Other regimes are six cycles of chemotherapy followed by radiation (sequential treatment) or concomitant chemoradiotherapy. There are no randomized trials comparing these regimes. In this chapter the authors evaluate the benefit of six cycles of chemotherapy followed by pelvic radiotherapy (sequential regime) in stage IIIC disease.

Rationale for Adjuvant Multimodal Treatment in Stage IIIC Endometrial Cancer

There are two recent randomized controlled trials assessing effects of combination therapy compared to radiotherapy alone in advanced-stage EC. In the first study (PORTEC-3) there was a significant overall survival advantage in 660 high-risk EC patients (295 had stage III disease) in favor of combination therapy compared to radiation alone. Radiation therapy alone was associated with 68% five-year overall survival, while this was 78% for those undergoing combination treatment. In the PORTEC-3 trial, the sequence of treatment was external beam pelvic radiotherapy (concomitant chemoradiotherapy) followed by adjuvant therapy in which there was a three-week break between two treatment modalities. Interestingly, a subgroup analysis of stage III patients receiving chemoradiotherapy had longer progression-free survival (PFS). The second study (GOG-258) included 715 patients diagnosed with stage III disease and compared the effect of radiotherapy alone to combination treatment. There was no difference with respect to PFS, however a significant toxicity in the combination arm of both studies was observed. In PORTEC-3 and GOG-258, radiotherapy was given along with cis-platin as a radiosensitizer followed by administration of four cycles of chemotherapy. Probably administration of chemotherapy in a radiosensitizer dose was not good enough to control systemic disease. Moreover, four cycles of adjuvant chemotherapy seem to be inadequate to prevent distant metastasis compared to six cycles. The potential effects of multi-modal treatment are systemic disease control by means of chemotherapy and local control of vaginal recurrences by radiotherapy. But up to now there is no prospective data regarding the optimal sequencing and timing of chemotherapy and adjuvant radiotherapy.

Series Comparing Different Treatment Schemes

Goodman et al. evaluated 5795 women diagnosed with stage III–IVA type I EC with various adjuvant treatment schemes of which 26% received chemotherapy followed by radiation therapy and 10% received radiation therapy followed by chemotherapy [1]. In multivariate analysis, chemotherapy followed by radiation therapy was associated with longer overall survival compared to other regimes including radiation therapy followed by chemotherapy, radiation therapy alone, or chemotherapy alone. Moreover, when the cohort of women diagnosed with IIIC disease were only included, chemotherapy followed by radiation therapy was associated with longer five-year overall survival compared to radiation therapy before chemotherapy. In a study with analysis of 105 patients with stage IIIC2 disease, different adjuvant treatment regimens were compared [2]. In this group of patients, the type of adjuvant therapy effected disease-free and overall survival. Patients having received chemotherapy plus radiation therapy had a better prognosis compared to either chemotherapy or radiation therapy as a sole treatment. The combination therapy included mainly chemotherapy followed by external beam radiation therapy. Particularly in endometrioid histology, combination therapy was associated with longer locoregional or distant disease-free survival. In another study in the United States, from the National Cancer Database, 6981 patients were identified with stage IIIC disease; 5116 received chemotherapy then radiation therapy, 696 radiation therapy before chemotherapy, and 1196 received concomitant chemoradiation between 2004–2015 [3]. Interestingly, the use of chemotherapy before radiation therapy increased significantly from 39% to 75% between 2004 to 2015. In a median follow-up of 43 months, there was no difference between chemotherapy-first (then radiation) or radiation therapy first regimes. To note, when compared to these two regimes, concomitant chemoradiation was associated with a 47% increased risk of mortality. Lu et al. evaluated 51 stage III EC patients receiving multimodal therapy (either in sandwich or sequential manner) [4]. The five-year overall survival, local, or distant progression-free survival were all comparable between two groups with similar toxicity profiles. Though not significant, there was a trend towards a higher grade III–IV hematologic toxicity in the sandwich group [4]. In a study with 25 patients with stage IIIC disease, sequential therapy was compared to the sandwich regime. More patients in the sandwich group experienced grade III–IV neurologic and hematologic toxicity and undesired breaks in the course of treatment compared to the sequential regime, particularly in IIIC2 disease [5].

Conclusion

Studies evaluating different combinations in locally advanced-stage EC are all heterogeneous. Large prospective studies are warranted to compare different combination regimes including sandwich and sequential regimes; but inclusion of only stage IIIC disease is not realistic as stage IIIC disease is relatively rare. Prognosis of stage IIIC disease is still poor, with a high rate of distant recurrences pointing out need for a better systemic therapy. As a conclusion, multimodal treatment should be given to all patients with stage III EC. Either sandwich therapy or a sequential regime seem to be reasonable approaches; but sequential regime, particularly for stage IIIC2, is well tolerated, with less toxicity and treatment breaks.

References

1. Goodman CR, et al. Association of chemotherapy and radiotherapy sequence with overall survival in locoregionally advanced endometrial cancer. *Gynecol Oncol* 2019;153(1):41–48.

2. Bogani G, et al. Role of adjuvant therapy in stage IIIC2 endometrial cancer. *Int J Gynecol Cancer* 2020;30(8):1169–1176.

3. Latham AH, et al. Sequencing of therapy in women with stage III endometrial carcinoma receiving adjuvant combination chemotherapy and radiation. *Gynecol Oncol* 2019;155(1):13–20.

4. Lu SM, et al. Sequential versus "sandwich" sequencing of adjuvant chemoradiation for the treatment of stage III uterine endometrioid adenocarcinoma. *Gynecol Oncol* 2015;137(1):28–33.

5. Dogan NU, et al. Comparison of "sandwich chemo-radiotherapy" and six cycles of chemotherapy followed by adjuvant radiotherapy in patients with stage IIIC endometrial cancer: a single center experience. *Arch Gynecol Obstet* 2013;288(4):845–850.

Should an Attempt at Debulking Grossly Metastatic Endometrial Cancer be Undertaken?
Yes

Brooke M. Lamparello and Joyce N. Barlin

Debate

Management of advanced endometrial cancer, including the role of surgical cytoreduction, remains controversial. Debulking surgery is widely utilized in metastatic cancer due to demonstrated physiologic and clinical survival benefits. Removal of large necrotic masses can facilitate drug delivery to smaller tumors that maintain a good blood supply. Debulking to minimal residual disease decreases the number of malignant cells present and improves the ability of chemotherapeutic agents to reach tumor centers, decreasing the likelihood of the development of drug-resistant cells. Further, by removing tumor burden that causes clinical sequelae, such as bowel obstruction, nutritional and immunologic status can be improved.

Owing to the low incidence and prevalence of stage IV endometrial cancer, research investigating the role of surgical cytoreduction is retrospective. A meta-analysis of 14 retrospective studies, comprising 672 patients with advanced and recurrent endometrial cancer of all histologies, showed a statistically significant association with median overall survival (OS) and the proportion of patients undergoing surgical cytoreduction. Each 10% increase in the percentage of patients undergoing complete cytoreduction improved survival by 9.3 months [1]. A retrospective study of 65 stage IVB endometrial cancer patients with mixed histologies undergoing primary surgical debulking showed a statistically significant survival advantage for optimal debulking compared to those who had residual disease, 34.3 months versus 11.0 months, respectively [2]. This improvement in survival retained statistical significance even when controlling for other factors, including age, performance status, tumor histology, and adjuvant therapy. In fact, the strongest predictor of survival was the volume of residual disease after debulking surgery [2]. In a more homogeneous population of 58 patients with stage IV endometrioid endometrial cancer and macroscopic disease, the extent of cytoreduction achieved was a statistically significant prognostic factor in progression-free survival (PFS) and OS [3]. Patients in this study with no residual disease had a median OS of 42.2 months compared with 19 months for patients with any residual disease, and 2.2 months for those that did not have cytoreductive surgery. Extent of residual disease and adjuvant chemotherapy were also independently associated with OS when analyzed on a multivariate level [3].

The paucity of advanced metastatic endometrial cancer patients prohibits the development of a randomized trial. In fact, many of the retrospective studies in metastatic endometrial cancer spanned several decades. In contrast to endometrial cancer, most ovarian cancer patients are diagnosed at an advanced stage, and surgical cytoreduction in advanced ovarian cancer has been widely investigated and established as a valuable cornerstone of treatment. The DESKTOP-III trial prospectively randomized 407 patients with recurrent ovarian cancer to surgery (n=206) followed by chemotherapy, or no surgery (n=201) with immediate chemotherapy. The median OS was 53.7 months versus 46.0 months in the surgery versus no surgery cohorts, respectively (95% CI: 0.58–0.96, p=0.02) [4]. Given the similarity in patterns of metastasis, prospective ovarian cancer data has been extrapolated to the advanced stage endometrial cancer population. This provides additional support and justification for cytoreductive surgery in stage IV endometrial cancer.

While the surgeon must consider the potential for surgical morbidity in a patient population with advanced disease and a high likelihood of comorbidities, this does not preclude these patients from the survival benefits of debulking surgery. In a retrospective multi-institutional study, 426 patients with stage IVB endometrial cancer were divided by initial treatment. One hundred and twenty-five patients underwent initial chemotherapy treatment due to their poorer performance status and higher rates of comorbidities [5]. These patients had a decreased OS of 12 months compared to 21 months in the primary surgery group (279 patients). However, 59 of the primary chemotherapy patients additionally underwent surgical cytoreduction, and their OS curves were the same as those patients in the primary surgery cohort. This suggests that patients who may be poor candidates for debulking can benefit from chemotherapy followed by surgery. This data is further validated by the numerous prospective randomized controlled trials within the advanced ovarian cancer population that have shown neoadjuvant chemotherapy followed by cytoreductive surgery as a valid therapeutic option for patients who are poor surgical candidates or initially have unresectable disease.

Conclusion

Optimal cytoreductive surgery in grossly metastatic endometrial cancer is supported by physiologic rationale and a clinically significant improvement in survival. The biological benefits include reduction of tumor burden to improve clinical status, increase in chemotherapy drug delivery to the tumor, and decrease in the development of drug resistance. Multiple retrospective studies have demonstrated an increased PFS and OS in stage IV endometrial cancer patients with varying histologic subtypes. A meta-analysis in advanced and recurrent endometrial cancer suggested that complete cytoreduction to no gross residual disease is associated with superior OS outcomes. In the absence of readily achievable prospective data in this rare cohort, results extrapolated from advanced-stage ovarian cancer offer additional support for the benefits of debulking surgery. Furthermore, of the prognostic factors favoring survival, the amount of residual tumor is the only factor that can be directly influenced by the surgeon. A randomized prospective trial in metastatic endometrial cancer to confirm or refute the clinical utility of surgical cytoreduction will require a tremendous multi-institutional effort. However, until this is achieved, the current data support surgical tumor debulking in advanced endometrial cancer in an effort to optimize outcomes and improve survival.

References

1. Barlin JN, et al. Cytoreductive surgery for advanced or recurrent endometrial cancer: a meta-analysis. *Gynecol Oncol* 2010;118:14–18.

2. Bristow RE, et al. Stage IVB endometrial carcinoma: the role of cytoreductive surgery and determinants of survival. *Gynecol Oncol* 2000;78(2):85–91.

3. Shih KK, et al. Surgical cytoreduction in stage IV endometrioid endometrial carcinoma. *Gynecol Oncol* 2011;122 (3):608–611.

4. Du Bois AA, et al. Randomized phase III study to evaluate the impact of secondary cytoreductive surgery in recurrent ovarian cancer: final analysis of AGO DESKTOP III/ENGOT-ov20. *J Clin Oncol* 2020;38:6000).

5. Eto T, et al. Status of treatment for the overall population of patients with stage IVB endometrial cancer, and evaluation of the role of preoperative chemotherapy: a retrospective multi-institutional study of 426 patients in Japan. *Gynecol Oncol* 2013;131(3):574–580.

34B

Should an Attempt at Debulking Grossly Metastatic Endometrial Cancer be Undertaken?

No

Frederick M. Howard and Gini F. Fleming

Debate

Interest in debulking surgery for advanced uterine cancer arose in the 1980s after publication of a number of case series demonstrating improved survival in women who had undergone optimal or complete cytoreductive surgery. A 2010 meta-analysis of 14 retrospective series (eight of which included women with stage IIIC disease, in whom outcomes are generally better regardless of surgery, and in whom optimal debulking is more likely to be achieved) evaluated the impact of extent of surgical debulking on outcomes in advanced or recurrent endometrial cancer, and found that both optimal and complete cytoreduction were associated with improved survival [1]. However, this should not be taken as evidence that debulking should be attempted for stage IV endometrial cancer patients with grossly metastatic disease, and may reflect a variety of confounders – in particular, optimally debulked patients likely had lower pre-surgical disease burden. The presence of confounders is highlighted by the finding of the same meta-analysis that receipt of chemotherapy was negatively associated with survival (a 10.4 month decrease in survival per 10% increase in patients receiving chemotherapy), which lies in direct conflict with data from randomized controlled trials.

In general, the fact that an improvement in survival is associated with positive outcomes from a particular intervention does not prove that the intervention improves outcomes, as outcomes of the intervention may be a surrogate marker for prognosis. For example, numerous studies randomizing patients with cervical cancer to neoadjuvant chemotherapy or no neoadjuvant chemotherapy found that while a good response to neoadjuvant chemotherapy among patients receiving neoadjuvant chemotherapy was associated with better outcomes, the group randomized to receive neoadjuvant chemotherapy nonetheless fared worse overall. Or, for a surgical example, results of the Gynecology Oncology Group (GOG) 213 (which randomly assigned women with platinum-sensitive recurrent ovarian cancer to undergo surgical cytoreduction followed by chemotherapy or to receive chemotherapy only) showed that among patients who underwent surgery, complete gross resection as compared to incomplete resection was associated with longer overall survival (56.0 months vs. 37.8 months) and longer progression-free survival. Yet overall, there was no benefit for the group receiving surgery versus the group receiving no surgery. Indeed, surgery was associated with a nonsignificant trend to worse overall survival (50.6 months vs. 64.7 months, p=0.08) [2].

Debulking surgery is utilized for a wide range of intraabdominal malignancies, including gastrointestinal stromal tumors, well differentiated neuroendocrine carcinoma, peritoneal mesothelioma, and ovarian cancer. Although tempo of disease varies with histology and grade, endometrial cancer generally is associated with a shorter survival than other malignancies where peritoneal debulking is routine. In a case control series, stage IIIC ovarian and stage IVB endometrial cancer patients undergoing primary cytoreduction were matched for age and residual disease. Survival was significantly inferior in the endometrial cancer patients with optimal cytoreductive surgery versus ovarian cancer patients with optimal cytoreductive surgery (overall survival 57% at two years vs. 82% at two years) [3].

Any possible benefit from debulking surgery must also be weighed against the mortality and morbidity of surgery. Relative to ovarian cancer, uterine cancer occurs in an older population with higher levels of obesity and increased operative risk. In one retrospective review of 85 patients with advanced endometrial cancer undergoing primary surgical cytoreduction, the rates of minor and major (including bladder, bowel, and vascular injury) postoperative complications were 36% and 13% respectively, and 4% of patients passed away within 30 days of surgery [4]. Only 19 patients had stage IV disease, and 17 had extrapelvic sites; the operative morbidity of achieving primary optimal cytoreduction in patients with stage IV grossly metastatic disease may be higher. Indeed, complications were more frequent in patients who had suboptimal cytoreduction, perhaps due to the higher proportion of stage IV disease in that subgroup. This series, which was included in the aforementioned meta-analysis, found a survival advantage to optimal versus suboptimal cytoreduction. However, the survival analysis included 39 patients with stage IIIC disease and only 19 with stage IV disease, and the authors found that after adjusting for stage the survival advantage for optimal cytoreduction was no longer statistically significant.

Conclusion

In carefully selected patients with few comorbidities, minimal extrapelvic disease that appears completely resectable, and slow growing tumors, complete cytoreduction may improve survival. Moreover, hysterectomy can potentially reduce the risk of massive pelvic hemorrhage, although radiation therapy and embolization can also palliate bleeding. Surgical morbidity is, of course, decreased by the use of chemotherapy prior to surgery. However, at this time we have no meaningful data supporting any survival benefit for the broad use of debulking surgery for patients with grossly metastatic endometrial cancer, and its routine use is not warranted in the absence of prospective randomized data.

References

1. Barlin JN, et al. Cytoreductive surgery for advanced or recurrent endometrial cancer: a meta-analysis. *Gynecol Oncol* 2010;118:14–18. https://doi.org/10.1016/j.ygyno.2010.04.005

2. Coleman RL, et al. Secondary surgical cytoreduction for recurrent ovarian cancer. *N Engl J Med* 2019;381:1929–1939. https://doi.org/10.1056/NEJMoa1902626

3. Landrum LM, et al. Stage IVB endometrial cancer: does applying an ovarian cancer treatment paradigm result in similar outcomes? A case-control analysis. *Gynecol Oncol* 2009;112:337–341. https://doi.org/10.1016/j.ygyno.2008.10.009

4. Lambrou NC, et al. Optimal surgical cytoreduction in patients with stage III and stage IV endometrial carcinoma: a study of morbidity and survival. *Gynecol Oncol* 2004;93:653–658. https://doi.org/10.1016/j.ygyno.2004.03.015

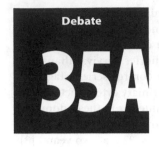

Debate

Should Secondary Cytoreduction be Performed for Recurrent Endometrial Cancer?

Sometimes

Lea A. Moukarzel, Kevin Espino, and Chris Awtrey

Debate

Endometrial cancer is the most common gynecologic malignancy in the United States. The primary form of treatment is surgical resection of the uterus, bilateral fallopian tubes and ovaries, with or without complete or sentinel lymph node dissection. After which the decision for adjuvant treatment is not only guided by stage, but most importantly by tumor characteristics, i.e., tumor grade, histology, myometrial invasion, and more recently molecular profiling. These factors also guide the decision on whether adjuvant therapy will entail locoregional radiotherapy, chemotherapy, immunotherapy (currently under investigation in the upfront setting), or a combination among them. Using these treatment paradigms there is an 11–14% rate of recurrence with a median survival after recurrence of 21–29 months [1,2].

One of the major challenges within the realm of treatment for endometrial cancer is that for recurrent disease. Recurrent endometrial cancer represents a heterogeneous cohort of cases with varying histologies, previous adjuvant therapy, time interval, as well as size and pattern of disease recurrence. Therapeutic options vary significantly, and include surgical resection, radiation therapy (RT), chemotherapy, hormonal therapy, immunotherapy, or a combination among them. Traditionally, surgical resection for recurrent endometrial cancer was limited to pelvic exenteration in previously irradiated patients presenting with central pelvic recurrences. This has gradually been replaced with literature demonstrating a utility in treating this disease with secondary cytoreductive surgery (SCS) for not only central pelvic, but also other sites of disease recurrence.

Legge et al. and Moukarzel et al. demonstrated that SCS, not involving pelvic exenterations, offers prolonged survival over other modalities of therapy when selected in the appropriate patient [1,2]. Moukarzel et al. demonstrated that patients treated with SCS had the longest median overall survival (OS) of 57.6 months (95% CI: 33.3–not reached) resulting in an 80.9% two-year OS rate. These patients required a median of one additional line of subsequent therapy. On multivariate analysis, after accounting for all significant factors that differed across treatment modalities, SCS was an independent predictor of improved survival. Compared with surgery, medical management with RT or chemotherapy with or without radiation portended worse survival (HR=2.1, 95% CI: 1.3–3.5, p<0.012), as did those treated with hormonal therapy (HR=2.3, 95% CI: 1.1–4.5, p=0.012).

Similar findings have been reported by others, suggesting that SCS for the treatment of recurrence, even when nonexenterative, confers a significant survival benefit. This observation is partially due to appropriate patient selection for SCS. Thus far, there remains no well-established prospectively validated selection criteria. However, findings from these retrospective studies can help guide decision making. One criterion that has been repeatedly shown in these studies to positively impact OS is achieving complete gross resection (CGR) or optimal cytoreduction. In a meta-analysis, Barlin et al. demonstrated that for each 10% increase in patients achieving CGR at debulking for advanced or recurrent EC, there was a significant improvement in survival of 9.3 months [3].

Unfortunately, data is not as clear when it comes to delineating other selection criteria for SCS. In their study, Moukarzel et al., proposed selection criteria based on factors that were significantly more common in the population of patients selected for SCS as compared to medical management [2]. They recommend that higher consideration for SCS should occur in patients with the following features from time of diagnosis: age ≤70, time to recurrence ≥19 months, grade 1/2 endometrioid or clear cell histology, early-stage (I/II) disease; the following features from primary surgery: no residual disease, short length of stay (LOS) (0–6 days), no more than two grade 3 complications, received adjuvant RT; and the following feature from time of recurrence: single-site disease. Features that did not differ statistically in distribution between patients selected for SCS versus medical management should merit less consideration. These include BMI at initial diagnosis, adjuvant chemotherapy after primary surgery, size of recurrent tumor, and distant site of recurrent disease. While the literature thus far can help guide decision making, due to the complexity of this decision and need for treatment personalization it is recommended that these cases undergo multidisciplinary tumor board assessment.

Summary and Recommendations

For vaginal recurrences in previously irradiated field, surgical resection should be considered as first-line therapy, followed by the consideration of adjuvant brachytherapy. Currently, literature demonstrates that SCS are effective and less morbid than pelvic exenterations. Vaginal recurrences in nonirradiated patients become more controversial, as traditionally these patients are salvaged with RT. In PORTEC-1, among cases of isolated vaginal recurrences in women without prior RT treatment, there was an 89% complete remission and 65% five-year survival when treated with RT. However surgical cytoreduction has also proven curative in this setting. Hardarson et al. showed comparable survival in patients with surgical resection and RT, in previously nonirradiated patients [4]. More specifically, surgical resection should be considered in large tumors, as tumor size significantly influences the effect of radiation. Therefore, in patients who decline RT or are not candidates for RT, SCS is a strong alternative in this setting.

As for women with locoregional-pelvic confined recurrences who are surgical candidates and complete or optimal cytoreduction is deemed technically feasible, then SCS should lead as primary modality of therapy with consideration of factors as previously discussed. PORTEC-1 demonstrated that when extra-vaginal extension or pelvic lymph involvement is present then RT no longer offers as promising results. If a patient is not deemed a good candidate for SCS then RT should be considered if no history of prior RT, while medical management would best suit those having already undergone RT. In addition, the role of immunotherapy as an alternative option should be considered.

Lastly, SCS can also play a role in the treatment of patients with distant disease, having shown a two-year progression-free survival of 77% in this setting [2]. Tangjitgamol et al. reported that the surgical resection of solitary, pulmonary, hepatic, and cerebral metastasis is feasible and reported prolonged survival in patients with good performance status, long disease-free interval, and clear margins [5].

Conclusion

In conclusion, the treatment of recurrent endometrial cancer remains a therapeutic challenge. However, it has become increasingly clear that with improved patient selection the role of SCS offers tremendous impact on survival. Importantly, with the advancements in the field of immunotherapy and the promising results for patients with endometrial cancer, an important next step is to investigate how best to integrate it into the treatment paradigm.

References

1. Legge F, et al. Clinical outcome of recurrent endometrial cancer: analysis of post-relapse survival by pattern of recurrence and secondary treatment. *Int J Gynecol Cancer* 2020;30(2):193–200. https://doi.org/10.1136/ijgc-2019-000822

2. Moukarzel LA, et al. Non-exenterative surgical management of recurrent endometrial carcinoma. *Gynecol Oncol* 2021;162(2):268–276. https://doi.org/10.1016/j.ygyno.2021.05.020

3. Barlin JN, et al. Cytoreductive surgery for advanced or recurrent endometrial cancer: a meta-analysis. *Gynecol Oncol* 2010;118 (1):14–18. https://doi.org/10.1016/j.ygyno.2010.04.005

4. Hardarson HA, et al. Vaginal vault recurrences of endometrial cancer in non-irradiated patients – radiotherapy or surgery. *Gynecol Oncol Rep* 2015;11:26–30. https://doi.org/10.1016/j.gore.2015.01.002

5. Tangjitgamol S, et al. Role of surgical resection for lung, liver, and central nervous system metastases in patients with gynecological cancer: a literature review. *Int J Gynecol Cancer* 2004;14(3):399–422. https://doi.org/10.1111/j.1048-891x.2004.14326.x

35B Should Secondary Cytoreduction be Performed for Recurrent Endometrial Cancer?

Never

Marcela G. del Carmen

Debate

Background

Treatment options available to patients with recurrent endometrial cancer, including use of systemic therapy and radiation, are selected based on patient- and tumor-related factors, as well as previously delivered treatment, including use of radiation therapy [1]. Historically, the role of surgical resection in the management of recurrent endometrial cancer was limited to total pelvic exenteration (TPE) in select cases of isolated vaginal apex recurrence and a previously irradiated area. Given that most patients who develop recurrent endometrial cancer have diffusely metastatic disease, and would not be appropriate candidates for TPE, many have adopted secondary debulking principles and extrapolated from the data pertinent to treatment of recurrent epithelial ovarian cancer (EOC) to support this strategy in the management of patients with metastatic recurrent endometrial cancer [1]. As in the case of secondary cytoreduction in patients with platinum-sensitive EOC, the data in recurrent endometrial cancer is limited to retrospective evidence and surgical effort intends to enhance response rates to salvage systemic therapy. Importantly, cytoreduction in this setting was adopted prior to the development of more promising adjuvant therapies, including innovation in targeted approaches.

Available Evidence

In 1998, Scarabelli et al. published the first study, inclusive of 20 patients, evaluating the role of cytoreductive surgery for recurrent endometrial cancer [2]. Complete microscopic resection was attained in 65% of patients, with a reported improvement in survival when compared to those with measurable disease after surgery (12 months vs. undefined; p<0.01). Two patients had major complications and two deaths were reported. In another retrospective study of 75 patients, cytoreduction to 1 cm or less was achieved in 75%, with an improvement in overall survival of 53 months, compared to 9 months in those with residual disease >1 cm (p<0.05). The investigators also reported a 31% rate of major complications and 8% mortality rate [3]. Bristow et al. reported on outcomes of 61 patients with recurrent endometrial cancer, including those managed with nonsurgical therapies [4]. When compared to the nonsurgical group, the 35 patients who underwent surgery had a longer median survival of 28 vs. 13 months, respectively (p<0.0001). In 66% of patients treated surgically, complete cytoreduction was attained and associated with improved median survival, when compared to patients with a sub-optimal debulking effort. In a study of 27 patients, 18 of whom had cytoreduction of recurrent endometrial cancer to <2 cm of residual disease, median disease-specific survival was 43 months, compared to 10 months in those with >2 cm residual disease [5]. In this study by Awtrey et al., there were no reported major perioperative complications or mortality.

Limitations of Available Evidence

Secondary cytoreduction for patients with recurrent endometrial cancer was adopted from the surgical treatment paradigm embraced by many as a management strategy for patients with recurrent, platinum-sensitive EOC. Two randomized studies have evaluated the role of secondary cytoreduction in the latter patient population with conflicting results. While DESKTOP III reported an improvement in progression-free survival benefiting patients randomized to cytoreductive surgery, data are not yet mature to inform on the impact on overall survival. The Gynecology Oncology Group (GOG) 213 failed to show an improvement in overall or progression-free survival benefitting patients with recurrent EOC randomized to secondary cytoreduction. This level of evidence remains lacking to inform on the utility of secondary debulking in patients with recurrent endometrial cancer. The available data have significant limitations.

Given that the studies informing on the role of secondary cytoreductive surgery in the treatment of patients with recurrent endometrial cancer are retrospective, inherent selection bias presents a significant limitation. Furthermore, many of these studies include small numbers of patients, from single institutions and have different definitions for achieved optimal surgical effort. Adjuvant therapies available to patients after secondary surgical debulking are not standardized, have changed over time, and may indeed have significant impact on patient overall and progression-free survivals. Lastly, most of these retrospective studies report significant morbidity and mortality rates, which also need to be considered in offering surgical therapy that carries an unlikely curative outcome.

With the emergence of new systemic therapeutic options in the treatment of patients with recurrent endometrial cancer, including discovery of molecular pathways offering targeted therapeutic approaches, secondary cytoreductive surgery, informed solely based on retrospective evidence and carrying a significant risk of perioperative morbidity and mortality, should be abandoned.

Conclusion

The role of secondary debulking surgery in the treatment of recurrent endometrial cancer is not justified based on the limited nature of available data and emergence of new systemic therapeutic options.

References

1. del Carmen MG, et al. Recurrent endometrial cancer. *Clin Obstet Gynecol* 2011;54(2):266–277.

2. Scarabelli C, et al. Maximal cytoreductive surgery as a reasonable therapeutic alternative for recurrent endometrial carcinoma. *Gynecol Oncol* 1998;70(1):90–93

3. Campagnutta E, et al. Surgical treatment of recurrent endometrial carcinoma. *Cancer* 2004;100(1):89–96.

4. Bristow RE, et al. Salvage cytoreductive surgery for recurrent endometrial cancer. *Gynecol Oncol* 2006;103(1):281–287.

5. Awtrey CS, et al. Surgical resection of recurrent endometrial carcinoma. *Gynecol Oncol* 2006;102:480–488.

36A

Is Hormonal Therapy the Best Therapy for Chemo-resistant Endometrial Cancer?

Yes

Roni Nitecki and Pamela T. Soliman

Debate

Based on the knowledge that the uterus is an endocrine organ and the observations that excess endogenous or exogenous estrogen was strongly linked to the development of endometrial cancer, gynecologic oncologists have been using hormonal agents for decades. The first report of progesterone as a therapeutic agent for endometrial cancer dates back to 1961. While hormonal therapy may be appropriate in different cancer stages for a variety of indications, in the case of chemo-resistant endometrial cancer it is important to understand the activity of hormonal therapy in the context of the existing therapeutic landscape.

Endometrial cancer is the most common gynecologic malignancy in the United States, accounting for an estimated 65,620 new cases in 2020. The incidence and mortality of uterine cancer have been on the rise for over a decade, but since 2009, the age-adjusted death rate has been rising at 1.9% per year – double the rise of the incidence rate. With a five-year relative survival of 81.2%, the majority of patients will have excellent prognosis. A subset, however, present with advanced and recurrent disease that is rarely curable. This subset may account for the rising death rate, as the majority of patients with advanced disease will progress after first-line chemotherapy, and thereafter, treatment options are limited.

In the absence of a standard regimen, the Gynecologic Oncology Group (GOG) created the 129 series, a group of phase II studies measuring response as the primary endpoint for patients with recurrent or persistent disease who received one prior chemotherapy regimen. Of this series, the only single agent considered active was paclitaxel with a response rate of 27% in 44 patients who were not exposed to prior taxane-based chemotherapy [1]. As the modern most utilized first-line regimen is carboplatin plus paclitaxel, other chemotherapeutic agents have been studied, and these have yielded disappointing response rates at the cost of significant toxicity. In this setting, hormonal agents have been found to be particularly useful given their moderate efficacy and favorable side-effect profile compared to cytotoxic chemotherapy. There are a variety of hormonal strategies that can be broadly categorized as progestins, selective estrogen receptor modifiers (SERMs, i.e., tamoxifen), aromatase inhibitors, and combination strategies. Hormonal therapy is well tolerated. Side effects are usually minor and include weight gain, edema, thrombophlebitis, possible venous-thromboembolic disease, headache, and occasional hypertension.

While initial clinical trials of hormonal agents in patients with advanced or recurrent endometrial cancer demonstrated response rates of 30–50%, larger studies with more specific response criteria demonstrated more modest response rates in the range of 11–24%. A meta-analysis specifically examining the effect of different standardized criteria on the association between hormonal therapies and response found that studies utilizing RECIST or WHO found a mean response rate of 9.2%, while studies using GOG criteria demonstrated an overall response rate of 20.5% [2]. In this setting, systematic reviews have demonstrated conflicting evidence of the efficacy of hormonal therapy for persistent or recurrent endometrial cancer, but the majority of evidence demonstrates better response than chemotherapy, particularly in patients with low-grade steroid hormone receptor positive (i.e., progesterone-receptor (PR) and estrogen-receptor (ER)) tumors [2–4].

In a systematic review, Kokka and colleagues pooled six randomized trials encompassing 542 women who received various forms and combinations of hormonal therapies and concluded that there was a dearth of evidence supporting hormonal therapy for advanced or recurrent endometrial cancer [4]. It is important to note, however, that only one included study compared hormonal therapy to chemotherapy, and three out of the six studies included different hormonal regimens in both arms of the trial. In addition, significant heterogeneity in stage of disease, prior treatment, histology, grade, and presence or absence of hormonal receptors limited the study. In a more recent and representative systematic review of 39 studies and 1937 patients, Ethier and colleagues combined randomized and observational studies to quantify the overall response rates to hormonal therapy in patients with advanced or recurrent endometrial cancer [2]. They found that hormonal therapy was associated with an overall response rate of 21.6% and a clinical benefit rate (inclusive of complete response, partial response, and stable disease) of 36.7%.

In comparing hormonal therapy regimens, Ethier and colleagues found that progestins, tamoxifen, and combinations of progestins and tamoxifen were all associated with similar response rates of 21–24%. The complete response rates appeared to be higher in tamoxifen-containing regimens compared to single-agent progestin. In three studies examining aromatase inhibitors the mean overall response rate was only 9%. Notably, in the included phase II trial of anastrozole, more than 25% of the patients had nonendometrioid histologic subtypes, the majority had grade 3 tumors, and only 22% of the patients had estrogen receptor (ER)- and progesterone receptor (PR)-positive tumors. In the subset of women with low-grade tumors with endometrioid histology, the response rate was 30%.

The importance of steroid hormone receptors was demonstrated in an analysis of seven studies (n=184) where the mean response rate was 26.6% in patients with ER-positive tumors as compared to just 9.2% in six studies (n=119) reporting on patients with ER-negative tumors [2]. Similarly, in pooled estimates of patients with PR-positive tumors receiving hormonal therapy, the mean response rate was 35.5% compared to just 12.1% in those with PR-negative tumors.

Finally, combination strategies including novel agents have shown promise. For example, combining hormonal agents such as letrozole with mTOR inhibitors (everolimus) had a reported response rate of 32% with a median duration of response of 12.5 months [5]. The addition of metformin to everolimus and letrozole has also demonstrated promise with a clinical benefit rate of 50% and overall response rate of 28% in 54 patients with advanced or recurrent endometrioid or mixed-endometrioid histology enrolled in a phase II study [6]. In this study, PR-positive tumor status was associated with 90% and 45% clinical benefit and overall response rate respectively. Finally, in a randomized placebo-controlled phase II trial, the addition of palbociclib, a CDK4/6 inhibitor, to letrozole resulted in a disease control rate at 24 weeks of 64% versus 38% in patients receiving palbociclib versus placebo [7].

Conclusion

Ultimately, while the majority of data support the use of hormonal therapy from both an efficacy and toxicity standpoint, the clinical benefit of endocrine therapy has not been completely defined, as the presence of steroid hormone receptors has not been fully incorporated in clinical trials and methods determining hormone receptor status have not been standardized. Because of the low toxicity profile and modest efficacy, hormonal agents should be considered in patients with recurrent endometrial cancer, particularly those who are not eligible for clinical trials with well-differentiated hormone receptor positive disease. In addition, histologic type should be considered in the decision making for recurrent therapy as response rates to hormonal therapy are higher in those with endometrioid tumors. With novel combination strategies of hormonal agents and improved stratification by presence of hormonal receptors, we expect hormonal agents to become even more valuable in the care of patients with chemo-resistant endometrial cancer.

References

1. Lincoln S, et al. Activity of paclitaxel as second-line chemotherapy in endometrial carcinoma: a Gynecologic Oncology Group study. *Gynecol Oncol* 2003;88:277–281. https://doi.org/10.1016/S0090-8258(02)00068-9

2. Ethier J-L, et al. Is hormonal therapy effective in advanced endometrial cancer? A systematic review and meta-analysis. *Gynecol Oncol* 2017;147:158–166. https://doi.org/10.1016/j.ygyno.2017.07.002

3. Decruze SB, et al. Hormone therapy in advanced and recurrent endometrial cancer: a systematic review, *Int J Gynecol Cancer* 2007;17:964–978. https://doi.org/10.1111/j.1525-1438.2007.00897.x

4. Kokka F, et al. Hormonal therapy in advanced or recurrent endometrial cancer. *Cochrane Database Syst Rev* 2010 (online). https://doi.org/10.1002/14651858.CD007926.pub2

5. Slomovitz BM, et al. Phase II study of everolimus and letrozole in patients with recurrent endometrial carcinoma. *J Clin Oncol* 2015;33:930–936. https://doi.org/10.1200/JCO.2014.58.3401

6. Soliman PT, et al. Metformin in women with advanced or recurrent endometrioid endometrial cancer: a multi-center, single arm, phase II study. *Clin Cancer Res* 2020;26:581–587. https://doi.org/10.1158/1078-0432.CCR-19-0471

7. Mirza MR, et al. LBA28 A randomised double-blind placebo-controlled phase II trial of palbociclib combined with letrozole (L) in patients (pts) with oestrogen receptor-positive (ER+) advanced/recurrent endometrial cancer (EC): NSGO-PALEO / ENGOT-EN3 trial. *Ann Oncol* 2020;31:S1160. https://doi.org/10.1016/j.annonc.2020.08.2258

Debate

Is Hormonal Therapy the Best Therapy for Chemo-resistant Endometrial Cancer?

No

Julianne Lima and Susana Banerjee

Debate

For recurrent/advanced endometrial cancer (EC), carboplatin in combination with paclitaxel remains the current first-line standard of care globally. In the NRG Oncology/GOG209 phase III trial, the median progression-free survival (PFS) and overall survival (OS) was 13 months and 37 months respectively (NRG/GOG209) [1]. Whilst hormonal therapy (HT) may be the preferred front-line systemic therapy for selected patients with low-grade EC carcinomas without rapidly progressive disease [2], we argue that the efficacy in advanced/recurrent EC post chemotherapy (i.e., chemo-resistant) is limited and alternative options should now be considered in clinical practice.

Endometrial cancer is a group of diseases harboring different biological features. Estrogen receptor (ER) was the first biomarker identified in EC with prognostic and potentially predictive implications. The first classification of EC divided into type I or type II tumors based primarily on ER positivity or negativity, respectively.

Response rates from different endocrine agents (HT) were reported in a meta-analysis of 39 studies (n=1837) showing a mean overall response rate (ORR) of 21.6%, clinical benefit rate (CBR) of 36.7%, median PFS of 2.8 months, and OS of 10.2 months in the first-line setting [3]. In the second-line setting, ORR and CBR were 18.5% and 35.8%, respectively. However, the CBR was found to be significantly impacted by different timing of radiological assessments ranging from four to 24 weeks. Although hormonal receptor positivity was associated with higher ORR particularly amongst those treated with tamoxifen (CBR >50%), these studies were highly heterogeneous in terms of outcomes and standard measurements of benefit [3]. For example, only three studies used RECIST criteria [4]. In a multivariate analysis, previous response to HT and tumors with grade 1 were found to be potential predictors of response to subsequent HT lines [3]. The association between previous HT and greater ORR raises the possibility of re-treatment of good responders to first-line hormonal therapy, influencing the clinical activity in subsequent lines. A prospective phase II single-arm study of anastrozole 1 mg/day for patients with endocrine-naïve ER and/or PR positive advanced/recurrent EC showed PFS of 3.2 months (95% CI: 2.8–5.4), 44% CBR (defined as objective response and stable disease of three months) (n=82) including 7% (n=6) who derived a partial response (PR) [5].

The concept of endocrine-sensitive EC has been taken further with the use of CDK4/6 inhibitors in combination with HT. The results of the PALEO/ENGOT-EN3, a phase II, randomized, placebo-controlled trial which evaluated the combination of letrozole and palbociclib in patients with ER+ endometrioid, EC post-progression to chemotherapy or ≤1 line of endocrine therapy (MPA/megestrol acetate), reported a significant PFS increase of five months for the combination compared to letrozole alone (8.3 vs. 3.0 months, HR=0.56, 95% CI: 0.32–0.98, p=0.041) [5]. It would be of interest to see the clinical activity according to molecular profile including mismatch repair/microsatellite instability (MMR/MSI) status. However, although the dualistic classification of EC has highlighted the concept of potentially endocrine-driven tumors, HT alone has not been shown to improve PFS or OS post first-line progression so far [6,7].

Limiting toxicities are less common with HT compared to other systemic treatment (e.g., vomiting, myelosuppression, hair loss), which in daily practice, makes hormonal therapy a valid option for patients with contraindications to other systemic therapies including chemotherapy and immunotherapy or among women whose performance status is 2 or greater.

The new molecular classification from The Cancer Genome Atlas (TCGA) has evolved the understanding of EC, reframing the classification of EC into four genomic categories, and incorporating new molecular biomarkers with prognostic and potentially predictive implications into practice [6].

The four molecular subtypes described are: p53-abnormal (p53abn), polymerase epsilon mutation (POLEmut), mismatch repair-deficient (MMRd), and nonspecific molecular profile (NSMP) [8]. Among those, endometrioid histology was the most common histotype found on MMRd tumors and NSMP subtype was associated with endometrioid grade 1 and 2, hormone-receptor positive tumors [6]. Of note, endometrioid histotypes were found to be related with estrogen/progesterone receptor pathways, less frequently described in serous-like subtypes, in which HER2 amplification was found in approximately 30% of cases.

MMRd or microsatellite instability-high (MSI-H) tumors represent 25–30% of EC. In recurrent/advanced EC post first-line chemotherapy, MMRd/MSI-H status is the first biomarker to be linked to approval of therapy based on the clinical activity of PD-1/-L1 inhibitors, changing clinical practice. The extent of clinical benefit reported with immuno-therapy so far is superior to HT alone as summarized below.

In the KEYNOTE-158 study, pembrolizumab monotherapy led to an ORR of 57% (8% complete responses) in MSI-H EC. The median duration of response was not reached (2.9 – 27.0+ months) [9]. In 2017, pembrolizumab received the approval from the Food and Drug Administration (FDA) as tissue-agnostic therapy for metastatic MSI-H/MMRd solid tumors which included endometrial cancer in post first-line progression setting.

Analysis of the phase I expansion cohort of the anti-PD1 inhibitor, dostarlimab, within the GARNET trial (NCT02715284) reported a response rate of 44.7% which included 10.7% with complete response in patients with MMRd EC who had progressed on first-line platinum-based chemotherapy and had not received more than two lines of therapy [7,10]. At the time of reporting (median follow-up 16.3 months), the median duration of response had not been reached. In 2021, FDA and European Medicines Agency (EMA) approved dostarlimab for women with MMRd recurrent or advanced endometrial cancer who have progressed on or following prior treatment with platinum-based chemotherapy.

In 2022, the results of the phase III, randomized trial of lenvatinib with pembrolizumab (KEYNOTE-775) set a new standard of care for patients with advanced/recurrent disease who have had prior chemotherapy. This study (n=827) showed superior PFS [6.6 vs. 3.8 months (HR=0.6, p<0.0001) in mismatch repair-proficient (MMRp) subgroup as well as the overall population 7.2 vs. 3.8 months (HR=0.56, p<0.001)] with lenvatinib and pembrolizumab versus physician's choice of chemotherapy (doxorubicin or weekly pacli-taxel). Similarly, OS was improved (17.4 vs. 12 months (HR=0.68, p<0.001)) for the MMRp subgroup and overall population (18.3 vs. 11.4 months (HR=0.62, p<0.001)) [11]. Subsequent analysis reported an improvement in PFS (10.7 vs. 3.7 months (HR=0.36, p<0.0001) and OS (HR=0.37, p<0.0001) for lenvatinib and pembrolizumab compared to chemotherapy in MMRd population as well. The benefit of this nonchemotherapy combin-ation was seen across endometrioid, serous, and clear cell histologies [12].

Anti-HER2 therapies have also shown encouraging results. A randomized phase II study of trastuzumab in combination with carboplatin and paclitaxel followed by maintenance, which included stage III/IV and recurrent HER-2 positive serous uterine carcinomas, reported a 54% reduction in the risk of disease progression compared to chemotherapy alone (HR=0.46; 90% CI: 0.28–0.76, p=0.005) and significantly longer OS with the addition of trastuzumab (29.6 months vs. 24.4 months (HR=0.58; 90% CI: 0.34–0.99; p=0.046). Among the subgroup of patients with recurrent disease (n=17), an improvement in median PFS (7.0 vs. 9.2 months, HR=0.12, 90% CI: 0.03–0.48, p=0.004) but not OS was noted.

Conclusion

In conclusion, post progression on chemotherapy, immunotherapy, and targeted therapies including endocrine agents are valid choices in clinical practice. However, the efficacy with approved immunotherapy approaches is higher than hormonal therapy alone and should be considered the preferred choice if available. The combination of pembrolizumab and lenvatinib is a new standard of care following first-line chemotherapy in MMRp EC (FDA and EMA approval) and MMRd EC (EMA). Dostarlimab monotherapy is approved for MSI-H/MMRd EC. HT is an option for patients with slow-growing disease, co-morbidities, or worse performance status. Clinical trials should be considered for all patients with recurrent EC who have received prior chemotherapy. Anti-HER2 options and other tar-geted therapies (e.g., ATR inhibitors) are under investigation. In the meantime, new strategies of endocrine manipulation under investigation are likely to open new horizons for therapeutic sequencing and redefine individualized management for EC patients, in particular post immunotherapy.

References

1. Miller DS, et al. Carboplatin and paclitaxel for advanced endometrial cancer: final overall survival and adverse event analysis of a phase III trial (NRG Oncology/GOG0209). *J Clin Oncol* 2020;38(33):3841–3850.

2. Concin N, et al. ESGO/ESTRO/ESP guidelines for the management of patients with endometrial carcinoma. *Int J Gynecol Cancer* 2021;31(1):12–39.

3. Ethier JL, et al. Is hormonal therapy effective in advanced endometrial cancer? A systematic review and meta-analysis. *Gynecol Oncol* 2017;147(1):158–166.

4. Mileshkin L, et al. Phase 2 study of anastrozole in recurrent estrogen (ER)/

progesterone (PR) positive endometrial cancer: The PARAGON trial–ANZGOG 0903. *Gynecol Oncol* 2019;154(1):29–37.

5. Mirza MR, et al. A randomised double-blind placebo-controlled phase II trial of palbociclib combined with letrozole (L) in patients (pts) with oestrogen receptor-positive (ER plus) advanced/recurrent endometrial cancer (EC): NSGO-PALEO/ENGOT-EN3 trial. *Ann Oncol* 2020;31(Suppl. 4):S1160. https://doi.org/10.1016/annonc/annonc325

6. Leon-Castillo A, et al. Molecular classification of the PORTEC-3 trial for high-risk endometrial cancer: impact on

prognosis and benefit from adjuvant therapy. *J Clin Oncol* 2020;38:3388e3397. https://doi.org/10.1200/JCO.20.00549

7. Oaknin A, et al. Clinical activity and safety of the anti-programmed death 1 monoclonal antibody dostarlimab for patients with recurrent or advanced mismatch repaire-deficient endometrial cancer: a nonrandomized phase 1 clinical trial. *JAMA Oncol* 2020;6v11:1766e1772. https://doi.org/10.1001/jamaoncol.2020.4515

8. Fader AN, et al. Randomized phase II trial of carboplatin-paclitaxel compared with carboplatin-paclitaxel-trastuzumab in advanced (stage III-IV) or recurrent uterine serous carcinomas that overexpress Her2/Neu (NCT01367002): updated overall survival analysis. *Clin Cancer Res* 2020;26(15):3928e3935.

9. Omalley D, et al. KEYNOTE 158. *Ann Oncol* 2019;30(Suppl. 5):

v403ev404. https://doi.org/10.1093/annonc/mdz25

10. Oaknin A, et al. Safety and antitumor activity of dostarlimab in patients with advanced or recurrent DNA mismatch repair deficient (dMMR) or proficient (MMRp) endometrial cancer (EC): results from GARNET. *Ann Oncol* 2020;31(Suppl. 4):S1142–S1215. 10.1016/annonc/annonc325

11. Makker V, et al. Study 309–KEYNOTE-775 Investigators. Lenvatinib plus pembrolizumab for advanced endometrial cancer. *N Engl J Med* 2022;386(5):437–448.

12. Colombo N, et al. Outcomes by histology and prior therapy with lenvatinib plus pembrolizumab vs treatment of physician's choice in patients with advanced endometrial cancer (Study 309/KEYNOTE-775). *Ann Oncol* 2021;32 (Suppl. 5):S725–S772. https://doi.org/10.1016/annonc/annonc703

Is there a Role for Using Immunotherapy in Endometrial Cancer?

37A

Yes

Ana Oaknin, Lorena Farinas-Madrid,
and J. Francisco Grau

Debate

Endometrial cancer (EC) is the most common gynecologic malignancy in post-menopausal women. Although early-stage disease is associated with an excellent prognosis, to date patients with advanced or recurrent disease have poor survival outcomes. While first-line chemotherapy based on carboplatin/paclitaxel regimen is well established, for those patients who progressed on or after this therapy, until recently, treatment alternatives (hormonal therapy and single-agent chemotherapy) have been limited and scarcely active. As current therapeutic alternatives do not satisfy the criteria to be defined as a "treatment of choice," new therapeutic approaches are needed in the setting of recurrent/advanced EC, and immune checkpoint inhibitors (ICI) seems to be one of the most promising.

The Cancer Genome Atlas (TCGA) Research Project, and subsequently the ProMisE classification, identified two EC subtypes as highly immunogenic: polymerase-ε (POLE) mutated (7% of EC) and microsatellite instability-high/mismatch repair-deficient (MSI-H/ MMRd) (30% of EC) subgroups [1,2]. The POLE mutated subtype (7%), characterized by hotspot mutations of the catalytic subunit of DNA POLE, and MMRd, featuring sporadic or hereditary alterations in mismatch repair system genes (MLH1, MSH2, MSH6, PMS2), harbor common distinctive biological features. Both of them feature higher mutational rates resulting in a large number of neoantigens, and a greater number of CD8+ tumor-infiltrating lymphocytes (TIL). This immune microenvironment leads to a tumoral adaptive immune-resistance response, which is defined by the upregulation of immune checkpoint proteins by tumor and immune cells, such as PD-(L)1/2. Beyond these two EC subtypes, other molecular subgroups with low mutation loads also display a TIL-high phenotype. This robust biological rationale has supported the clinical development of immunotherapy in advanced or recurrent EC, regardless of the molecular subtypes.

Following early evidence of pembrolizumab activity in MMRd tumors that led to its approval by the FDA, the open-label multi-cohort study KEYNOTE-158 confirmed pembrolizumab's efficacy in MMRd EC patients [3].

Subsequently, several phase 1 and 2 clinical trials have assessed different anti-PD-1/PD-L1 antibodies in the advanced/recurrent setting.

The GARNET trial, the largest EC patient dataset treated with ICI to date, evaluated the efficacy of dostarlimab (anti-PD-1 antibody) in 108 patients with MMRd and 156 with mismatch repair-proficient (MMRp) recurrent or advanced EC, respectively. The confirmed objective response rate (ORR) was 43.5% and 14.1% in patients with MMRd and MMRp, respectively. Both median overall survival (mOS) and median progression-free survival (mPFS) have not yet been reached in either cohort [4]. The dostarlimab efficacy outcomes have led to its approval by the FDA and EMA for MSI-H/MMRd EC that has progressed after prior platinum-based therapy. Besides, other anti-PD-(L)1 monotherapies, namely durvalumab and avelumab, have demonstrated consistent clinical activity in MMRd EC patients, with an ORR of 43% and 26.7%, respectively.

While the efficacy of anti-PD-(L)1 agents in MMRd EC has been clearly demonstrated, their activity is not encouraging in the MMRp population. Therefore, new venues have been explored to increase the anti-PD-(L)1 agents' efficacy, such as the combination with anti-angiogenic agents.

In this context, mature clinical data on the combination of pembrolizumab and the oral multikinase inhibitor lenvatinib in women with previously treated EC have been already reported in the randomized phase 3 study KEYNOTE-775/Study 309. This trial compared the lenvatinib and pembrolizumab regimen with physician's choice chemotherapy. A total of 827 patients with advanced or recurrent EC (84% had MMRp/Microsatellite stable tumors) who had received at least one prior platinum-based regimen were enrolled. For the MMRp cohort and the all-comers population, the combination of lenvatinib and pembrolizumab was statistically and clinically superior to chemotherapy for both primary end-points (PFS and OS). mPFS was 6.6 versus 3.8 months (Hazard Ratio (HR)=0.60, 95% Confidence Interval (CI): 0.50–0.72, p<0.001), and 7.2 versus 3.8 months (HR=0.56, 95% CI: 0.47–0.66, p<0.001); and mOS was 17.4 versus 12.0 months (HR=0.68; 95% CI: 0.56–0.84; p<0.001) and 18.3 versus 11.4 months (HR=0.62; 95% CI: 0.51–0.75, p<0.001) in the MMRp and overall population, respectively. An exploratory analysis in the MMRd population also demonstrated better outcomes in favor of the combination. Interestingly, the confirmed ORR in this cohort was 40.0% (95% CI: 28–53%), which, acknowledging the limitations of cross-trials comparisons, seems to be similar to that achieved with ICI monotherapy in an akin patient population [5]. Based on KEYNOTE-775 outcomes, the pembrolizumab and lenvatinib regimen was FDA Fapproved for patients with previously treated advanced EC that are not MSI-H/MMRd and by the EMA, for all-comers.

Beyond these clinical activity outcomes, introducing immunotherapy in the EC landscape treatment is somehow part of the precision oncology. Predictive biomarkers as MMR deficiency determined by immunohistochemistry and Tumor Mutational Burden status seem to correlate significantly with objective responses. Nevertheless, about half of patients with MMRd/MSI-H tumors do not derive yet any benefit from anti-PD-(L)1 antibodies or combination therapies.

Selecting the most appropriate approach for advanced/recurrent EC requires a balance in activity and safety profile. In this regard, the rate of immunotherapy discontinuation due to adverse events ranges from 10% to 18% depending on monotherapy or combination regimens. However, the broader knowledge in the immune-related adverse events and their management is leading to a better tolerability.

Conclusion

The arrival of immunotherapy in the recurrent/advanced EC treatment landscape is leading to a shift in the therapeutic paradigm of this poor prognosis population and should currently be considered as a treatment of choice after failure to platinum therapy, regardless of MMR status. Further investigation on predictive biomarker is mandatory to uncover potential mechanisms of immune escape and better select the candidates to ICI.

References

1. Kandoth C, et al. Cancer Genome Atlas Research Network,Integrated genomic characterization of endometrial carcinoma. *Nature* 2013;497 (7447):67–73.

2. Talhouk A, et al. Confirmation of ProMisE: a simple, genomics-based clinical classifier for endometrial cancer. *Cancer* 2017; 123 (5):802–813.

3. O'Malley DM, et al. Pembrolizumab in patients with microsatellite instability-high advanced endometrial cancer: results from the KEYNOTE-158 Study. *J Clin Oncol* 2022;40(7):752–761.

4. Oaknin A, et al. Clinical activity and safety of the anti-programmed death 1 monoclonal antibody dostarlimab for patients with recurrent or advanced mismatch repair-deficient endometrial cancer: a nonrandomized phase 1 clinical trial. *JAMA Oncol* 2020;6(11):1766–1772.

5. Makker V, et al. Lenvatinib plus pembrolizumab for advanced endometrial cancer. *N Engl J Med* 2022;386(5):437–448.

Is there a Role for Using Immunotherapy in Endometrial Cancer?

No

William A. Zammarrelli III and Vicky Makker

Debate

Immune checkpoint blockade (ICB) therapy has emerged as a valuable treatment modality for previously treated advanced or metastatic endometrial cancer (EC) that is mismatch repair deficient (dMMR) or microsatellite instability-high (MSI-H), with impressive and durable response rates seen in a significant proportion of patients. Conversely, a substantial proportion of patients with dMMR/MSI-H EC will not derive benefit from these therapies. It is vitally important to understand the mechanisms behind these disparate responses, as a one-size-fits-all approach, even within the dMMR/MSI-H EC subgroup, cannot be employed. Responses to ICB therapy in mismatch repair proficient (pMMR) or microsatellite stable (MSS) EC have been disappointing, and ICB monotherapy in this setting has not shown efficacy. Additional disadvantages of ICB therapy for the management of EC include the following: a lack of more definitive biomarkers predictive of response; the potential for long-term toxicity, which can necessitate the need for lifelong hormone replacement; a risk of serious sequalae (e.g., colitis, insulin-dependent diabetes mellitus); and extensive financial cost. Caution is warranted when considering this class of therapeutics for patients with EC, as there are still unanswered questions regarding their optimal use.

Approximately 2–4% of all cancers are dMMR, and only 17–33% of advanced or recurrent ECs are dMMR/MSI-H [1,2]. Studies of the anti-PD-1 (anti-programmed cell death protein 1) monoclonal antibodies pembrolizumab and dostarlimab have shown efficacy in dMMR EC, with objective response rates (ORR) of 45–57% and median durations of response (mDORs) not reached at data cut-off [2,3]. The anti-PDL-1 (anti-programmed death ligand 1) agents avelumab (ORR=27%) and durvalumab (objective tumor response rate, 47%) have also shown efficacy in dMMR EC [4,5]. However, most recurrent ECs are pMMR, and response rates to ICB therapy in this setting have ranged from 3–13%, indicating a clear lack of efficacy when used as monotherapy [3–5].

Our understanding of the optimal use of immune checkpoint inhibitors in the treatment of EC is confounded by the lack of definitive biomarkers of response, which is of paramount importance in order to maximize efficacy and minimize toxicity. Tumor mutational burden (TMB) and tumor-infiltrating leukocytes (TILs) do not uniformly correlate with response to ICB therapy, and while mutations in Janus kinase 1 (JAK1) and ß2-microglobulin (B2 M) may correlate with resistance, a clearer understanding of the chief mechanisms of response and resistance are needed [5]. The identification of molecular and tumor microenvironment factors that correlate with response is also imperative, as ICB therapy is associated with grade 3 or higher immune-related adverse events in up to 19% of patients [2–5]. Other important issues to address include the optimal timing and length of ICB therapy; ICB rechallenge after initial response and progression; and racial disparities in access to ICB treatment, treatment response, and adverse events.

Although chemotherapy may induce tumor vulnerability to immunotherapy secondary to apoptosis and increased tumor antigen presentation, diminished response to ICB mono-therapy after increasing lines of previous therapy have been shown in EC and other malignancies. In the PHAEDRA study, the ORR of durvalumab treatment in patients with EC was higher after first-line compared to second-line or beyond treatment (57% vs. 38%, respectively) [4]. The timing of ICB therapy may impact response, and exposure to prior therapies may lead to changes in the tumor microenvironment, with a reduction of host immune response, all leading to lower responses to ICB therapy. This is an important consideration, as there are now multiple front-line phase 3 trials evaluating platinum-taxane-based chemotherapy in combination with ICB therapy.

While ICB monotherapy appears to be a promising option for a select group of patients with dMMR advanced or metastatic EC, the lack of efficacy in a significant proportion of both dMMR and pMMR patients highlights the need to explore combination therapeutic approaches. In the phase 3 KEYNOTE-775/Study 309 trial, one such combination – lenvatinib plus pembrolizumab – compared to physician's choice demonstrated statistically significant improvements in overall survival (17.4 vs. 12 months, respectively), progression-free survival (6.5 vs. 3.8 months, respectively), and ORR (30% vs. 15%, respectively) following platinum-based chemotherapy and regardless of MMR status [6]. Based on these findings, this combination was recently FDA approved for the treatment of patients with advanced EC that is not MSI-H or dMMR who experience disease progression following prior systemic therapy in any setting [6]. This landmark development has ushered in a new era of therapeutics for EC.

Conclusion

As the incidence and disease-related mortality of this heterogeneous disease continue to rise, ICB combination therapies exploiting signaling pathways that dominate the genetics of EC must be more thoroughly explored and identified.

References

1. Cortes-Ciriano I, et al. A molecular portrait of microsatellite instability across multiple cancers. *Nat Commun* 2017;8:15180.

2. Marabelle A, et al. Efficacy of pembrolizumab in patients with noncolorectal high microsatellite instability/mismatch repair-deficient cancer: results from the phase II KEYNOTE-158 Study. *J Clin Oncol* 2020;38(1):1–10.

3. Oaknin A, et al. Safety and antitumor activity of dostarlimab in patients (pts) with advanced or recurrent DNA mismatch repair deficient (dMMR) or proficient (MMRp) endometrial cancer (EC): results

from GARNET. *J Immunother Cancer* 2022 (online). https://doi.org/10.1136/jitc-2021-003777

4. Antill Y, et al. Clinical activity of durvalumab for patients with advanced mismatch repair-deficient and repair-proficient endometrial cancer. A nonrandomized phase 2 clinical trial. *J Immunother Cancer* 2021;9(6):e002255.

5. Konstantinopoulos PA, et al. Phase II study of avelumab in patients with mismatch repair deficient and mismatch repair proficient recurrent/persistent endometrial cancer. *J Clin Oncol* 2019;37(30):2786–2794.

6. Makker V, et al. A multicenter, open-label, randomized phase 3 study to compare the efficacy and safety of lenvatinib in combination with pembrolizumab vs treatment of physician's choice in patients with advanced endometrial cancer: Study 309/KEYNOTE-775. Society of Gynecologic Oncology 2021 Virtual Annual Meeting on Women's Cancer. Abstract 37/ID 11512. Presented March 19, 2021.

38A

What is the Best Chemotherapy Regimen for Uterine Carcinosarcoma?
Carboplatin/Paclitaxel

Domenica Lorusso

Debate

Uterine carcinosarcoma (UCS), previously known as mixed mesodermal tumor, is a rare (2–3% of uterine cancers) endometrial neoplasm in which both the adenomatous as well as the stromal (mesenchymal) elements of the endometrium are malignant. The most frequent epithelial element consists of a poorly differentiated serous carcinoma and the most common sarcomatous component is represented by high-grade stromal sarcoma. For several years mixed mullerian tumors were considered biphasic tumors with epithelial and mesenchymal components; the current concept is that most UCSs are monoclonal epithelial neoplasms with metaplastic degeneration. Accordingly, the precursor (stem) cell is the origin of both the epithelial and mesenchymal components during histogenesis, but the dominant epithelial component dictates the behavior of the tumor, thus suggesting that drugs with proven efficacy against uterine epithelial tumors should represent the first treatment choice [1].

The clinical behavior of UCS resembles that of Grade 3 endometrial endometrioid adenocarcinoma with a worse prognosis. Disease stage is the most important prognostic factor: only 40–60% of women with carcinosarcoma present with stage I or II disease, and even when tumor is apparently confined to the uterus, metastases can be found in up to 60% [1].

Adjuvant chemotherapy is indicated in all stages of UCS even in stage I, as the recurrence rate is as high as 50%. Adjuvant pelvic external irradiation or brachytherapy reduces the rate of local recurrences without impacting on overall survival (OS) because the recurrences are mostly distally [2].

Traditionally, when UCS was considered a biphasic neoplasm, the most common chemotherapy agents used were platinum and ifosfamide with the aim of using the most active available drugs against the epithelial and mesenchymal component of the neoplasia, respectively. Unfortunately, in the metastatic setting, the combination registered moderate activity with short progression-free survival (PFS) and duration of response, and impressive toxicity particularly in terms of leukopenia, gastrointestinal and neurologic toxicity [2].

Subsequently, paclitaxel was introduced in the treatment strategy. A GOG prospective randomized phase III trial in 214 stage III–IV persistent or recurrent UCS patients reported a significant five-month increase in OS for the ifosfamide-paclitaxel combination compared to ifosfamide alone [3] with a 31% decrease in the hazard ratio (HR) for death and a 29%

decrease in HR for progression, consecrating ifosfamide-paclitaxel combination as the new standard treatment.

Several studies found that carboplatin-paclitaxel is an effective regimen when used either in the metastatic setting, where up to 54% objective response rate (ORR) was reported, or as adjuvant treatment where a four-year PFS and OS of 67.9% and 76.0 %, respectively, were reported. In all the published trials, the authors commonly concluded that the combination of paclitaxel and carboplatin was a feasible and effective therapy for patients with UCS and presented better tolerability and response rates compared with previous reports of ifosfamide/cisplatin or ifosfamide/paclitaxel doublets [3].

A retrospective cohort study evaluated the activity and toxicity of cisplatin-ifosfamide (group A) and carboplatin-paclitaxel (group B) as adjuvant treatments in 65 patients with UCS. At a median follow-up of 30 months, the median PFS was 11.6 and 16.6 months (p=0.20), and the median OS was 17.1 months and 35.1 months (p=0.14) for groups A and B, respectively. No differences were identified among heterologous or homologous components according to chemotherapy treatment and toxicity profiles widely differ between treatment arms favoring the carboplatin-paclitaxel combination. The authors concluded that because of the super imposable activity and the better toxicity profile, carboplatin-paclitaxel could be considered a suitable alternative to cisplatin-ifosfamide in the treatment of UCS [4].

At ASCO 2019 the results of a randomized phase III trial comparing paclitaxel-carboplatin versus paclitaxel-ifosfamide in 449 patients with stage I–IV uterine and ovarian CS were reported [5]. In the primary UCS cohort, median OS was 37 and 29 months for patients receiving paclitaxel/carboplatin and paclitaxel/ifosfamide, respectively (HR=0.87, p<.01 for noninferiority). Additionally, the median PFS was 16 and 12 months for women who received paclitaxel/carboplatin and paclitaxel/ifosfamide, respectively (HR=0.73; p=<.01 for noninferiority). The investigators reported increased hematologic toxicity for the paclitaxel/carboplatin treatment, while neurologic toxicity and genitourinary hemorrhage were significantly worse with paclitaxel/ifosfamide combination. During treatment, both groups experienced a similar decline in quality of life and increased neurotoxicity symptoms. A similar trend was observed in the smaller, secondary cohort of patients with ovarian carcinosarcoma, with a 30-month median OS in the paclitaxel/carboplatin arm versus 25 months in the paclitaxel/ifosfamide arm and 15-month median PFS for the paclitaxel/carboplatin arm versus 10 months for the paclitaxel/ifosfamide arm. The authors concluded that paclitaxel/carboplatin was not inferior to paclitaxel/ifosfamide based on the primary end-point OS, and paclitaxel/carboplatin was associated with longer PFS and a more manageable toxicity profile when compared with paclitaxel/ifosfamide and should be considered the new standard treatment.

Conclusion

In conclusion, the epithelial nature of the tumor (suggesting that drugs with proven activity toward epithelial cells should represent the first choice when establishing treatment), the efficacy data coming from retrospective and prospective trials, the manageable toxicity profile, and the comfortable 3-weekly schedule given in an outpatient setting, prompt the author to conclude that carboplatin-paclitaxel should be considered the standard of care in UCS treatment strategy.

References

1. Denschlag D, et al. Uterine carcinosarcomas – diagnosis and management. *Oncol Res Treat* 2018;41(11):675–679.

2. Menczer J. Review of recommended treatment of uterine carcinosarcoma. *Curr Treat Options Oncol* 2015;16(11):53

3. Berton-Rigaud D, et al. Gynecologic Cancer InterGroup (GCIG) consensus review for uterine and ovarian carcinosarcoma. *Int J Gynecol Cancer* 2014;24(9 Suppl. 3): S55–60.

4. Lorusso D, et al. Carboplatin-paclitaxel versus cisplatin-ifosfamide in the treatment of uterine carcinosarcoma: a retrospective cohort study. *Int J Gynecol Cancer* 2014;24 (7):1256–1261.

5. Powell MA, et al. A randomized phase 3 trial of paclitaxel (P) plus carboplatin (C) versus paclitaxel plus ifosfamide (I) in chemotherapy-naive patients with stage I–IV, persistent or recurrent carcinosarcoma of the uterus or ovary: an NRG Oncology trial. *JCO* 2019;37 (15):5500.

Debate

What is the Best Chemotherapy Regimen for Uterine Carcinosarcoma?
The Case for "Other" Regimens

Sara Bouberhan, Whitfield B. Growdon, and Richard T. Penson

Debate

Carcinosarcomas have fascinated pathologists and clinicians alike since they were first described by Virchow in 1863. Improved understanding of the molecular underpinnings of these rare tumors has led to a treatment paradigm shift for women with uterine carcinosarcoma away from a sarcoma-focused approach to that of a high-grade, metaplastic carcinoma. In this regard, the reported Gynecologic Oncology Group (GOG)-261 clinical trial established carboplatin and paclitaxel as the standard first-line treatment for women with uterine carcinosarcoma (UCS). The doublet combination of carboplatin and paclitaxel was well-tolerated and demonstrated favorable progression-free survival (PFS) and overall survival (OS) when compared to ifosfamide and paclitaxel [1]. We agree that carboplatin and paclitaxel should be strongly considered as a first-line treatment regimen for all women with UCS.

While the combination of carboplatin and paclitaxel gives us another option for the treatment of UCS, it provides only incremental benefits and does not improve OS. In the primary uterine carcinosarcoma cohort of GOG-261, median OS, while numerically better for paclitaxel/carboplatin, was not statistically different from paclitaxel/ifosfamide (HR=0.87, p<.01 for noninferiority, p>.1 for superiority). While grade ≥3 toxicities occurred in 90% of subjects receiving carboplatin/paclitaxel as opposed to 65% receiving ifosfamide/paclitaxel, formal evaluations of quality of life were not different. The results of GOG-261 confirm the observation that no advance in the last 10 years has resulted in a meaningful improvement in OS for patients with UCS [1,2] highlighting the desperate need for the development of alternative treatment approaches to improve outcomes for women with this rare disease.

Molecular characterization of UCS commonly reveals several potentially actionable mutations, including alterations in the phosphatidylinositol 3-kinase (PI3K) pathway, *ARID1A/B, ATM, BRCA2, ERBB2, and ERBB3* [3,4]. While *TP53* is the most common genetic aberration (>90%), approximately half of UCS have mutations in at least one PI3K pathway genes [3]. Biomarker-driven combination studies with CDK inhibitors and PI3K inhibitors show promise and could be applied to UCS in future studies. Alterations of chromatin remodeling genes (*ARID1A/B*) or in histone *H2A* and *H2B* genes [4] suggest that epigenetic modifiers may be effective, and we are presently investigating PLX2853 as an orally active, small molecule inhibitor of BET bromodomain-mediated interactions in

ARID1A mutated tumors. Perhaps the most exciting development has been the increase in understanding of the epithelial-mesenchymal transition (EMT) that may be at the heart of the metaplastic transformation of carcinomas into carcinosarcoma. We eagerly await advances in therapeutics targeting the EMT process.

Tissue-of-origin agnostic treatment approaches may be another underexplored strategy to treat UCS. While rare, microsatellite instability and *POLE* mutations have been reported in UCS [3]. These patients may be candidates for treatment with pembrolizumab, and testing for both microsatellite instability and tumor mutation burden is reasonable in the recurrent disease setting. Several emerging treatment approaches studied in other tumor types could be applied to UCS. Enhancer of zeste homolog 2 (EZH2) works as a master regulator of cell cycle progression, autophagy, and apoptosis and may be a very good target in carcinosarcoma. The role for immunotherapy in UCS has not yet been established, but agents such as defactinib which targets FAK and PYK2 may reduce tumor survival signals and make cold tumors immunologically hot.

Conclusion

The current status of therapy for carcinosarcomas is clearly inadequate and we cannot be complacent about ineffective standards of care. We must apply advances from bench-to-bedside research to develop a better regimen than carboplatin and paclitaxel. The lack of clinical data to support regimens other than platinum-taxane and ifosfamide-based chemotherapy is notable. The rarity of UCS and its aggressive clinical course have made development of carcinosarcoma-specific trials challenging. Moreover, many trials of novel and targeted therapies all too often exclude UCS patients, focusing rather on the activity of novel therapies in endometrioid or serous histology tumors. If new therapeutic strategies are to emerge, women with UCS must be enrolled in dedicated clinical trials that seek to exploit the various molecular signatures that are prevalent in these complex, metaplastic carcinomas.

References

1. Powell MA, et al. A randomized phase 3 trial of paclitaxel (P) plus carboplatin (C) versus paclitaxel plus ifosfamide (I) in chemotherapy-naive patients with s-IV, persistent or recurrent carcinosarcoma of the uterus or ovary: an NRG Oncology trial. *J Clin Oncol* 2022;40(9):968–977.

2. Berton-Rigaud D, et al. Gynecologic Cancer InterGroup (GCIG) consensus review for uterine and ovarian carcinosarcoma. *Int J Gynecol Cancer* 2014;24(9 Suppl. 3): S55–60.

3. Cherniack AD, et al. Integrated molecular characterization of uterine carcinosarcoma. *Cancer Cell* 2017;31 (3):411–423. https://doi.org/10.1016/j .ccell.2017.02.010

4. Zhao S, et al. Mutational landscape of uterine and ovarian carcinosarcomas implicates histone genes in epithelial-mesenchymal transition. *Proc Natl Acad Sci U S A* 2016;113 (43):12238–12243. https://doi.org/10.1073/ pnas.1614120113

What is the Best Management for Premenopausal Women with Early-stage Uterine Leiomyosarcoma Status Post Hysterectomy for Presumed Uterine Leiomyomas?

39A

Oophorectomy

Anastasios Tranoulis, Kavita Singh, and Janos Balega

Debate

Oophorectomy Should be Considered as Standard for Patients with Estrogen-/Progesterone- positive Leiomyosarcoma

Surgery represents the mainstay of treatment for uterine leiomyosarcomas (u-LMS) [1]. Resection of disease without fragmentation and with negative surgical margins seemingly provides survival advantage [1]. For macroscopically uterus-limited disease, total abdominal hysterectomy (TAH) should be considered as the standard management of choice [1]. Uterine leiomyosarcomas usually are discovered as incidental findings after hysterectomy or myomectomy for presumed benign pathology (e.g., fibroid uterus). For peri-menopausal or post-menopausal women, routine bilateral salpingo-oophorectomy (BSO) is usually performed; however, amongst pre-menopausal women with uterus-limited disease, the role of ovarian preservation (OP), as part of the staging process, remains to date a field of contention. The Gynecologic Cancer InterGroup (GCIG) recommends that BSO is reasonable and could also be offered in pre-menopausal women with apparent uterine-limited LMS [1].

Overall, the risk of ovarian metastasis has been reported 4%, although most cases coexist with peritoneal spread [1,2]. Recurrence rates even for early-stage disease are high, ranging from 53% to 71% [2]. Estrogen and/or progesterone receptors have been found to be positive in 40% to 70% of u-LMS [2]. The Memorial Sloan Kettering Cancer group reported that the majority of u-LMS expressed estrogen (ER), progesterone (PR), and androgen (AR) receptor [3]. After adjusting for stage, PR and AR status was found to be predictive of a lower risk of recurrence. However, ER, PR, and AR were not found to be associated with overall survival (OS) after adjustment for stage [2]. In a more recent study from the same group, ER/PR expression was found to be associated with survival outcomes in 43 women with high-grade uterine-limited LMS [4]. PR expression was associated with both improved progression-free survival (PFS) and OS in the overall cohort analysis, whilst ER expression was not statistically associated with either PFS or OS. Nonetheless, after adjusting for stage (disease confined to the uterine body), ER expression was associated with improved PFS but not OS, while PR expression maintained its association with PFS and approached significant association with OS [4].

These findings suggest that ER/PR activation may play an important role in tumor development in u-LMS. There is a growing body of evidence on the role of hormonal treatment – especially of aromatase inhibitors – on patients with low disease burden u-LMS [1,2]. Several studies have shown objective response rates and improvement in PFS amongst women with u-LMS treated with aromatase inhibitors such as anastrozole or letrozole [1,2]. ER/PR appear to have a pivotal role in regulating the growth and remodeling of uterine smooth muscle, thus, necessitating a shift in the focus of future research into understanding the potential role of targeting steroid hormone receptors as therapeutic options in u-LMS. To this end, better understanding of the role of ER/PR may also guide clinicians to decipher the circumstances under which oophorectomy may benefit the outcome.

On the other hand, a retrospective review of 1395 u-LMS patients showed that OP did not have a significant impact on OS, whilst independent predictors for PFS included age, race, stage, grade, and primary surgery [5]. In their SEER (Surveillance, Epidemiology, and End Results) review, Nasioudis et al. sought to ascertain the prognostic role of OP amongst 800 women with apparent FIGO stage I u-LMS [6]. The authors reported that approximately one third of all women did not undergo oophorectomy and that OP was not associated with either worse OS or PFS. These findings are also supported from smaller retrospective studies; yet, these are constrained by the small number of women included in addition to the lack of controlling for age, FIGO stage, and adjuvant treatment [6].

Conclusion

Currently, there is no consensus on the prognostic significance of OP in women with early-stage u-LMS. In light of the limited quality of the available data, deriving only from retrospective studies, the risks and benefits of OP should be thoroughly discussed with the patient and OP may be offered only in selected cases with documented negative endocrine receptor status until more robust evidence becomes available.

References

1. Hensley ML, et al. Gynecologic Cancer InterGroup (GCIG) consensus review: uterine and ovarian leiomyosarcomas. *Int J Gynecol Cancer* 2014;9(Suppl. 3): S61–66.

2. Zivanovic O, et al. A nomogram to predict post resection 5-year overall survival for patients with uterine leiomyosarcoma. *Cancer* 2012;118:660–669.

3. Leitao MM, et al. Tissue microarray immunohistochemical expression of estrogen, progesterone, and androgen receptors in uterine leiomyomata and leiomyosarcoma. *Cancer* 2004;101:1455.

4. Leitao MM, et al. O outcomes in patients with newly diagnosed uterine leiomyosarcoma. *Gynecol Oncol* 2012;124:558–562.

5. Kapp DS, et al. Prognostic factors and survival in 1396 patients with uterine leiomyosarcomas: emphasis on impact of lymphadenectomy and oophorectomy. *Cancer* 2008;112:820–830.

6. Nasioudis D, et al. Safety of ovarian preservation in premenopausal women with stage I uterine sarcoma. *J Gynecol Oncol* 2017;28(4):e46.

39B
What is the Best Management for Premenopausal Women with Early-stage Uterine Leiomyosarcoma Status Post Hysterectomy for Presumed Uterine Leiomyomas?
Ovarian Preservation

Melissa K. Frey and Ryan M. Kahn

Debate

Uterine sarcomas are a rare subgroup of malignancies that comprise 3–7% of uterine neoplasms and just nearly 1% percent of all gynecologic cancers [1]. Leiomyosarcomas (LMS) of the uterus, which arise from the smooth muscle of the myometrium, are aggressive malignancies with high rates of recurrence. Uterine LMS has been historically difficult to diagnose pre-operatively. Both uterine leiomyoma and LMS share common presenting symptoms including abnormal uterine bleeding, large pelvic masses, lower abdominal pain, and abdominal distension. Because of this, the diagnosis of uterine LMS is commonly made upon pathology evaluation after myomectomy or hysterectomy for suspected benign disease.

The mainstay of local treatment for uterine LMS is complete tumor resection with surgical excision. As the median age of diagnosis for uterine LMS is relatively young (54 years), many newly diagnosed women are premenopausal and must decide on ovarian preservation [1]. Uterine LMS commonly expresses estrogen (ER) and progesterone (PR) receptors; therefore, many have supported iatrogenic menopause through bilateral oophorectomy to reduce the possibility of tumor recurrence and growth from stimulation of endogenous steroid hormones. However, given the rarity of this tumor and inconclusive data, the role of oophorectomy in premenopausal women with uterine LMS remains controversial.

One of the initial studies investigating the prevalence of ER and PR receptors in uterine LMS demonstrated that steroid receptor expression showed no significant association with clinicopathologic outcomes [2]. Bodner et al. [2] reviewed 21 patients with uterine LMS and found ER and PR positivity exhibited in 57% and 43% of cases, respectively. Although a large portion of LMS cases exhibited positive ER and PR expression, the presence of steroid receptors was not associated with any of the factors studied including age of diagnosis, clinical stage, vascular involvement, disease recurrence, disease-free survival, and overall survival (p>0.05). That lack of association between receptor and prognosis has led to the hypothesis that ER and PR are not the driving receptors for these malignancies.

Similarly, Giuntoli et al. [3] evaluated the surgical management and associated outcomes for uterine LMS. This case-control study comprised of 25 patients who maintained ovarian function versus 25 matched cases who underwent bilateral salpingo-oophorectomy (BSO). Kaplan–Meier analysis of disease-specific survival among the matched ovarian preservation cases (mean >30 years) compared to controls (mean >30 years) demonstrated no significant difference (p=0.49) [3]. Likewise, mean recurrence-free survival between ovarian preservation compared to the BSO cohort demonstrated no significant difference (p=0.97) [3]. However, it should be noted that the exclusion criteria for the case group included adjuvant pelvic radiation therapy, whereas 24% (6/25) of women in the control group received some form of radiation therapy. This difference could have led to potential bias favoring oophorectomy.

Nearly 15 years later, Nasioudis et al. [4] performed a large population-based study, using the National Cancer Institute's Surveillance, Epidemiology, and End Results database, evaluating survival differences between uterine LMS patients undergoing ovarian preservation versus BSO among premenopausal women diagnosed with stage I disease. The search identified 800 women, aged <50 years, diagnosed between the timeframe of 1988–2013, with LMS limited to the uterus. Within this cohort, women with ovarian preservation had better five-year overall survival (OS) rates as compared to the oophorectomy group (72.8% vs. 68.9%). Likewise, women with ovarian perseveration had greater cancer-specific survival (CSS) rates as compared to oophorectomy (74.2% vs. 70.8%). However, these rates were not statistically significant (OS, p=0.078; CSS p=0.098). Additionally, after controlling for age and FIGO staging, ovarian preservation was not associated with a change in overall survival as compared to BSO (p=0.23) or cancer-specific mortality (p=0.34) [4].

Another large-scale observational cohort study – conducted by Seagle et al. [1] investigated 7455 cases of uterine LMS from the National Cancer Database reported between 1998–2013 [1]. Among all patients, 762 underwent hysterectomy without oophorectomy (10.2%) [1]. Women with ovarian preservation were younger (median 46 years) as compared to those with oophorectomy (median 55 years) (p<0.001). Ovarian preservation demonstrated no difference in survival in event time ratio among women <51 years old at diagnosis when compared to bilateral oophorectomy (p=0.48) [1]. This study demonstrates that removal of bilateral ovaries may be safely omitted for early-stage uterine LMS.

Conclusion

Based on the current literature, there appears to be no added benefit of removing bilateral ovaries following the diagnosis of early stage uterine LMS in premenopausal women. In addition, there remains minimal data demonstrating any increased risk of recurrence or tumor growth following ovarian preservation in this patient population. Given this, the 2019 European Society for Medical Clinical Practice Guidelines for uterine LMS recommend that the added value of BSO is not established, particularly in pre-menopausal women [5]. This form of management must be balanced with shared decision making and extensive counseling. If the ovaries are preserved, close long-term follow-up is vitally important.

References

1. Seagle BL, et al. Prognosis and treatment of uterine leiomyosarcoma: a National Cancer Database study. *Gynecol Oncol* 2017;145 (1):61–70.

2. Bodner K, et al. Estrogen and progesterone receptor expression in patients with uterine smooth muscle tumors. *Fertil Steril* 2004;81 (4):1062–1066.

3. Giuntoli RL, et al. Retrospective review of 208 patients with leiomyosarcoma of the uterus: prognostic indicators, surgical management, and adjuvant therapy. *Gynecol Oncol* 2003;89 (3):460–469.

4. Nasioudis D, et al. Safety of ovarian preservation in premenopausal women with stage I uterine sarcoma. *J Gynecol Oncol* 2017;28(4):e46. https://doi.org/10.3802/jgo .2017.28.e46

5. ESMO/European Sarcoma Network Working Group. Soft tissue and visceral sarcomas: ESMO clinical practice guidelines for diagnosis, treatment and follow-up. *Ann Oncol* 2014;25(Suppl. 3):iii102–112.

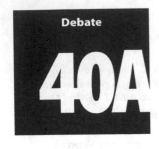

Debate

Should Primary Debulking Surgery be Performed for Metastatic Leiomyosarcoma?

Yes

Sumer K. Wallace and Jamie N. Bakkum-Gamez

Debate

Surgical resection is the standard of care in the setting of early stage uterine leiomyosarcoma (uLMS). Additionally, hysterectomy is often also the primary diagnostic procedure for uterine-confined LMS given the limitations of imaging in the diagnostic setting and the lack of any other biomarkers that differentiate uLMS from the more common benign uterine leiomyoma. Although the majority of patients with uLMS have uterine-confined disease, 30–40% of patients will have extrauterine disease at the time of presentation [1–3]. Limited ability to discern uLMS preoperatively on imaging may lead to encountering unanticipated metastatic abdominopelvic disease. This may lead to consideration of additional surgery for debulking of extrauterine disease discovered either during surgery or on postoperative imaging. Primary surgery for uLMS consists of, at minimum, hysterectomy and bilateral salpingectomy with consideration of bilateral oophorectomy, although uLMS are typically not hormone-responsive sarcomas. Lymph node basins should be evaluated for lymphadenopathy, but systematic lymphadenectomy is not required as the rate of uLMS metastasis to lymph nodes is <5% [2]. Ideally, primary surgery would be performed after a comprehensive workup such that all sites of uLMS metastases are known. This also ensures that a primary surgical approach is appropriate for the patient. However, as previously noted, apparent early stage uLMS is most often diagnosed after hysterectomy for presumed benign leiomyomata. In this setting, operative details and postoperative imaging will guide whether further surgical intervention is recommended, as stage is the most accurate measure of prognosis [1,3].

Due to the poor prognosis for uLMS, adjuvant treatment is often recommended despite the limited efficacy and paucity of overall survival (OS) benefit. Observation is the current standard of care for stage I uLMS following R0 resection and it remains unknown whether systemic therapy improves survival in stage I uLMS. Multi-modality treatment with surgery, chemotherapy, and/or radiation is often utilized in the management of advanced stage uLMS. Cytotoxic chemotherapy agents, such as doxorubicin, docetaxel, gemcitabine, and ifosfamide, are active in uLMS and often recommended for treatment of advanced stage disease; however, recurrence rates remain high despite adjuvant chemotherapy with no demonstration of improved OS in the current literature [1,4]. Similarly, while adjuvant radiation may improve local control, it has not been shown to increase OS [5]. As such innovative and progressive therapeutic modalities that address frequent sites of spread, such as metastases to the liver and lung, are important in the uLMS armamentarium.

Given the potential survival advantage associated with debulking, resection to R0 remains an essential prognostic component of treatment planning for uLMS. However, the risks of surgical complications and morbidity need to be balanced with the potential oncologic benefits. In the setting of oligometastatic disease, surgery may only require a low complexity operation. However, given the hematogenous spread pattern of LMS, surgical debulking may require resection of hepatic or pulmonary metastases to achieve R0 resection. A recent review of the literature confirmed the importance of complete surgical resection, when feasible, prior to considering further treatment with chemotherapy or radiation [4]. This review reiterated the lack of efficacy of chemotherapy and radiation in improving survival in uLMS patients, and discussed the importance of surgical management for patients in which R0 resection can be achieved. Additionally, based on retrospective and limited prospective data solely in uLMS, women with disease that is amenable to complete surgical resection appear to fare better from the oncologic standpoints of progression-free survival (PFS), OS and even cure [2,4]. Surgical clinical trial data in uLMS alone is limited, with the majority of available data being retrospective due to the rare nature of the disease. Therefore, primary surgical resection data in the setting of metastatic uLMS is often extrapolated from clinical studies that include heterogeneous uterine sarcoma histologies or LMS from various primary tissue origins. Burt et al. demonstrated that resection of pulmonary metastases from primary LMS yielded improved OS when compared to non-LMS sarcoma metastases (69.9 months and 23.9 months, respectively). Uterine LMS comprised 42% of this study population, and pulmonary metastases from LMS were relatively indolent in nature compared to other types of sarcoma metastases which may have contributed to the improved OS [6]. While OS outcomes appear mixed, in good surgical candidates who are deemed to have resectable disease, a maximal surgical cytoreduction effort that achieves an R0 resection offers improved PFS outcomes and potentially extends OS [2,3].

It is also important to recognize that there may be a role for palliative hysterectomy in those with known metastatic disease and uterine symptoms of pain and/or bleeding in which quality of life could be improved with hysterectomy. Such surgical management requires weighing benefits with surgical risks, mode of hysterectomy, and assessment as to whether surgery will impact the timing of initiation of systemic therapy for unresectable disease.

Conclusion

In summary, multimodality management of uLMS is often recommended with the goal of optimizing OS in this highly lethal cancer. While current adjuvant therapy options seem to have limited impact, and novel active systemic agents are desperately needed for metastatic uLMS, upfront surgical excision of advanced stage uLMS amenable to R0 resection appears to extend PFS and OS. Therefore, a comprehensive workup for metastatic disease is critical in the setting of a new uLMS diagnosis so that individualized treatment, which may include upfront aggressive surgical resection, can be considered.

References

1. Hensley ML, et al. Adjuvant gemcitabine plus docetaxel for completely resected stages I–IV high-grade uterine leiomyosarcoma: results of a prospective study. *Gynecol Oncol* 2009;112:563.

2. Dinh TA, et al. The treatment of uterine leiomyosarcoma. Results from a 10-year experience (1990–1999) at the Massachusetts General Hospital. *Gynecol Oncol* 2004;92:648–652.

3. Leitao MM Jr, et al. Surgical cytoreduction in patients with metastatic uterine leiomyosarcoma at the time of initial diagnosis. *Gynecol Oncol* 2012;125 (2):409–413.

4. Friedman CF, et al. Options for adjuvant therapy for uterine leiomyosarcoma. *Curr Treat Options Oncol* 2018;19(2):7.

5. Reed NS, et al. Phase III randomized study to evaluate the role of adjuvant pelvic radiotherapy in the treatment of uterine sarcomas stage I and II: a European Organisation for Research and Treatment of Cancer Gynaecological Cancer Group Study (protocol 55874). *Eur J Cancer* 2008;44:808–818.

6. Burt BM, et al. Repeated and aggressive pulmonary resections for leiomyosarcoma metastases extends survival. *Ann Thorac Surg* 2011;92:1207.

Should Primary Debulking Surgery be Performed for Metastatic Leiomyosarcoma?

No

Beatrice Seddon

Debate

Gynecological sarcomas are rare tumors, with tumors of uterine origin being the most common. Leiomyosarcoma is the most common subtype of uterine sarcoma, with 2383 new diagnoses in England between 1985 and 2008 (approximately 100 cases per year), accounting for 54% of all uterine sarcomas and 86% of all gynecological leiomyosarcomas. Other rarer sites of origin include leiomyosarcoma of the vulva, vagina, cervix, broad ligament and ovary. The age-specific incidence rates are highest in women aged 50 to 64 years [1]. Approximately two thirds of women present with FIGO stage I disease, and approximately 20% with distant metastatic disease [2].

For patients presenting with localized disease, the most important component of treatment is surgery, which for the commonest group of uterine tumors is a hysterectomy [3]. Incidence of lymph node or ovarian metastases is low such that routine lymphadenectomy and removal of ovaries are not mandatory, and indeed do not improve survival [2]. For patients with gynecological sarcomas presenting with metastatic disease, the question arises as to whether these patients should have surgery to remove the primary tumor at diagnosis, or whether they should receive palliative chemotherapy or radiotherapy for their metastases. There is some evidence that for patients with metastatic disease undergoing surgical cytoreduction of disease at diagnosis, surgery is associated with improved progression-free survival compared with patients not undergoing surgery [4].

There are arguments for and against surgery to remove the primary tumor in the metastatic setting. Outcomes for patients presenting with metastatic disease are poor, with median survival of 12 to 18 months, often less for patients with aggressive disease. Therefore the priority for patients with rapidly progressing disease is often to start chemotherapy as soon as possible, in order to try to achieve some stability of the metastatic disease, and thereby to prolong survival [5]. There may be the option following chemotherapy to consider local therapy to the primary tumor, such as palliative radiotherapy. However, primary tumors are frequently large and bulky, causing symptoms such as pelvic pain, vaginal bleeding, and offensive vaginal disease, and these symptoms can be very difficult to palliate, with either chemotherapy, or with radiotherapy as local therapy. For this reason, if a patient presents with small-volume metastatic disease that is not obviously progressing rapidly, consideration may be given to surgery to remove the primary tumor, and then to consider chemotherapy postoperatively to treat the metastatic disease. The balance between the need to remove the primary tumor surgically, and to treat progressing metastatic disease in the first instance can be fine, and the judgement as to optimal treatment for an individual patient difficult.

It is clear however, that surgery should only be undertaken if the disease can be completely removed, with no macroscopic residual disease, as a debulking procedure leaving overt residual disease gives the worst of both worlds, in that the disease will very frequently grow back rapidly while the patient is recovering from surgery such that the procedure has achieved nothing other than exposing the patient to a futile and potentially morbid surgical procedure, and in the meantime the metastatic disease continues to grow. There is also a risk that the patient is debilitated by surgery to the extent that they may no longer be fit for palliative chemotherapy.

Conclusion

The key therefore is careful patient selection for surgical removal of the primary tumor at diagnosis in the metastatic setting. This can be considered for patients with small-volume metastatic disease that is not obviously progressing rapidly, for whom it is judged that complete macroscopic removal of the primary disease can be achieved. However, patients with rapidly progressing metastatic disease, and those for whom complete macroscopic removal of the primary tumor is not possible, are unlikely to benefit from such surgery, which should be avoided, and priority given to treatment with palliative chemotherapy or radiotherapy.

References

1. Francis M, et al. Incidence and survival of gynecologic sarcomas in England. *Int J Gynecol Cancer* 2015;25 (5):850–857.

2. Kapp DS, et al. Prognostic factors and survival in 1396 patients with uterine leiomyosarcomas: emphasis on impact of lymphadenectomy and oophorectomy. *Cancer* 2008;112 (4):820–830.

3. Ghirardi V, et al. Role of surgery in gynaecological sarcomas. *Oncotarget* 2019;10(26):2561–2575.

4. Leitao MM Jr., et al. Surgical cytoreduction in patients with metastatic uterine leiomyosarcoma at the time of initial diagnosis. *Gynecol Oncol* 2012;125(2):409–413.

5. George S, et al. Soft tissue and uterine leiomyosarcoma. *J Clin Oncol* 2018;36 (2):144–150.

41A

Should Secondary Cytoreductive Surgery be Offered to all Patients that are Surgical Candidates with Optimally Resectable Recurrent Uterine Leiomyosarcoma?

Yes

Giovanni Aletti

Debate

Uterine sarcomas are rare gynecologic malignancies, being 3–7% of all uterine malignant tumors, and approximately 1% of all female gynecologic cancers. Leiomyosarcomas (LMS) encompass approximately 1% of all the uterine cancers. Leiomyosarcoma is the most common uterine sarcoma, with an extremely aggressive clinical behavior. Consequently, this neoplasm is associated with a poor prognosis and very high risk of recurrence even among women with early-stage disease. The reported recurrence rates range between 45% and 73%. The main sites of these recurrences are the abdomen or the pelvis; a high proportion of uterine LMS will recur in the lung, with pulmonary metastases. Typically, survival for patients with recurrent disease is extremely poor. Unfortunately, the best management strategy for patients with recurrent uterine LMS has yet to be defined. Management options for recurrent disease include additional resection in operable patients, ablation, chemotherapy, radiation therapy, hormonal therapy in selected patients, or a combination of these. The decision of the treatment strategy should be taken in an interdisciplinary setting, involving gynecologic oncologists, medical oncologists, radiation therapists, interventional radiologists, and all specialists (thoracic surgeons, oncologic surgeons, etc.) involved in all the different therapeutic options. Due to the paucity of data, and the different clinical presentations of patients with recurrent LMS, treatment is proposed to each patient on an individual basis, trying to maximize the potential benefits of each treatment by individualizing the strategy. The main factors that guide the multidisciplinary team in this choice are represented by the number of metastases and the anatomical locations of metastases, the patient's disease-free interval, the disease burden, the organ function, the different prior therapies, the patient's clinical condition and performance status, and the patient's preferences.

245

The question posed in the present chapter underlies two main issues:

- What is the rationale of secondary cytoreduction in recurrent uterine LMS?
- How can we define surgical candidates with optimally resectable recurrent uterine LMS?

After elucidating these topics, we can definitely answer "yes" to the question posed in the present chapter:

- Should secondary cytoreduction be offered to all patients with optimally resectable recurrent uterine LMS?

Rationale for Secondary Cytoreduction in Recurrent Uterine Leiomyosarcoma

The prognosis for patients with recurrent disease is poor, with five-year overall survival (OS) of 40–60% [1,2]. Management options in this setting are limited and poorly defined.

Options for Chemotherapy in Recurrent Disease

Patients with recurrent uterine LMS will often receive chemotherapy. Systemic chemotherapy is often advocated for the treatment of recurrent uterine LMS, and doxorubicin is the most active drug for this malignancy, with a reported response rate of 25%. Different options for recurrent disease (depending also on previous chemotherapy regimens utilized) include a combination of anthracycline with ifosfamide or dacarbazine or trabectedin, The combination of gemcitabine and docetaxel, or single agents doxorubicin, trabectedin, dacarbazine, pazopanib, high-dose ifosfamide, paclitaxel, etoposide. Unfortunately, these regimens have been associated with modest activity in treating patients with recurrent uterine LMS.

Due to these poor results, the first reason to consider secondary surgery for candidates with resectable uterine LMS is the extremely poor alternative demonstrated in patients with recurrent disease managed by non-surgical approaches.

Secondary Surgery in Patients with Recurrent Leiomyosarcoma

Pulmonary Metastasectomy

The concept of resection of isolated pulmonary metastases from uterine malignancies (pulmonary metastasectomy) was introduced in 1930 by Torek, and has been validated by several retrospective cohorts.

For example, in a relatively large retrospective study published by the Thoracic Surgery Group at the Brigham and Women's Hospital in Boston, 31 patients underwent pulmonary metastasectomy for metastases from LMS, of which 15 patients (48%) underwent repeated pulmonary metastasectomy. They compared the outcome of these patients to a group of patients with pulmonary metastases from sarcomas non LMS. Patients with LMS metastases had an improved overall survival as opposed to those with non-LMS pulmonary metastases, with an overall survival of 70 months versus 24 months (p=0.049). Furthermore, it is relevant to notice that a long-term survival can be achievable for patients with isolated metastases from uterine LMS localized in the lung/s. Several studies confirmed the feasibility and the benefits o pulmonary metastasectomy in selected groups of patients with recurrent uterine LMS. Overall, resection of isolated lung metastases in patients with recurrent uterine LMS has been associated with five-year survival of approximately 40%.

Secondary Cytoreduction

In this chapter we take into consideration patients with extra-pulmonary metastases from uterine LMS, who are surgical candidates for secondary surgery.

Leitao and the Gynecologic Oncology Group at Memorial Sloan Kettering Cancer Center [2] demonstrated the benefits of optimal resection of recurrent uterine LMS. They retrospectively analyzed 41 patients with recurrent uterine LMS (17 local pelvic, 18 distant, six both), who underwent surgical resection at time of first recurrence. A pulmonary metastasectomy alone was performed in 13 cases. The disease-specific two-year survival for all 41 patients was 71.2%. In univariate analysis, time to first recurrence and optimal resection were significantly associated with longer overall survival. This study underlines the importance of a complete resection of the distant metastases, even when they are localized in the abdomen.

Giuntoli and the group at the Mayo Clinic [3] analyzed 128 patients with recurrent uterine LMS. Management included secondary cytoreductive surgery in 63% (80/128) of patients, chemotherapy in 55% (71/128) of patients and included radiation therapy (discounting palliative radiation) in 26% (33/128) of patients. At univariate analysis, secondary cytoreductive surgery was associated with significantly improved disease-specific survival from time of first recurrence (p<0.001). Other factors including greater than six-month disease-free interval, either local or distant recurrence, and complete response were also associated with significantly improved outcome in uni-variate analysis. At multivariate analysis, the presence of both distant and local recurrence, the utilization of surgery for treatment of recurrent disease, and recur-rence time greater than six months, were independently correlated with disease-specific survival from the time of first recurrence (p≤0.05). They also reported that optimal secondary surgical resection was associated with a significantly improved survival.

Cybulska et al. recently reported the outcomes of patients with recurrent uterine LMS treated again at Memorial Sloan Kettering Cancer Center [4]. In this study, the authors analyzed the outcomes of patients who underwent secondary surgery, by different sites of recurrence and by different surgical outcomes in terms of complete gross resection (CGR). They identified 62 patients: 29 with abdominal/pelvic recur-rence only, 30 with lung recurrence only, three with both sites of recurrences. Median time to first recurrence was 15.8 months for patients with abdominal/pelvic recur-rence, and 24.1 months lung-only recurrence (p=0.03). The median OS was 37.7 months for patients with abdominal/pelvic recurrence; 78.1 months for lung recur-rence (p=0.02). Complete gross resection was obtained in 58 cases (93%), with gross residual between 1–2 cm in two cases (3.5%) and RD > 2 cm in two cases (3.5%). Median OS based on residual disease was 54.1 months, 38.7 months, 1.7 months, respectively (p<0.001). The results of this study underlie the role and benefits of secondary surgical resection of recurrent uterine LMS when a complete resection is feasible.

Furthermore, lung-only recurrences were associated with a more favorable outcome, and the resection of lung recurrence/s should definitely be considered as the best option when the patient is amenable to complete surgical resection.

Surgical Candidates for Optimally Resectable Recurrent Uterine Leiomyosarcoma

Given the rationale and the results of secondary cytoreduction for patients with recurrent uterine LMS, the main issue is to define the subgroup of patients with two specific characteristics:

1. High chance of performing a secondary complete gross resection
2. Minimizing peri-operative morbidity and mortality, avoiding a deterioration in the quality of life.

In 2016, the Trans-Atlantic Retroperitoneal Sarcoma Working Group published a consensus approach in the management of recurrent retroperitoneal sarcoma (RPS) [5]. While uterine LMS recurrences were not included in the statements, the approach described can be extrapolated to patients with recurrent uterine LMS. Before considering secondary cytoreduction, patients with recurrent RPS should be discussed at a multidisciplinary meeting, involving surgical oncologists, medical oncologists, radiation oncologists, pathologists, and radiologists with expertise in sarcoma (in this case in uterine LMS). The following data should be reviewed in detail:

- Specimens of the previous surgery
- Previous surgery/ies, systemic treatments, radiation therapy
- Current localization of the recurrence/s: the use of CT scan, and MRI as an ancillary modality, are recommended
- Patient's evaluation for symptoms, performance status

In case of intra-abdominal metastases, a complete resection is difficult to predict based on imaging.

Extra peritoneal oligo metastatic recurrence/s, especially in the lung, can be better assessed for complete resection. The delicate balance between the likelihood of completely resecting the recurrence/s versus the risk of surgical complications and mortality should be carefully considered on an individual basis in a multidisciplinary setting, in order to offer the best option to each patient.

Conclusion

Secondary cytoreductive surgery should be offered to patients with recurrent uterine LMS who are amenable of complete resection for these reasons:

1. In the case of complete resection, a survival advantage can be achieved. This is particularly evident for lung-only recurrences.
2. Systemic treatments have shown discouraging results in recurrences that are not manageable with surgery.

A careful multidisciplinary selection is of paramount importance to determine the best approach on an individual basis.

References

1. Burt BM, et al. Repeated and aggressive pulmonary resections for leiomyosarcoma metastases extends survival. *Ann Thorac Surg* 2011;92:1202–1207.

2. Leitao MM, et al. Surgical resection of pulmonary and extrapulmonary recurrences of uterine leiomyosarcoma, *Gynecol Oncol* 2002;87: 287–294.

3. Giuntoli RL, et al. Secondary cytoreduction in the management of recurrent uterine leiomyosarcoma. *Gynecol Oncol* 2007;106:82–88.

4. Cybulska P, et al. Secondary surgical resection for patients with recurrent uterine leiomyosarcoma. *Gynecol Oncol* 2019;154 (2):333–337.

5. Trans-Atlantic RPS Working Group. Management of recurrent retroperitoneal sarcoma (RPS) in the adult: a consensus approach from the Trans-Atlantic RPS Working Group. *Ann Surg Oncol* 2016; 23 (11):3531–3540.

Should Secondary Cytoreductive Surgery be Offered to all Patients that are Surgical Candidates with Optimally Resectable Recurrent Uterine Leiomyosarcoma?

No

Félix Blanc-Durand, Amandine Maulard, and Patricia Pautier

Debate

After complete cytoreductive surgery of uterine leiomyosarcomas (uLMS), the risk of recurrence within two years is around 40% and once metastatic, treatment has often been palliative due to the dismal overall survival rates. Nearly 80% of all recurrences involve an extra pelvic site (including lung and abdominal metastases) and overall prognosis is similar for both pelvic and extra pelvic recurrences. It is well established that surgery of isolated pulmonary recurrences offers improved overall survival and should be encouraged [1]. However, whether patients with recurrent uLMS benefit also from secondary cytoreductive surgery (SCS) of extrapulmonary sites is not known.

Small retrospective studies have suggested that resection of extrapulmonary metastases may also be beneficial for patients. Leitao et al. [2] reported on 37 patients with recurrent uLMS who had undergone SCS with or without adjuvant chemotherapy and/or radiotherapy. Importantly, the large majority of patients (29/37) had only pelvic or lung recurrences and half of the population (18/37) received adjuvant therapy. In this heavily selected population, with heterogeneous management, six patients (16.2%) had prolonged remission without evidence of disease after a median follow-up of 25 months. Two out of these six patients received adjuvant therapy and whether they subsequently developed extensive or localized recurrences was not reported. Conversely, Nakamura et al. in 2018, in a small subset of LMS(n=3) out of 18 uterine sarcomas, reported that two patients had prolonged remission after SCS. Both presented with pelvic recurrences and benefited from complete cytoreductive surgery. In this report, data on adjuvant treatment was not provided. Hoang et al. [3] reported on three (13%) uLMS patients with complete remission after SCS. Details on the type of recurrence and surgery were not reported but overall, the extent of surgical resection, and the time to recurrence, were significantly associated with outcome. Bonvalot et al., in 2005, reported a small randomized trial of intraperitoneal chemotherapy (with doxorubicin and cisplatin) versus observation in patients with completely resected peritoneal sarcomatosis in which half of the population had visceral sarcoma. Interestingly, median local relapse-free survival was 12.5 months in both groups. Compared to median progression-free survival (PFS) observed in metastatic LMS (around six months) we can acknowledge the benefit of optimal SCS in this selected population [4]. Finally, Díaz-Montes et al. [5] reported numerically superior median disease-free survival for patients treated with SCS (n=14) versus nonsurgical treatments (n=5) (5.3 months vs. 2.4 months respectively) and notably, two uLMS patients with pelvic recurrences had long-term complete remission after SCS + chemotherapy.

Beside these encouraging observations in heavily selected populations, most of these studies agreed that recurrence within 12 months after initial treatment and suboptimal surgical cytoreduction, as defined in the management of epithelial ovarian carcinomas, are major prognostic markers associated with significantly worse disease-free and overall survival rates. Moreover, patients with suboptimal surgery appear to have similar survival rates compared to patients who do not have surgery [6]. Therefore, they may not be the best candidates for SCS, especially considering surgical morbidity.

Most of these studies do not report on the use of chemotherapy (CT) after SCS that may have biased the results. Systemic CT, in particular doxorubicin-containing regimens, achieve overall response rates of 30% with median PFS of nine months. However, this landscape is rapidly evolving. Very recently, at ESMO 2021, first-line doxorubicin + trabectidine used for recurrent/metastatic uLMS and soft-tissue LMS demonstrated improved overall response rates of 38% and disease control rate of 92% over doxorubicin monotherapy, as well as significantly prolonged PFS (13.5 months vs. 7.4 months). To date, this trial is the first one demonstrating significant survival benefit over the gold standard doxorubicin for recurrent/metastatic uLMS. In this regard, the optimal place for extensive extrapulmonary SCS versus standard systemic therapy is unknown. Regarding the activity of a doxorubicin doublet, we can anticipate that "neoadjuvant" systemic therapy may better select the best candidates for SCS, improving optimal resection rates as well as converting primary unresectable diseases. Yet it should be stressed that response rates are not similar to what is observed in ovarian carcinomas and some patients may progress under chemotherapy and miss the opportunity for complete surgery. Moreover, chemotherapy for sarcoma diseases is associated with significant toxicity and secondary surgery may be challenging. Nevertheless, preoperative chemotherapy appears feasible and promising but reports concerning its efficacy are scarce and limited to case reports. On the other hand, active CT done on minimal residual disease may have a greater chance to be effective. In this regard, three randomized trials tested adjuvant chemotherapy after initial surgery and two of them demonstrated increased cure rates and one did not observe any benefit. Herein, this strategy remains highly controversial.

Conclusion

To conclude, secondary cytoreductive surgery should be restricted to selected recurrent uLMS, after multidisciplinary discussion, since the greatest benefit appears to be observed in patients with localized pelvic and/or lung disease, late (>12 months) recurrence, in whom optimal resection is considered. In addition, the best use of systemic therapy in this situation is unclear and dedicated prospective clinical trials comparing these sequences are needed. Neoadjuvant chemotherapy may be an option for patients who cannot benefit from upfront complete resection and this approach, along with complementary CT after surgery, should also be discussed in specialized tumor boards depending on the number of metastatic intraabdominal sites, and previous CT in the adjuvant or metastatic setting.

References

1. van Geel AN, et al. Surgical treatment of lung metastases: the European Organization for Research and Treatment of Cancer-Soft Tissue and Bone Sarcoma Group study of 255 patients. *Cancer* 1996;77:675–682. https://doi.org/10.1002/(sici)1097-0142(19960215)77:4<675::aid-cncr13>3.3.co;2-h

2. Leitao MM, et al. Surgical resection of pulmonary and extrapulmonary recurrences of uterine leiomyosarcoma. *Gynecol Oncol* 2002;87:287–294. https://doi.org/10.1006/gyno.2002.6840

3. Hoang HLT, et al. Prognostic factors and survival in patients treated surgically for recurrent metastatic uterine leiomyosarcoma. *Int J Surg Oncol* 2014;2014:919323. https://doi.org/10.1155/2014/919323

4. Bonvalot S, et al. Randomized trial of cytoreduction followed by intraperitoneal chemotherapy versus cytoreduction alone in patients with peritoneal sarcomatosis. *Eur J Surg Oncol* 2005;31(8):917–923. https://doi.org/10.1016/j.ejso.2005.04.010. PMID: 15975759

5. Díaz-Montes TP, et al. Efficacy of hyperthermic intraperitoneal chemotherapy and cytoreductive surgery in the treatment of recurrent uterine sarcoma. *Int J Gynecol Cancer* 2018;28:1130–1137. https://doi.org/10.1097/IGC.0000000000001289

6. Aalders J, et al. Postoperative external irradiation and prognostic parameters in stage I endometrial carcinoma: clinical and histopathologic study of 540 patients. *Obstet Gynecol* 1980;56:419–427.

Debate

42A

Is there a Role for Minimally Invasive Radical Hysterectomy for Management of Cervical Cancer?

Yes

Vanna Zanagnolo, Francesco Multinu, and Stefano Bogliolo

Debate

The introduction of a minimally invasive (MIS) approach has had a dramatic impact on health care management of gynecologic oncology patients, mainly for those with endometrial and cervical cancer. Before the Laparoscopic Approach to Cervical Cancer (LACC) [1] trial results became available, there was a paucity of adequately powered, prospective trials evaluating oncological outcomes of MIS in cervical cancer patients. Guidelines from the National Comprehensive Cancer Network (NCCN) and European Society of Gynaecological Oncology (ESGO) indicated that either laparotomy or MIS were acceptable approaches to radical hysterectomy (RH) in patients with early-stage cervical cancer.

In the LACC randomized trial, the investigators found a significant oncologic inferiority (disease-free survival, pelvic recurrences) of minimally invasive radical hysterectomy compared with open radical hysterectomy. The results were highly unexpected. Some speculated that the use of intrauterine manipulators, the CO_2 gas, or intra-corporeal colpotomy might have accounted for those surprising outcomes. Nevertheless, since we are now dealing with level I evidence, we have to learn from these results, starting by critically analyzing our own data, trying to understand what could have gone wrong with the MIS approach, what can be modified to prevent the negative impact of such an approach, and whether there is still room for another, better designed, randomized trial.

Since the dissemination and publication of the LACC trial, guidelines from NCCN and ESGO have changed and laparotomy is now recommended as the standard approach to radical hysterectomy in patients with early-stage (IA2 to IIA) cervical cancer. The MIS approach can still be performed for those patients with negative margins on their conization specimen and it can still be considered after a thorough discussion with the patients of the available data.

A few recent studies have been published, all retrospective, mostly large series that confirmed that the open approach was better than MIS in terms of progression-free survival (PFS) and overall survival (OS), however in some of these studies OS was not significantly different.

Different results were observed in a recently published Swedish nationwide population-based cohort study [2]. The aim of the study was to compare OS and disease-free survival (DFS) after open and robotic RH for women with cervical cancer stage IA1–IB who underwent RH from January 2011 to December 2017; 864 women (236 open and 628 robotic) were included in the study. The five-year OS was 92% and 94% and DFS was 84% and 88% for the open and robotic cohorts, respectively. The recurrence pattern was similar in both groups.

Based on these results, the authors designed and have opened to accrual the Robot-assisted Approach to Cervical Cancer (RACC) study, a multi-centre open-label randomized non-inferiority trial of robot-assisted laparoscopic surgery versus laparotomy in women with early-stage cervical cancer (FIGO stage IB (IB3 excluded), IIA1) [3]. This trial aims to compare the oncologic safety of robotic RH to conventional laparotomy and RH with the primary outcome being five-year recurrence-free survival and secondary outcome being OS.

An International European Cohort Observational Study [4] comparing MIS versus open surgery in patients with stage IB1 (FIGO 2009) cervical cancer was recently published. This study included 1116 patients who underwent surgery in 126 centers from 29 ESGO countries from 2013–2014. The primary outcome was 4.5 years DFS. With a median follow-up of 59 months, the risk of relapse in the MIS group was significantly higher in patients with cervical cancer stage IB1. The use of a uterine manipulator worsened the outcomes among MIS patients. Patients with tumors <2 cm and those with a previous cone biopsy did not demonstrate any difference in DFS. Patients who underwent MIS without use of a manipulator had the same outcome as those undergoing open surgery. Protective maneuvers to avoid tumor spillage at the time of the vaginal colpotomy in MIS improved the DFS in these patients.

In agreement with these results, Kohler at al. published a retrospective study [5] of 389 consecutive patients with initial FIGO stages identical to the LACC trial who underwent combined laparoscopic-vaginal RH, with vaginal creation of a tumor covering vaginal cuff without the use of any uterine manipulator. With a median follow-up period of >8 years, the three-year OS and three-year DFS were 98.5% and 96.8%, respectively. These oncologic data are nearly identical to the excellent results of open radical hysterectomy in the LACC trial, but should be validated in further randomized trials.

Conclusion

Based on these results and the Swedish nationwide population-based cohort study, we can speculate that the possible explanations for the findings in the LACC study could be the use of intrauterine manipulators and the lack of implementation of protective procedures to prevent cancer seeding at the time of colpotomy. But these speculations remain conjectures and until further evidence becomes available, we are in a position that the only level I evidence favors open surgery. As clinicians, the options we have now to contemplate are: (1) a complete return to open surgery, (2) defining selection criteria for those who can safely be treated with MIS with the implementation of protective measures to prevent cancer seeding, or (3) participating in further clinical trials, such as the RACC study. With further studies, selection criteria could be developed, based on the presence or absence of risk factors, such as tumor size, previous cervical conization with negative margins, and histotype, that would allow safe selection of those patients who can safely be treated with MIS.

References

1. Ramirez PT, et al. minimally invasive versus abdominal radical hysterectomy for cervical cancer. *N Engl J Med* 2018;379 (20):1895–1904.

2. Alfonzo E, et al. No survival difference between robotic and open radical hysterectomy for women with early-stage cervical cancer: results from a nationwide population-based cohort study. *Eur J Cancer* 2019;116:169–177.

3. Falconer H, et al. Robot-assisted approach to cervical cancer (RACC): an international multi-center, open-label randomized controlled trial. *Int J Gynecol Cancer* 2019;29 (6):1072–1076.

4. Chiva L, et Al. SUCCOR study. An international European cohort observational study comparing minimally invasive surgery versus open abdominal radical hysterectomy in patients with stage IB1 (FIGO 2009, <4 cm) cervical cancer operated in 2013–2014. *Int J Gynecol Cancer* 2020;30:1269–1277.

5. Kohler C, et al. Laparoscopic radical hysterectomy with transvaginal closure of vaginal cuff – a multicenter analysis. *Int J Gynecol Cancer* 2019;29(5):845–850.

Is there a Role for Minimally Invasive Radical Hysterectomy for Management of Cervical Cancer?

42B

No

Pedro T. Ramirez

Debate

The current recommended treatment for patients with early-stage cervical cancer is radical hysterectomy with pelvic lymphadenectomy or sentinel lymph node mapping. Traditionally, an approach by laparotomy was considered the standard until the introduction of the minimally invasive approach either by laparoscopy or robotic surgery. Retrospective data on minimally invasive radical hysterectomy had shown better perioperative results when compared to the open approach with no compromise in oncologic outcomes. However, there are a number of flaws in these retrospective studies including small sample size, comparisons to historical controls, unbalanced groups pertaining to oncologic risk factors and follow-up times.

The only prospective randomized trial comparing open versus minimally invasive radical hysterectomy (LACC trial) was published in October 2018 [1]. In that study, patients with FIGO 2009 stage IA1 (LVSI)-IB1 cervical cancer and histologic subtype of squamous cell carcinoma, adenocarcinoma, or adenosquamous carcinoma, were included. The two groups were similar with regards to histologic subtypes, rate of lymphovascular invasion, rates of parametrial and lymph node involvement, tumor size, tumor grade, and use of adjuvant treatment. The primary outcome was the rate of disease-free survival at 4.5 years. The investigators found that the rate of disease-free survival was 86% with minimally invasive surgery and 96.5% with open surgery. In addition, minimally invasive surgery was also associated with a lower rate of overall survival (three-year rate, 93.8% vs. 99%). Of note, of the patients assigned to minimally invasive surgery, 84.4% underwent laparoscopy and 15.6% robot-assisted surgery. A subsequent study by Melamed et al. [2] evaluated 2461 patients (1236 open surgery vs. 1225 minimally invasive surgery) in determining the effect of minimally invasive surgery on all-cause mortality among women undergoing radical hysterectomy for cervical cancer. Over a median follow-up of 45 months, the four-year mortality was 9.1% among women who underwent minimally invasive surgery and 5.3% among those who underwent open surgery (p=0.002). The adoption of minimally invasive surgery coincided with a decline in the four-year relative survival rate of 0.8% per year after 2006 (p=0.01 for change of trend).

In a subsequent study, data from the LACC trial was evaluated to compare the incidence of adverse events after minimally invasive versus open radical hysterectomy. In that study, Obermair et al. [3] found that the incidence of intraoperative grade ≥2 adverse events was 12% in the minimally invasive group and 10% in the open surgery group (p=0.45) and the overall incidence of postoperative grade ≥2 adverse events was 54% in the minimally invasive group versus 48% in the open group (p=0.14). Of note, 1.4% of patients in the minimally invasive group had wound complications versus 6% in the open surgery group (p=0.004). However, the overall incidence of adverse events was similar between the groups. Lastly, the most recent publication from LACC trial data was reported by Frumovitz et al. [4], where the investigators reported on the quality-of-life comparison between the open versus minimally invasive radical hysterectomy. Eligible patients completed validated quality-of-life and symptom assessments one and six weeks before surgery and at one and at three and six months after surgery, with one tool (Functional Assessment of Cancer Therapy-Cervical [FACT-Cx]) also completed at additional timepoints up to 54 months after surgery. The authors found no difference in the measures of quality of life between open versus minimally invasive radical hysterectomy in the early (≤6 weeks) or late (≥3 months) phase of recovery.

Most recently, Nitecki et al. [5] published a systematic review and meta-analysis of observational studies comparing minimally invasive (laparoscopic or robotic) and open radical hysterectomy in patients with early cervical cancer. Study quality was assessed using the Newcastle-Ottowa Scale with scores of at least 7 points that controlled for confounders by tumor size or stage. In 9499 patients, the pooled hazard of recurrence or death was 71% higher among patients who underwent minimally invasive radical hysterectomy compared to those who underwent open surgery (HR=1.71, 95% CI: 1.36–2.15, p<0.001) and the hazard of death was 56% higher (HR=1.56, 95% CI: 1.16–2.11, p=0.004). These results provided further evidence to support the survival benefit associated with open radical hysterectomy.

Conclusion

As a result of these studies, the National Comprehensive Cancer Network Guidelines (NCCN), European Society of Gynecologic Oncology (ESGO) Guidelines, European Society of Medical Oncology (ESMO) Guidelines, and the FIGO Guidelines have all provided concrete recommendations indicating that open radical hysterectomy should be the current standard of care in the management of patients with early cervical cancer.

References

1. Ramirez PT, et al. Minimally invasive versus abdominal radical hysterectomy for cervical cancer. *N Engl J Med* 2018;379:1895–1904.

2. Melamed A, et al. Survival after minimally invasive radical hysterectomy for early-stage cervical cancer. *N Engl J Med* 2018;379:1905–1914.

3. Obermair A, et al. Incidence of adverse events in minimally invasive vs open radical hysterectomy in early cervical cancer: results of a randomized controlled trial. *Am J Obstet Gynecol* 2020;222:249.e1–249.e10

4. Frumovitz M, et al. Quality of life in patients with cervical cancer after

open versus minimally invasive radical hysterectomy (LACC): a secondary outcome of a multicentre, randomised, open-label, phase 3, non-inferiority trial. *Lancet Oncol* 2020;21:851–860.

5. Nitecki R, et al. Survival after minimally invasive vs open radical hysterectomy for early-stage cervical cancer: a systematic review and meta-analysis. *JAMA Oncol* 2020;6:1019–1027. https://doi.org/10.1001/jamaoncol.2020.1694

43A

Is Radical Surgery or Parametrectomy Needed for Early-stage FIGO IA2 and Microscopic IB1 Cervical Cancer?

Yes

Joo-Hyun Nam and Jeong-Yeol Park

Debate

Approximately 80% of cases of cervical cancer are diagnosed at an early stage, when it is amenable to perform radical surgery. Radical surgery is characterized by parametrectomy, which involves the excision of parametrial tissues, including the ventral (the vesicouterine and vesicovaginal ligaments), lateral (the cardinal ligament), and dorsal (the uterosacral and rectovaginal ligaments) parts of parametrial or paracervical tissues. Insufficient excision is associated with an increased risk of cancer recurrence, whereas excessive excision is associated with an increased risk of surgical morbidity. The extent of parametrectomy should be tailored according to the extent of the cancer.

It is unclear whether parametrectomy should be performed in stage IA2 and microscopic IB1 cervical cancer because parametrectomy is associated with increased surgical morbidity and the frequency of parametrial invasion is very low in small cancers. However, the surrounding tissues are excised during cancer surgery not only because the tumor has invaded the surrounding tissues but also because a sufficient tumor-free resection margin must be secured. A sufficient tumor-free resection margin cannot be secured by removing only the cervix, even in stage IA2 and microscopic IB1 cervical cancer. Therefore, the current treatment guidelines recommend parametrectomy for stage IA2 and microscopic IB1 cervical cancer.

The extent of parametrectomy can be adjusted according to tumor size and the degree of cervical stromal invasion [1]. In stage IA2 and microscopic IB1 cervical cancer, type 2 or type B hysterectomy is mainly performed. The rates of gastrointestinal and urologic complications after type 2 or type B hysterectomy are much lower than those after type 3 or type C hysterectomy [1]. Therefore, surgery-related complications are not generally a concern after type 2 or type B hysterectomy in stage IA2 and microscopic IB1 cervical cancer.

Recent studies have reported the results of predicting the presence or absence of parametrial invasion by a combination of factors such as tumor size, cervical stromal invasion depth, lymphovascular space invasion, and lymph node metastasis [2]. However, it is difficult to exactly determine these predictive factors before surgery. Another form of parametrial involvement is parametrial lymph node metastasis or parametrial lymphovascular space invasion, which differs from direct parametrial invasion and cannot be confirmed before surgery.

The absence of parametrial invasion and the need for parametrectomy are different problems in small cervical cancers. The purpose of parametrectomy is to excise tumor invasion and secure a sufficient tumor-free resection margin. Therefore, parametrectomy is recommended for stage IA2 and microscopic IB1 cervical cancer without suspected parametrial invasion. Sufficient tumor-free resection margins should not be ignored, even in small cervical cancers.

Thus far, no prospective randomized study has evaluated whether simple hysterectomy is a safe treatment for stage IA2 and microscopic IB1 cervical cancer. In retrospective studies, the prognosis of stage IA2 and small IB1 cervical cancer, discovered incidentally after simple hysterectomy, was poor without additional parametrectomy or radiotherapy [3]. The largest retrospective study reported significantly lower survival after simple hysterectomy (92.4%) than after radical hysterectomy (95.3%) in stage IB1 cervical cancer (<2 cm; hazard ratio (HR)=1.55, 95% confidence interval (CI): 1.18–2.03) [4]. A recent meta-analysis also suggested that simple hysterectomy in women with stage IB1 cervical cancer may adversely affect survival [5]. Thus, simple hysterectomy or trachelectomy are insufficient for the treatment of stage IB1 cervical cancer.

Conclusion

One recently completed clinical trial (the CONCERV trial) evaluated the safety of less radical surgery in low-risk, early-stage cervical cancer, which is also being evaluated in the following three ongoing clinical trials: the SHAPE trial (ClinicalTrials.gov, NCT01658930), GOG-278 (ClinialTrials.gov, NCT01649089), and the LESSER trial (ClinialTrials.gov, NCT02613286). In the CONCERV trial, the recurrence rate was 3% in 100 patients with stage IA2–IB1 cervical cancer (<2 cm) with no lymphovascular space invasion and depth of invasion <10 mm after a median follow-up of 25 months (range 0–71 months). In the LACC trial, the recurrence rate was 0.7% in stage IB1 cervical cancer after open radical hysterectomy [6]. A 3% difference may be statistically or clinically significant. However, some surgeons may argue that the increase in morbidity due to radical hysterectomy is not justified for a survival benefit of 3%. However, the morbidity of type 2 or type B hysterectomy is much less than that of type 3 or type C hysterectomy; thus, if the survival benefit is considered, tailored radical hysterectomy with small parametrectomy is an appropriate treatment for stage IA2 or microscopic IB1 cervical cancer.

References

1. Panici PB, et al. Tailoring the parametrectomy in stages IA2-IB1 cervical carcinoma: is it feasible and safe? *Gynecol Oncol* 2005;96:792–798.

2. Frumovitz M, et al. Parametrial involvement in radical hysterectomy specimens for women with early-stage cervical cancer. *Obstet Gynecol* 2009;114:93–99.

3. Park JY, et al. Management of occult invasive cervical cancer found after simple hysterectomy. *Ann Oncol* 2010;21:994–1000.

4. Sia TY, et al. Trends in use and effect on survival of simple hysterectomy for early-stage cervical cancer. *Obstet Gynecol* 2019;134:1132–1143.

5. Wu J, et al. Less-radical surgery for early-stage cervical cancer: a systematic review. *Am J Obstet Gynecol* 2021;224 (4):348–358.e5.

6. Ramirez PT, et al. Minimally invasive versus abdominal radical hysterectomy for cervical cancer. *N Engl J Med* 2018;379:1895–1904.

Debate

Debate

43B
Is Radical Surgery or Parametrectomy Needed for Early-stage FIGO IA2 and Microscopic IB1 Cervical Cancer?

No

Zibi Marchocki and Allan Covens

Debate

Radical hysterectomy or radical trachelectomy with lymph node assessment are considered the treatment of choice in patients with stages IA2 and IB1 cervical cancer (depending on fertility wishes) [1]. However, not only is there no level 1 evidence to support this recommendation, but also radical procedures are associated with significant morbidity. Complications, including perioperative blood loss, bladder, rectal, and sexual dysfunction, as well as fistula formation, adversely affect quality of life. All of those are mainly attributed to the parametrectomy causing destruction of blood vessels and nerve plexuses. As cervical cancer is diagnosed earlier, and women postpone pregnancy until later in life, the need for less radical and fertility-sparing surgery has become more important. Traditionally the rationale for parametrectomy has been to achieve clear margins or to remove potential sites of tumor spread. However, controversy exists as most patients with lymph node involvement and a high proportion of those with tumor invasion >10 mm will receive adjuvant treatment regardless of the radicality of surgery. Prior studies demonstrated that in patients with favorable factors such as tumor size ≤2 cm, depth of stromal invasion <10 mm, absence of lymphovascular space invasion and lymph node involvement, the risk of parametrial involvement is less than 1% [2]. Therefore, it questions the need and role for radical surgery (parametrectomy) in this group of patients. A number of retrospective studies have demonstrated that in selected cases a less radical approach (without parametrectomy) is a safe alternative.

Using the Surveillance, Epidemiology and End Results (SEER) database, Tseng and colleagues compared 807 patients with stage IB1 cervical cancer treated with conization, trachelectomy, or simple hysterectomy to 1764 patients treated with modified radical or radical hysterectomy (lymph node assessment was performed in all groups) [3]. The authors showed a very similar 10-year disease-specific survival between the two groups (93.5% for less radical vs. 92.3% for more radical surgery, p=0.511). The largest retrospective study to date, consisting of 1530 patients with stage IA and 3931 patients with stage IB1 treated with simple and radical hysterectomies, compared simple and radical hysterectomy for stage IA2 and showed no difference in five-year survival rate (simple hysterectomy 97.6% vs. radical 95.1%, hazard ratio (HR)=0.70, 95% confidence interval (CI): 0.41–1.20) [4]. Interestingly patients with stage IB1 disease had a 55% greater risk of death (HR=1.55, 95% CI: 1.18–2.03) after simple hysterectomy compared with radical hysterectomy, with a five-year survival rate of 92.4% and 95.3%, respectively. However, the increased hazard risk of 55% represented a five-year survival difference of 2.9%, which is below the threshold used in most noninferiority oncologic trials (margins typically 5–8%). Additionally, many important prognostic factors and survival outcomes were either missing or incomplete, rendering the final study conclusion questionable. The standard-of-care pelvic lymphadenectomy was omitted in 19% and 2% of stage IB1 patients treated by simple and radical hysterectomy respectively, and more patients received adjuvant chemotherapy and radiation after simple hysterectomy compared with radical hysterectomy (16% vs. 7% for chemotherapy, 9% vs. 3% for radiation). After adjusting for nodal assessment and receipt of adjuvant therapy, the difference in survival was not statistically significant.

More recently Li and colleagues in a small retrospective study, examined 40 patients with low-risk criteria (IA1 with lymphovascular space invasion (LVSI) to IB1, tumor size<2 cm on the diagnostic specimen and no gross visible tumor at preoperative assessment, no radiological evidence of metastasis, (squamous and adenocarcinoma or adeno-squamous histology) treated with simple conization with pelvic lymphadenectomy and demonstrated a two-year recurrence-free period in 97.5% of patients [5]. This is in line with the findings from a prospective, multicenter trial (ConCerv) with 100 patients (IA2–IB1, no LVSI, depth of invasion <10 mm and cone biopsy with negative margins) post-cervical conization or simple hysterectomy and pelvic lymph node assessment [6]. The trial showed that after a median follow-up of 25 months (range 0–71), recurrent disease was diagnosed in only three patients (3%).

Gynecologic Oncology Group (GOG) 278 (NCT01649089) and SHAPE (NCT01658930) are "Gynecologic Oncology Group (GOG) 278 (NCT01649089) and SHAPE (NCT01658930) are both closed to accrual and awaiting results." accrual. GOG 278 is a prospective cohort study evaluating the physical function and quality of life pre- and post-surgery in patients with stage I (IA1 with positive LVSI) and IA2–IB1 ≤2 cm (with no radiological signs of metastases) cervical cancer treated with nonradical surgery. In the SHAPE trial, women with early-stage cervical cancer are randomized to radical or simple hysterectomy. Reassuringly, both trials have been promising, with no safety concerns raised by the data safety monitoring committees so far. Results from both trials are expected this year.

Conclusion

The recent trend towards less radical surgery represents the paradigm shift towards a less radical approach. This is based on the growing evidence suggesting that in patients with a low risk of parametrial involvement (tumor size ≤2 cm, depth of stromal invasion <10 mm, absence of lymphovascular space invasion and lymph node involvement) non-radical surgery (conization, trachelectomy, or hysterectomy) with lymph node assessment is a safe alternative to radical surgery (parametrectomy).

References

1. National Comprehensive Cancer Network. NCCN guidelines in oncology: cervical cancer. Available at: www.nccn.org/profes sionals/physician_gls/pdf/cervical.pdf. Retrieved September 11, 2020.

2. Covens A, et al. How important is removal of the parametrium at surgery for carcinoma of the cervix? *Gynecol Oncol* 2002;84 (1):145–149. https://doi.org/10.1006/gyno .2001.6493

3. Tseng JH, et al. Less versus more radical surgery in stage IB1 cervical cancer: a population-based study of long-term survival. *Gynecol Oncol* 2018;150:44–49.

4. Sia TY, et al. Trends in use and effect on survival of simple hysterectomy for early-stage cervical cancer. *Obstet Gynecol* 2019;134:1132–1143.

5. Li X, et al. Simple conization and pelvic lymphadenectomy in early-stage cervical cancer: a retrospective analysis and review of the literature. *Gynecol Oncol* 2020;158(2):231–235. https://doi.org/10.1016/j.ygyno.2020.05.035

6. Schmeler K, et al. Concerv: a prospective trial of conservative surgery for low-risk early-stage cervical cancer *Int J Gynecol Cancer* 2019;29: A14–A15.

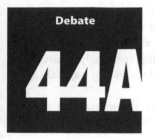

What is the Best Management Option for Young Women with Stage IB2 Cervical Cancer Who Wish to Preserve Fertility?

Abdominal Radical Trachelectomy

Michael Frumovitz

Debate

In 1998, Michel Roy and Marie Plante published the oft-cited criteria identifying appropriate candidates for radical trachelectomy in women with cervical cancer [1]. These criteria included:

1. Desire to preserve fertility
2. No clinical evidence of impaired fertility
3. Stage IA2 to IB (International Federation of Gynecology and Obstetrics)
4. Lesion size <2 cm
5. Limited endocervical involvement at colposcopic evaluation
6. No evidence of pelvic node metastasis

Over the last two decades, these "criteria" have transformed into guidelines and, for some, into dogma. These criteria were originally developed to assess patients for possible vaginal radical trachelectomy. Some of these factors are now routinely ignored such as "no clinical evidence of impaired fertility" as many seemingly infertile patients have achieved pregnancy after radical trachelectomy with assisted reproductive technologies. Others such as "limited endocervical involvement on colposcopic evaluation" have been replaced by preoperative imaging such as magnetic resonance imaging (MRI). MRI has a sensitivity of 82% and a specificity of 93% in predicting an endocervical margin of ≤ or >5 mm between the tumor and the internal os in radical trachelectomy candidates [2].

The "hard" cut-off of tumors <2 cm has been retained by many who perform the procedure. However, this size limitation was proposed by those performing vaginal radical trachelectomies likely due to the smaller amount of parametrium resected and the difficulty achieving an adequate endocervical margin during the vaginal approach. As surgeons recognized that an abdominal approach allowed for larger parametrial resections and easier assessment of where to transect the cervix to obtain a tumor-free margin while retaining enough cervical stump for re-anastomosis, they began to include women with tumors >2 cm in size.

Even with the ability to perform surgery that is more "radical" by the abdominal approach, many believe performing this procedure in women with stage IB2 leads to compromised oncologic outcomes. Although only retrospective data exist, systematic reviews show an overall recurrence rate of 7% after abdominal radical trachelectomy for women with tumors 2–4 cm in size which is comparable to that seen after radical hysterectomy for women with similarly sized tumors [3]. Furthermore, it is seemingly equivalent to the 10% recurrence rate seen after neoadjuvant chemotherapy followed by vaginal radical trachelectomy in women with stage IB2 disease.

In 2006, Alexander Burnett proposed updated criteria that summarize the decision making that most undertake when choosing appropriate candidates for radical trachelectomy for tumors 2–4 cm [4].

1. Can the cancer be safely and completely removed?
2. Does the woman wish to retain her uterus?
3. Is she informed of the risks, benefits, and alternatives to this procedure?

The main criteria of "can the cancer be safely and completely removed" truly focuses on achieving the expected oncologic outcomes that are equivalent to radical hysterectomy in these patients. The National Comprehensive Cancer Network (NCCN) guidelines acknowledge that radical trachelectomy is "most validated" for tumors < 2 cm but also stipulates that abdominal radical trachelectomy is an option for appropriately selected women with stage IB2 tumors. In other words, NCCN guidelines state abdominal radical trachelectomy is a reasonable fertility-sparing option in women with cervical cancers 2–4 cm in size in whom the cancer can "be safely and completely removed."

To these three criteria proposed by Burnett, I would add, "Does preoperative evaluation (exam, pathology, and imaging) suggest little risk for completion hysterectomy or postoperative radiotherapy?" Although achieving optimal oncologic outcomes is the primary consideration when making therapeutic recommendations to women with early-stage cervical cancer, the "raison d'être" for performing fertility-sparing surgery is (obviously) to spare fertility. A patient who is likely to have high-risk factors (positive margins, positive nodes, or positive parametrium) or have intermediate risk factor (Sedlis Criteria) for postoperative radiation should not be considered for either abdominal radical trachelectomy or neoadjuvant chemotherapy followed by vaginal radical trachelectomy. When evaluating 246 patients from 10 published studies on abdominal radical trachelectomy in women with stage IB2 cervical cancer, van Kol et al. [3] found that 204 (83%) ultimately had a fertility-sparing procedure completed. This compared favorably to 69 (75%) out of 92 patients with stage IB2 cervical cancer who retained their uterus and ovaries and did not need adjuvant radiation therapy after neoadjuvant chemotherapy followed by vaginal radical trachelectomy.

That said, fertility-sparing procedures do not necessarily mean patients can still get pregnant. For example, patients may encounter infertility due to cervical stenosis or Asherman's syndrome after a radical trachelectomy or decreased ovarian reserve and ovulation after neoadjuvant chemotherapy. In this manner, there may be an improvement in pregnancy rates for patients who undergo neoadjuvant chemotherapy and vaginal radical trachelectomy when compared to abdominal radical hysterectomy. In one large review of the literature, 19 (70%) of 27 women who attempted to conceive achieved pregnancy after neoadjuvant chemotherapy followed by vaginal radical trachelectomy compared to pregnancies achieved in only 17 (21%) of 82 women who attempted to conceive after abdominal radical trachelectomy [3]. Once pregnancy is achieved, however, pregnancy outcomes such as term births and live births are similar between the two approaches. It is important to note that these are very small sample sizes from retrospective studies so these results must be interpreted with great caution.

Conclusion

Fortunately, we will have good prospective data on neoadjuvant chemotherapy and vaginal radical trachelectomy. The CONTESSA/NEOCON-F study is currently enrolling 90 women with stage IB2 cervical cancer in a prospective, phase II trial of neoadjuvant chemotherapy followed by vaginal radical trachelectomy [5]. Outcomes include success rate of completing fertility-sparing surgery without the need for radiation, response rate to chemotherapy, overall survival, and pregnancy rates among other endpoints. The study is expected to complete accrual in 2022 and report in 2025.

References

1. Roy M, et al. Pregnancies after radical vaginal trachelectomy for early-stage cervical cancer, *Am J Obstet Gynecol* 1998;179:1491–1496.

2. Bhosale PR, et al. Is MRI helpful in assessing the distance of the tumour from the internal os in patients with cervical cancer below FIGO Stage IB2? *Clin Radiol* 2016;71:515–522.

3. van Kol KGG, et al. Abdominal radical trachelectomy versus chemotherapy followed by vaginal radical trachelectomy in stage 1B2 (FIGO 2018) cervical cancer. A systematic review on fertility and recurrence rates. *Gynecol Oncol* 2019;155:515–521.

4. Burnett AF. Radical trachelectomy with laparoscopic lymphadenectomy: review of oncologic and obstetrical outcomes, *Curr Opin Obstet Gynecol* 2006;18:8–13.

5. Plante M, et al. FIGO 2018 stage IB2 (2–4 cm) Cervical cancer treated with Neo-adjuvant chemotherapy followed by fertility Sparing Surgery (CONTESSA); Neo-Adjuvant Chemotherapy and Conservative Surgery in Cervical Cancer to Preserve Fertility (NEOCON-F). A PMHC, DGOG, GCIG/CCRN and multicenter study. *Int J Gynecol Cancer* 2019;29:969–975.

Debate

44B What is the Best Management Option for Young Women with Stage IB2 Cervical Cancer Who Wish to Preserve Fertility?

Neo-adjuvant Chemotherapy Followed by Fertility-sparing Surgery

Marie Plante

Debate

Upfront Radical Trachelectomy

The radical trachelectomy (RT) procedure is feasible but technically challenging in patients with larger size lesions. Recurrence rates are clearly higher following the vaginal or laparoscopic approach (17–21%). Abdominal and robotic approaches appear to be better options in terms of radicality. However, there is increasing concern over the minimally invasive (MIS) approach in view of the reported increased risk of recurrence and death compared to abdominal approach when a radical hysterectomy is performed (LACC trial). Logically, the same concerns would apply if RT is performed by MIS particularly in the face of a macroscopic cervical lesion. Therefore, upfront abdominal RT (ART) appears to be the best option for patients with lesions >2 cm.

However, the reported rates of positive nodes in lesions measuring 2–4 cm is in the range of 10–15%. Therefore, following upfront ART, the probability of patients requiring adjuvant treatment because of positive nodes, or because of positive margins or parametrium (Peters criteria) or in the presence of intermediate risk factors (Sedlis criteria) identified on the final pathology of the trachelectomy specimen is significant (up to 26%). In most centers, these patients would receive adjuvant (chemo)/radiation which would not only ruin fertility potential but also ruin ovarian function in this young patient population. In a large series of 333 ART of which 132 had lesions >2 cm, up to 48% of patients required adjuvant treatment because of unfavorable pathological findings.

Neo-adjuvant Chemotherapy Followed by Fertility-sparing Surgery

The rationale to offer neo-adjuvant chemotherapy (NACT) to women with larger cervical cancer is to "cytoreduce" the size of the lesion in order to perform a less radical fertility sparing surgery (FSS), reduce the chances of requiring adjuvant treatment, and improve fertility and obstetrical outcome. The concept is based on the fact that cervical cancer is a chemo-sensitive cancer with reported response rate >70%. Prior to initiating NACT, a pelvic MRI is essential to carefully assess the size of the lesion and exclude extracervical/extrauterine extension. In general, three cycles of platinum/paclitaxel combination are given followed by a pelvic MRI to assess tumor response. In patients with complete or optimal response (i.e., residual tumor <2 cm) a less radical FSS is performed (large conization or simple trachelectomy). There is no clear evidence that more radical procedures in good responders is associated with better oncologic outcomes. Considering the trend towards less radical surgery in patients with small-volume tumors, it makes sense to offer this option to patients with optimal response following NACT, considering its lower surgical morbidity and excellent obstetrical results. Data from 264 cone/simple trachelectomies shows a recurrence rate of 1.7% and live birth rate of 73% [1]. Conversely, patients with suboptimal response to chemotherapy, (residual tumor >2 cm following NACT) have poorer outcome, higher rates of recurrence, and should be treated more aggressively (definitive chemoradiation or radical hysterectomy).

Available data on NACT/FSS for women with lesions measuring 2–4 cm remains limited to small retrospective series [1]. A standardized approach with regards to the optimal management of these patients will be conducted through a recently initiated prospective international phase II trial (Contessa/Neocon-F trial) [2].

Comparison between the Two Options

A recent literature review comparing NACT/ Vaginal Radical Trachelectomy (VRT) versus upfront ART specifically in patients with lesions measuring 2–4 cm was recently published and confirms that both options have comparable oncologic outcome, but NACT/FSS is definitively superior in terms of obstetrical outcome (Table 44B.1) [3].

Morbidity

The surgical morbidity of upfront ART is clearly superior compared to less radical procedures (simple trachelectomy or conization). In addition to higher risks of infection and bleeding, very serious complications such as uterovaginal anastomosis dehiscence and

Table 44B.1 Comparative oncologic and obstetrical outcome between NACT/VRT versus ART in women with cervical cancer measuring 2–4 cm

	NACT/VRT n=92	ART n=246
Attempts to conceive	39%	40%
Chances of getting pregnant	21%	7%
Successful pregnancy	70%	21%
Live birth rate	63%	42%
Recurrence rate	10%	6.9%
Death rate	2.9%	3.4%

From van Kol et al. [3]

uterine necrosis have been reported following ART. Extensive parametrial excision can also impair fallopian tube motility, malfunction, or cause obstruction. Lastly, uterine atrophy (secondary to uterine arteries ligation) may lead to Asherman's syndrome and cervical stenosis, all of which are associated with lower fertility and worse obstetrical outcome [4].

Oncologic Outcome

The oncologic outcome between the two options is actually comparable. In the van Kol review, the recurrence rate was 10% versus 6.9% and the death rate was 2.9% versus 3.4% for the NACT/FSS versus ART respectively (Table 44B.1) [3]. Fokom et al. calculated a recurrence rate and mortality rate following NACT/FSS of 8.5% and 2.1% respectively [1]. Bentivegna et al. also conducted an extensive systematic review and reported comparable recurrence rates of 4.3% versus 3.8% between the two procedures [5].

Fertility Outcome

Fertility preservation is better following NACT/FSS (ranging from 80–100%) compared to ART. In a recent large series of 211 ART, only 17.4% of women who attempted to conceive succeeded (fertility rate of only 7.2%); most infertility problems were related to cervical stenosis and fallopian tube obstruction [4]. According to van Kol et al., chances of getting pregnant following NACT/FSS were 21% compared to 7% following ART [3]. In Bentivegna's review, pregnancy rate was 77% following NACT/FSS versus 44% following ART [5]. Although there is a potential risk of premature ovarian insufficiency following NACT, this does not appear to be a major issue in most studies in terms of fertility.

Obstetrical Outcome

Obstetrical outcomes are clearly superior following NACT/FSS compared to ART. As can be seen in Table 44B.1, successful pregnancy rate following NACT/FSS is 70% compared to 21% for ART with a live birth rate of 63% versus 42% in favor of NACT/FSS [3]. Pregnancies following ART are associated with higher rates of obstetrical complications such as premature rupture of membranes and premature labor compared to simple trachelectomy or cone. Obstetrical outcome according to the type of FSS shows a prematurity rate of 57% following ART versus 15% after NACT/FSS [5].

Conclusion

A literature review comparing NACT/VRT versus upfront ART specifically in patients with lesions measuring between 2–4 cm was recently published and confirms that both options have comparable oncologic outcome, but NACT/FSS is definitively superior in terms of obstetrical outcome (Table 44B.1) [3]. Since the ultimate objective of these young patients is precisely to preserve fertility, NACT/FSS appears to be the best option. Even though upfront ART is technically doable, it is associated with higher surgical morbidity and worse obstetrical outcome.

Since a prospective randomized trial comparing both options is unlikely to ever be conducted considering the rarity of those cases and the number of patients that would be required to see a meaningful difference in outcome, we must currently rely on very heterogeneous retrospective data with a variable level of evidence to guide management. It is hoped that the Contessa/Neocon-F trial will provide solid data as to the oncologic safety, fertility preservation, and obstetrical outcome with the NACT/FSS approach [2].

References

1. Fokom Domgue J, et al. Conservative management of cervical cancer: current status and obstetrical implications. *Best Pract Res Clin Obstet Gynaecol* 2019;55:79–92.

2. Plante M, et al. FIGO 2018 stage IB2 (2–4 cm) cervical cancer treated with neo-adjuvant chemotherapy followed by fertility sparing surgery (CONTESSA); neoadjuvant chemotherapy and conservative surgery in cervical cancer to preserve fertility (NEOCON-F). *Int J Gynecol Cancer* 2019;29:969–975.

3. van Kol KGG, et al. Abdominal radical trachelectomy versus chemotherapy followed by vaginal radical trachelectomy in stage 1B2 (FIGO 2018) cervical cancer. A systematic review on fertility and recurrence rates. *Gynecol Oncol* 2019;155:515–521.

4. Li X, et al. Reproductive and obstetric outcomes after abdominal radical trachelectomy (ART) for patients with early-stage cervical cancers in Fudan, China. *Gynecol Oncol* 2020;157:418–422.

5. Bentivegna E, et al. Fertility results and pregnancy outcomes after conservative treatment of cervical cancer: a systematic review of the literature. *Fertil Steril* 2016;106:1195–1211(e5).

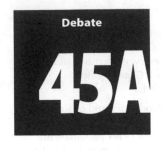

Debate

Should Adjuvant Hysterectomy be Performed for Patients with Locally Advanced Cervical Cancer Treated with Concurrent Chemoradiotherapy?

Yes

Dib Sassine, Alexandra Diggs, and Yukio Sonoda

Debate

The utility of adjuvant hysterectomy (AH) after concurrent chemo-radiation (CCRT) for the management of locally advanced cervical cancer (LACC) has been the subject of debate for over 20 years. Up to 64% of hysterectomy specimens in patients who have received CCRT have evidence of residual disease on pathology. In this setting, many gynecologic oncologists see a benefit in AH to decrease rates of local recurrence [1].

In 2003, Keys et al. evaluated the role of AH in patients who received pelvic radiation only for FIGO 1998 stage IB bulky cervical cancer. It demonstrated that patients with a large tumor burden having lesions 4–6 cm may benefit from AH after pelvic radiation, without increasing the rate of grade 3 or 4 adverse events [2].

To our knowledge, since these earlier studies, there have only been two additional randomized controlled trials (RCTs) comparing the outcomes of CCRT alone versus CCRT followed by AH [3,4].

A French trial attempted to investigate the therapeutic impact of AH after CCRT. The trial included patients with stage IB2 and stage II who had received external beam radiation therapy with concomitant cisplatin, followed by brachytherapy. Patients were randomized AH versus no AH. It did not show any difference between both arms in terms of recurrence and overall survival (OS). However, it is worth mentioning that the trial was underpowered as it suffered from a failure of accrual, and had to close early after enrollment of only 61 of the 320 planned patients [3].

A randomized trial from Mexico from 2014 aimed in turn to demonstrate that AH after CCRT radically improved survival outcomes when compared with standard brachytherapy. The study failed to show any difference in survival between both arms. The authors acknowledged that the study design many have over-estimated the potential benefit of radical hysterectomy and thus was underpowered. However, the trial did demonstrate both the safety and feasibility of AH following CCRT [4].

Owing to the scarcity of well-designed RCTs showing a benefit to AH, most of the available literature consists of retrospective data as well as single institution data.

A meta-analysis by Shim et al. published in *Gynecologic Oncology* in 2018, which included the aforementioned RCTs and six observational studies, demonstrated that AH following CCRT significantly decreased the risk of local recurrence by 44% (OR=0.56, 95% CI: 0.33–0.96, p=0.034), but had no effect on rates of distant metastasis. This benefit was again demonstrated in patients receiving combination external beam radiation therapy and vaginal brachytherapy, with a pooled OR of 0.58 (95% CI: 0.41–0.83, p<0.05) favoring CCRT + AH [5]. The same meta-analysis also concluded that there was no significant difference in late adverse events (grade 3 or higher) between the two groups.

A more recent meta-analysis by Lu et al. in *Oncology Letters* (2021), including 12 retrospective studies and the aforementioned RCTs, reported no significant differences in the cancer stage distribution between the two groups [6]. The CCRT + AH group had a significantly improved OS and disease-free survival than the CCRT alone group (HR=0.72, 95% CI: 0.56–0.91, p=0.007, and HR=0.72, 95% CI: 0.56–0.93, p=0.01, respectively). The incidence of recurrence was also significantly reduced in the CCRT + AH group compared to CCRT alone (17.14% vs. 26.96%, OR=0.61, 95% CI: 0.47–0.79, p=0.0002). Importantly, all of these statistically significant differences were observed only in pooled analyses of the retrospective studies [6].

The majority of the locally advanced cervical cancers in the previously mentioned studies were squamous cell carcinoma (SCC), as compared to adenocarcinoma, which may be both more chemo-resistant and radio-resistant.

A retrospective study by Yang et al., looking at locally advanced adenocarcinoma of the cervix, showed a significant improvement in PFS as well as OS in the group of patients who underwent CCRT + AH compared to CCRT alone, (median PFS 48 months vs. 10 months, HR=0.3431, 95% CI: 0.152–0.772, p=0.0097 and median OS 58 months vs. 36 months, HR=0.3667, 95% CI: 0.139–0.964, p=0.0419 respectively [7].

Conclusion

Currently, retrospective data and subsequent meta-analyses are the only available data to support the use of AH after CCRT for LACC. This data supports the practice of adjuvant hysterectomy in patients with residual disease after CCRT, especially in the chemo-radio-resistant and less common tumors such as AC. That being said, special attention should be paid to assessing for distant metastases in these patients prior to proceeding with definitive surgical management.

References

1. Yang J, et al. Completion hysterectomy after chemoradiotherapy for locally advanced adeno-type cervical carcinoma: updated survival outcomes and experience in post radiation surgery. *J Gynecol Oncol* 2020;31 (2):e16.

2. Keys HM, et al. Radiation therapy with and without extrafascial hysterectomy for bulky stage IB cervical carcinoma: a randomized trial of the Gynecologic Oncology Group. *Gynecol Oncol* 2003;89(3):343–353.

3. Morice P, et al. Results of the GYNECO 02 study, an FNCLCC phase III trial comparing hysterectomy with no hysterectomy in patients with a (clinical and radiological) complete response after chemoradiation therapy for stage IB2 or II cervical cancer. *Oncologist* 2012;17(1):64–71.

4. Cetina L, et al. Brachytherapy versus radical hysterectomy after external beam chemoradiation with gemcitabine plus cisplatin: a randomized, phase III study in IB2-IIB cervical cancer patients. *Ann Oncol* 2013;24(8):2043–2047.

5. Shim SH, et al. Impact of adjuvant hysterectomy on prognosis in patients with locally advanced cervical cancer treated with concurrent chemoradiotherapy: a meta-analysis. *J Gynecol Oncol* 2018;29(2):e25.

6. Lu W, et al. Chemoradiotherapy alone vs. chemoradiotherapy and hysterectomy for locally advanced cervical cancer: a systematic review and updated meta-analysis. *Oncol Lett* 2021;21(2):160.

7. Yang J, et al. Extrafascial hysterectomy after concurrent chemoradiotherapy in locally advanced cervical adenocarcinoma. *J Gynecol Oncol* 2016;27(4):e40.

45B Should Adjuvant Hysterectomy be Performed for Patients with Locally Advanced Cervical Cancer Treated with Concurrent Chemoradiotherapy?

No

Philippe Morice, Sebastien Gouy, and Cyrus Chargari

Debate

Concomitant chemoradiation (CRT) followed by brachytherapy (BT) is considered as the standard treatment for locally advanced cervical cancers in many countries. Adjuvant hysterectomy in patients treated with primary radiation therapy had been the aim of endless discussions. Adjuvant hysterectomy after such treatment had been widely used and evaluated in numerous retrospective analyses during the last two decades. The theoretical advantage is to remove any potential residual disease after CRT, thereby improving survival.

In a randomized trial conducted by Keys et al. comparing CRT and adjuvant hysterectomy versus external radiation therapy (ERT) and adjuvant hysterectomy, the rate of residual disease was lower in patients who received CRT compared to those treated with ERT but was still reported to be 48% (vs. 59% in patients treated without concurrent chemotherapy) [1]. This "high" rate should be evaluated with caution because it is strongly correlated with the technical modalities of external radiation therapy and BT and also with the timing of the surgery after the end of radiation therapy. Nevertheless, such a result was the theoretical basis to consider a routine hysterectomy in this context to remove potential residual cells that could explain recurrence or treatment failure.

Such a trial had been done before the major technical evolution of BT procedures and development of 3D image-guided adaptive BT that is now the standard of care for this technique, allowing dose escalations, which yield excellent local control while shielding organs [2]. The other major issue that needs to be integrated in the evaluation of adjuvant hysterectomy in this context is the morbidity of the pelvic surgery in this previously irradiated area. In a prior study on morbidity caused by radical hysterectomy via laparotomic approach after external radiation therapy for stage I or II cervical cancer, the rate of major morbidity was almost 25% [3]. This rate was correlated with the radicality of the hysterectomy (parametrial dissection) [3]. Such systematic radical hysterectomy should then surely be abandoned at least in patients with a "complete" clinical and radiological response. In such cases, a "simple" hysterectomy is theoretically sufficient but even with such a procedure, urological or intestinal morbidities could be observed due to the combination of the previous treatment and an additional pelvic dissection and de-vascularization of the pelvic organs. The use of a laparoscopic approach could reduce the morbidity rate, however, even lowering the morbidity rate does not justify the indication for this surgery from an oncological point of view.

Only randomized trials could evaluate accurately the therapeutic impact of completion surgery after radiation therapy. One randomized trial (carried out before the era of CRT) compared patients treated with initial radiation therapy and randomly allocated to hysterectomy versus no hysterectomy (whatever the presence of residual disease) but failed to demonstrate any benefit for overall survival with adjuvant hysterectomy [4].

Fifteen years ago, we conducted a phase III trial in patients with "complete" response following CRT and BT (evaluated between six to eight weeks after the end of the treatment) comparing hysterectomy versus no hysterectomy, but the trial had to be closed after three years due to lack of recruitment (only 61 patients were randomized). Nevertheless, despite the lack of power for this study, hysterectomy had no impact on survival rate [5].

According to the potential morbidity of adjuvant hysterectomy and unproved therapeutic impact of such a procedure, many teams and countries considered that such a strategy is now obsolete and should be abandoned at least in patients having a "complete" response after CRT and BT in locally advanced cervical cancer. Such surgery could be potentially considered in countries having no or low access to high quality BT [6]. But this should not be an argument to abandon BT and to increase the use of hysterectomy (and/or the dose of external radiation therapy) to replace it because such management will have an impact on overall morbidity rates and furthermore recent major data from the United States demonstrated clearly that omission of BT impacts negatively the survival of patients in locally advanced cervical cancer [2].

Is there potentially a subgroup of patients in whom hysterectomy would be helpful? This could be theoretically the case for patients with residual disease at the end of CRT and BT. This situation of "real" residual tumor with remaining disease >1 cm is rare with the modern techniques of external radiation therapy and BT (<10%). Thus, this surgery, in such a context of residual disease, should be considered as a "salvage" surgery and not simply as an adjuvant hysterectomy due to the possibly or requiring a radical hysterectomy or even pelvic exenteration (with higher rates of major postoperative morbidities), in order to optimize the rate of free surgical margins.

Additionally, patients who have a more "chemo-radio-resistant" disease also have a higher rate of concurrent extra-cervical disease (nodal involvement, peritoneal disease), explaining the high rate of (pelvic and extra pelvic) recurrences in patients with bulky residual disease following completion surgery at the end of treatment. This is why, even if salvage surgery should be considered in these latter cases, we strongly recommend a repeated complete radiological work-up is used (including new PET/CT imaging, even if done initially before CRT is begun) to select the best candidates and to exclude patients with obvious distant disease before such potentially radical surgery

Conclusion

Finally, these considerations also raise the question of the best modalities to accurately evaluate the presence of residual disease. Post-brachytherapy imaging, particularly using magnetic resonance imaging (MRI), is the conventional approach with which to evaluate it, but with the risk of false positives results. PET imaging or cone biopsies have also been proposed to increase this accuracy, but the main issue for PET imaging is the delay in using it after the end of treatment. Concerns regarding cone biopsies include morbidity (secondary bleeding) and accuracy. Currently, we have not yet determined the most accurate procedure or combination of techniques to optimally predict the quality of response after CRT and BT.

References

1. Keys HM, et al. Cisplatin, radiation and adjuvant hysterectomy compared with radiation and adjuvant hysterectomy for bulky stage Ib cervical carcinoma. *N Engl J Med* 1999;341:708.

2. Chargari C, et al. Brachytherapy: an overview for clinicians. *CA Cancer J Clin* 2019;69:386–401.

3. Touboul C, et al. Prognostic factors and morbidities after completion surgery in patients undergoing initial chemoradiation therapy for locally advanced cervical cancer. *Oncologist* 2010;15:405–415.

4. Keys HM, et al. Gynecologic Oncology Group. Radiation therapy with and without extrafascial hysterectomy for bulky stage IB cervical carcinoma: a randomized trial of the Gynecologic Oncology Group. *Gynecol Oncol* 2003;89:343–353.

5. Morice P, et al. Results of the GYNECO 02/108 phase III trial. Results of the GYNECO 02 study, an FNCLCC phase III trial comparing hysterectomy with no hysterectomy in patients with a (clinical and radiological) complete response after chemoradiation therapy for stage IB2 or II cervical cancer. *Oncologist* 2012;17:64–71.

6. Cetina L, et al. Brachytherapy versus radical hysterectomy after external beam chemoradiation with gemcitabine plus cisplatin: a randomized, phase III study in IB2-IIB cervical cancer patients. *Ann Oncol* 2013;24:2043–2047.

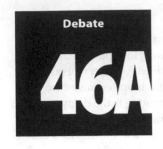

Debate

What is the Best Initial Treatment for Stage IB3 to IIB Cervical Cancer?
Neoadjuvant Chemotherapy Followed by Radical Hysterectomy

Jolien Haesen, Rawand Salihi, and Ignace B. Vergote

Debate

Neo-adjuvant chemotherapy (NACT) for cervical cancer reduces preoperatively the tumor size and metastatic spread. In addition, long-term adverse events of radiochemotherapy (CCRT), such as early menopause, dyspareunia, radio-enteritis and fistulas can be avoided.

A meta-analysis showed a significant benefit of neoadjuvant chemotherapy (NACT) followed by surgery compared with radiotherapy alone. In addition, a better five-year survival was observed with a short cycle (<14 days) NACT than with three-weekly regimens. Two randomized phase III trials compared NACT followed by surgery with radiochemotherapy (CCRT), and showed similar overall survival with both treatment strategies. In both studies the disease-free survival for FIGO stage IB3 and stage IIA were also similar.

In conclusion, NACT followed by surgery can be considered as a valuable alternative for CCRT in patients with cervical cancer FIGO stage IB3 or IIA, especially in premenopausal patients.

Locally advanced cervical cancer, including FIGO IB3–IVA, is mainly treated by CCRT followed by brachytherapy. Although in patients with stage IB3–IIB there is some evidence that NACT followed by a radical hysterectomy (RH) might be an alternative.

By adding NACT to the treatment regimen, the tumor size can be reduced, making inoperable tumors operable. In addition, better control of micro-metastatic disease can be achieved. A meta-analysis showed a significant benefit of NACT followed by RH compared with radiotherapy (without chemotherapy). In addition, a better five-year survival was observed with a short cycle (<14 days) NACT than with three-weekly regimens [1].

Recently, two large randomized phase III studies compared NACT + RH versus CCRT in cervical cancer FIGO stage IB3–IIB [2–3]. The first large single-center randomized controlled trial reported by Gupta et al. included 635 patients randomized to NACT with three-weekly carboplatin/paclitaxel followed by RH versus CCRT, and showed a five-year disease-free survival of 69.3% and 76.7%, respectively (HR=1.38, p=0.038) [2]. However overall survival was 75.4% and 74.7%, respectively. Subgroup analyses of patients with FIGO stage IB3 or IIA patients showed a similar disease-free survival with both treatment strategies. The delayed toxicities at 24 months or later after treatment completion in the

NACT + RH group versus the CCRT group were rectal (2.2% vs. 3.5%, respectively), bladder (1.6% vs. 3.5%, respectively), and vaginal (12.0% vs. 25.6%, respectively).

The EORTC 55994 study randomized 626 patients with cervical cancer FIGO stage IB3, IIA2, and IIB between cisplatin-based NACT (in total at least 225 mg/m² cisplatinum) followed by RH versus CCRT (80 Gy to high-risk PTV, with brachytherapy performed in 97% of patients). The primary endpoint, overall survival, was similar in both groups. Progression-free survival at five years was 56.9% and 65.6% for NACT and CCRT, respectively (p=0.021). However, in patients with FIGO stage IB3 (HR=0.89) NACT tended to be better than CCRT. In addition, in patients younger than 50 years old, the progression-free survival was similar with both treatment strategies. Long-term toxicity was lower in the NACT + RH group (15%) versus the CCRT group (20%), with more specifically excess of Chassagne grade 3–4 small bowel, colon, and vaginal complications in the CCRT group [3].

Although several studies have investigated the performance of different regimens of NACT for locally advanced cervical cancer, the ideal regimen, number, and dosage of NACT-courses remains uncertain. Paclitaxel – ifosfamide – cisplatinum three-weekly (TIP) as NACT regime has been shown to be one of the most efficient, however, the hematologic and nonhematologic toxicity is substantial [4]. As mentioned before, a meta-analysis showed that short cycles (<14 days) should be preferred. Therefore, we investigated a regimen with nine weekly dosages of paclitaxel (60 mg/m²) and carboplatin (AUC 2.7) and observed similar response rates and a better tolerability than with the TIP regimen [5].

Conclusion

In conclusion, NACT followed by surgery can be considered as a valuable alternative for CCRT in patients with cervical cancer FIGO stage IB3 or IIA, especially in premenopausal patients. In addition, in regions with no or not enough radiotherapy resources, NACT followed by surgery can be a valuable alternative for CCRT in FIGO IB3–IIB cervical cancer.

References

1. Tierney J. Neoadjuvant chemotherapy for locally advanced cervical cancer: a systematic review and meta-analysis of individual patient data from 21 randomised trials. *Eur J Cancer* 2003;39:2470–2486.

2. Gupta S, et al. Neoadjuvant chemotherapy followed by radical surgery versus concomitant chemotherapy and radiotherapy in patients with stage IB2, IIA, or IIB squamous cervical cancer: a randomized controlled trial. *J Clin Oncol* 2018;36(16):1548–1555.

3. Kenter G, et al. Results from neoadjuvant chemotherapy followed by surgery compared to chemoradiation for stage Ib2–IIb cervical cancer, EORTC 55994. *J Clin Oncol* 2019;37(15):5503.

4. Buda A, et al. Randomized trial of neoadjuvant chemotherapy comparing paclitaxel, ifosfamide, and cisplatin with ifosfamide and cisplatin followed by radical surgery in patients with locally advanced squamous cell cervical carcinoma: the SNAP01 (studio neo-adjuvante portio) Italian collaborative study. *J Clin Oncol* 2005;23:4137–4145.

5. Salihi R, et al. Neoadjuvant weekly paclitaxel-carboplatin is effective in stage I–II cervical cancer. *Int J Gynecol Cancer* 2017;27(6):1256–1260.

What is the Best Initial Treatment for Stage IB3 to IIB Cervical Cancer?

Primary Chemoradiation

Sudeep Gupta, Amita Maheshwari, and Supriya Chopra

Debate

The worldwide burden of cervical cancer continues to be high, with a substantial proportion of patients presenting with locally advanced disease. These are either large tumors and/or those which have infiltrated into vagina, parametrium, or other pelvic organs.

Historically, the first definitive treatment for invasive cervical cancer was radical hysterectomy. The classical indications of an unresectable tumor are infiltration of pelvic side walls and/or fixed pelvic lymph nodes. It is also known that radiation doses that are possible to be safely delivered using a combination of external beam radiotherapy (EBRT) and brachytherapy can cure many patients with advanced-stage cancer. One of the most important advances in cervical cancer was the demonstration, about two decades ago, that platinum-based chemotherapy delivered concurrently with radiotherapy could significantly improve disease-free survival (DFS) and overall survival (OS) in patients with locally advanced cervical cancer [1]. These results made concurrent chemoradiation (CTRT) the standard of care [2].

Another promising treatment strategy that has been studied in patients with FIGO stage IB2 (current stage IB3), IIA, and IIB disease, is neoadjuvant chemotherapy followed by surgery (NACT-surgery). The results of two randomized phase III trials comparing CTRT with NACT-surgery have now been presented [3,4]. Both studies have several similarities and a few notable differences. The control arm of both studies was CTRT using weekly cisplatin at a dose of 40 mg/m^2 and radiotherapy delivered in appropriate doses and durations. The investigational treatment in the Tata Memorial Hospital (TMH) study [3] was three cycles of paclitaxel and carboplatin followed by type III radical hysterectomy, with protocol defined cross-over to CTRT in case of suboptimal response. The investigational treatment in the EORTC study [4] was neoadjuvant cisplatin-based chemotherapy, with minimum cumulative planned dose of cisplatin $>/= 225$ mg/m^2, followed by surgery. Remarkably, 57% of the patients in both studies had stage IIB disease. The primary endpoint of the TMH study was DFS while that of the EORTC study was OS, and both studies have been reported with sufficient follow-up.

The results of both studies showed significantly higher five-year DFS with CTRT compared with NACT-surgery, with absolute differences of 7.4% and 8.6% in TMH and EORTC studies, respectively (Figure 46B.1). The DFS curves split apart early and stayed apart during the entire course of follow-up. OS was not significantly different between the

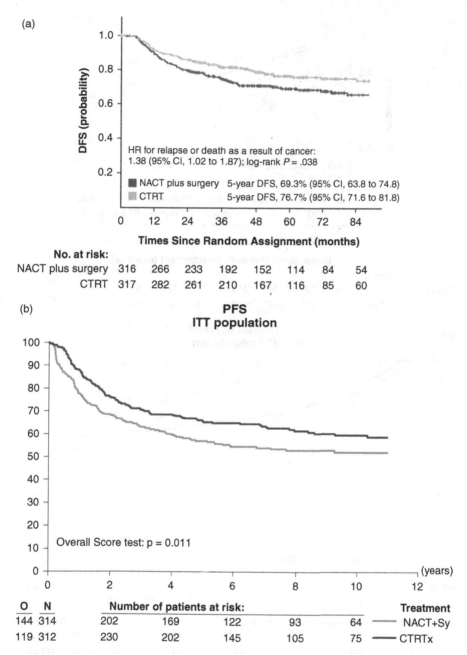

Figure 46B.1 (A–D) Disease-free and overall survival in the TMH (A & C) and EORTC (B & D) studies [3,4].

wo arms in both studies but there was a numerically superior (3.8%) five-year OS favoring
CTRT in the EORTC study (Figure 46B.1).

Subgroup analyses suggested that superior outcome with CTRT was concentrated in
patients with stage IIB disease. In terms of toxicity, the standout difference between the two

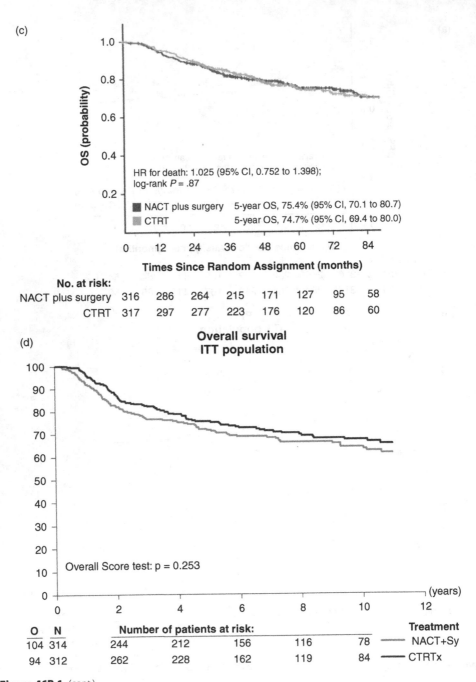

(c)

HR for death: 1.025 (95% CI, 0.752 to 1.398);
log-rank $P = .87$

■ NACT plus surgery   5-year OS, 75.4% (95% CI, 70.1 to 80.7)
▨ CTRT   5-year OS, 74.7% (95% CI, 69.4 to 80.0)

Times Since Random Assignment (months)

No. at risk:

NACT plus surgery	316	286	264	215	171	127	95	58
CTRT	317	297	277	223	176	120	86	60

(d)

**Overall survival
ITT population**

Overall Score test: p = 0.253

O	N	Number of patients at risk:					Treatment
104	314	244	212	156	116	78	── NACT+Sy
94	312	262	228	162	119	84	── CTRTx

Figure 46B.1 (cont.)

arms was higher vaginal toxicity in the CTRT arm after completion of treatment in both
studies and the higher gastrointestinal, bone marrow, and neurological toxicities during
treatment in the NACT-surgery arm in the EORTC study. Of note, in the NACT-surgery

arms of both studies, 24–28% of patients did not receive surgery while 27–44% patients received radiotherapy or CTRT, as protocol-defined cross-over or adjuvant treatment.

The results of these two well conducted large randomized studies are remarkably consistent and, in aggregate, suggest that CTRT results in superior outcomes compared with NACT-surgery. Importantly, both studies were planned to prove the superiority of NACT-surgery over CTRT and both failed to prove this in terms of their primary and secondary endpoints. Further, almost one fourth of patients planned for NACT-surgery are unable to undergo surgery and nearly one third or more require radiotherapy. While there have been few, if any, advances in chemotherapy and surgery for cervical cancer, the techniques of radiotherapy have rapidly progressed, and it is likely that in the current era, the results would be tilted even more in favor of CTRT. Notably, with currently practiced radiotherapy techniques, the incidence of short- and long-term toxicities is considerably lower than that reported in these two studies [5]. The choice of platinum drug (carboplatin or cisplatin) ultimately proved to be unimportant as was correctly speculated by us [3].

These results would ordinarily be sufficient to acknowledge CTRT as the standard of care, which it is in most parts of the world. However, some centers have a long and well entrenched practice of surgery in cervical cancer, even in advanced stages. To change practice and give up long-held beliefs is difficult but must be done in the face of overwhelming evidence. It is often argued that radiotherapy resources are constrained in some countries and therefore NACT-surgery is an acceptable alternative. This is an untenable argument for two reasons. First, surgical expertise is equally scarce, if not more so, in these same countries. Second, a considerable fraction of patients treated with NACT-surgery strategy end up requiring radiotherapy and it would be a disservice to them to plan partial and incomplete therapy. It would be more appropriate to enhance radiotherapy infrastructure and to implement referral networks that enable evidence-based treatment.

It has also been suggested that the superiority of CTRT is confined to patients with stage IIB disease and that NACT-surgery is an appropriate alternative in stage IB2 (current stage IB3) cancer. This is again untenable for two reasons. First, a substantial proportion (35.1%) of stage IB2 patients in the NACT-surgery arm of the TMH study [Gupta S, personal communication] ended up receiving radiotherapy, suggesting that NACT-surgery is often inadequate in these patients. Second, the burden of proof in current era is on the advocates of NACT-surgery and there is no indication from subgroup analysis of either study that this treatment is superior in patients with stage IB2 cancer.

Conclusion

It is likely that the current ceiling of 70–75% DFS in stage IB3 and stage II cervical cancer will be broken by integration of new treatments, like immunotherapy, with CTRT. Until this is achieved, we should focus on increasing the accessibility and delivery of good quality standard CTRT to these patients.

References

1. Chemoradiotherapy for Cervical Cancer Meta-Analysis Collaboration. Reducing uncertainties about the effects of chemoradiotherapy for cervical cancer: a systematic review and meta-analysis of individual patient data from 18 randomized trials. *J Clin Oncol* 2008;26:5802–5812.

2. Koh WJ, et al. Cervical Cancer, Version 3.2019, NCCN Clinical Practice Guidelines

in Oncology. *J Natl Compr Canc Netw* 2019;17(1):64–84.

3. Gupta S, et al. Neoadjuvant chemotherapy followed by radical surgery versus concomitant chemotherapy and radiotherapy in patients with stage IB2, IIA, or IIB squamous cervical cancer: a randomized controlled trial. *J Clin Oncol* 2018;36 (16):1548–1555.

4. Kenter G, et al. Results from neoadjuvant chemotherapy followed by surgery compared to chemoradiation for stage Ib2–IIb cervical cancer, EORTC 55994. 2019 ASCO Annual Meeting; May 31 to June 4, 2019; Chicago, IL: American Society of Clinical Oncology. Abstract 5503.

5. Tan LT, et al. Image-guided adaptive radiotherapy in cervical cancer. *Semin Radiat Oncol* 2019;29(3):284–298.

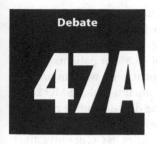

Debate

47A Is there a Role for Immunotherapy in Treatment of Cervical Cancer?
Yes

Chrisann Kyi and Dmitriy Zamarin[1]

Debate

Introduction

Cervical cancer (CC) is the most common gynecologic cancer worldwide. In the United States annually, more than 13,800 new cases are diagnosed and 4290 expected to succumb to the disease (SEER database, 2020). While early-stage disease CC can be cured with surgery or chemoradiation, patients with metastatic and recurrent CC have poor prognosis and limited treatment options after standard-of-care front-line platinum- and taxane-based chemotherapy and bevacizumab. New treatment modalities and paradigms are needed. Several immunotherapeutic approaches have emerged as promising new strategies in the treatment of CC.

Rationale behind Immunotherapy in Cervical Cancer

Cervical Cancer is a Virally Driven Cancer

Cervical cancer is driven by high-risk human papillomavirus (HPV) infection, with oncogenic HPV viral subtypes 16 and 18 accounting for more than ~70% of cases. While the majority of individuals clear the initial infection, persistence of the viral oncoproteins E6 and E7 leads to inactivation of p53 and RB, resulting in progression through cell cycle and carcinogenesis. As HPV-derived proteins represent a source of foreign antigens, HPV-transformed cancer cells theoretically exhibit high immunogenicity, prompting recognition and elimination by the immune system. However, HPV-related cancers have evolved multiple mechanisms of evading the immune system, generating rationale for therapeutic approaches targeting the mechanisms of immune evasion such as immune checkpoints or therapies directed against HPV proteins.

Immune Checkpoint Inhibition in Cervical Cancer

Clinical trials have demonstrated clinical efficacy of PD-1 inhibition (pembrolizumab and nivolumab) in the treatment of advanced and recurrent CC. KEYNOTE-158 was a phase II study of pembrolizumab in metastatic and recurrent CC. Overall response rate (ORR) was 12.2% with responses observed only in PD-L1 positive (CPS≥1) cases. Based on these results, the FDA approved pembrolizumab in recurrent and unresectable advanced

---

This study was supported in part by the MSK Cancer Center Support Grant P30 CA008748.

PD-L1+ CC in June 2018 [1]. CheckMate 358 was a phase I/II study of nivolumab in virus-associated tumors, with ORR of 26.3% reported in CC [2]. Expansion cohorts of CheckMate 358 presented at the ESMO 2019 meeting demonstrated promising results of nivolumab in combination with ipilimumab (CTLA-4 inhibitor), with ORR of 45.8% in patients with no prior treatment and 36.4% in patients with prior systemic treatment, with median progression-free survival of 8.5 months and 5.8 months, respectively (Naumann et al., ESMO 2019), highlighting that the utilization of immunotherapy earlier in the disease course may have a potential to benefit a larger percentage of patients and possibly even prevent disease recurrence. Ongoing or planned immune checkpoint inhibitor studies in CC are investigating combination with existing therapies (radiation therapy or chemotherapy) or combination therapy with other molecularly targeted drugs.

Immunotherapies Targeting HPV-related Genes

The viral oncoproteins E6 and E7 represent attractive targets for therapeutic cancer vaccination. In patients with precancerous lesions (CIN 2/3), vaccination with VGX-3100, a synthetic plasmid targeting HPV-16/HPV-18 E6 and E7 proteins, resulted in histopathologic regression of CIN lesions in 48.2% of VGX-3100 recipients, compared with 30% regression in the subjects treated with placebo (p=0.034) [3]. Unfortunately, various HPV-directed vaccination strategies to date have not demonstrated a consistent signal of efficacy, suggesting that in advanced disease, additional mechanisms of immune evasion (e.g., immune checkpoints) may need to be targeted to augment vaccine efficacy.

Adoptive cell therapies (ACT) refer to infusion of large numbers of ex vivo-expanded antigen-specific T cells into patients and thus bypass the need for generation of HPV-specific T cells in vivo. Several ACT approaches have been evaluated for therapy of CC, including tumor infiltrating lymphocyte (TIL) therapy and therapy with engineered T cells targeting HPV E6. In a study of nine patients with metastatic CC who received a single infusion of TILs selected for HPV E6 and E7 reactivity, two patients experienced a complete response, sustained for 22 and 15 months, and one patient experienced a partial response [4]. Similarly, an ACT trial of engineered T cells expressing HPV-16 E6-targeted TCR demonstrated two responses in 12 treated patients, providing a proof of concept that HPV-targeted approaches can be an effective strategy in this disease [5].

Conclusion

Cervical cancers are in large part driven by HPV infection and their progression requires acquisition of various immune evasion mechanisms. Though immunotherapies in CC to date have benefited a minority of patients, the depth and durability of responses highlight the power of the immune system to control and even eliminate this disease. New immune checkpoint blockade combinations, ACT approaches, and utilization of these strategies earlier in the disease setting will extend the benefit of these therapies in most if not all CC patients

References

1. Chung HC, et al. Efficacy and safety of pembrolizumab in previously treated advanced cervical cancer: results from the phase II KEYNOTE-158 study. *J Clin Oncol* 2019;37:1470–1478.

2. Naumann RW, et al. Safety and efficacy of nivolumab monotherapy in recurrent or metastatic cervical, vaginal, or vulvar carcinoma: results from the phase I/II Check Mate

358 Trial. *J Clin Oncol* 2019;37:2825–2834.

3. Trimble CL, et al. Safety, efficacy, and immunogenicity of VGX-3100, a therapeutic synthetic DNA vaccine targeting human papillomavirus 16 and 18 E6 and E7 proteins for cervical intraepithelial neoplasia 2/3: a randomised, double-blind, placebo-controlled phase 2b trial. *Lancet* 2015;386:2078–2088.

4. Stevanovic S, et al. Complete regression of metastatic cervical cancer after treatment with human papillomavirus-targeted tumor-infiltrating T cells. *J Clin Oncol* 2015;33:1543–1550.

5. Doran SL, et al. T-cell receptor gene therapy for human papillomavirus-associated epithelial cancers: a first-in-human, phase I/II study. *J Clin Oncol* 2019;37:2759–2768.

Debate

Is there a Role for Immunotherapy in Treatment of Cervical Cancer?
No

Fernando Cotait Maluf, Daniele Xavier Assad, and Angelica Nogueira-Rodrigues

Debate

Cervical cancer is responsible worldwide for 569,847 new cases and 311,365 deaths annually, more than 85% of the deaths occurring in low- and middle-income countries. So far, few advances have been seen in the treatment of locally advanced and metastatic disease. Immuno-oncology, including adoptive T-cell therapy and immune checkpoint inhibition (anti-CTLA-4 and anti-PD-1 and PD-L1), has emerged as a novel strategy to improve outcomes in patients with many solid tumors including gynecologic malignancies such as endometrial cancer. The role of immunotherapy is evolving in cervical cancer patients, either in first-line for locally advanced and metastatic disease or as salvage therapy after failure to platinum-based therapy. Based on evidence of human papillomavirus (HPV)-induced immune evasion, immunotherapy may be an attractive strategy in this disease. However, currently available data is limited and restricted to patients with metastatic or recurrent (M/R) disease in the salvage setting.

Ipilimumab, a human monoclonal IgG1 k antibody against CTLA-4, was evaluated in a phase I/II study in 42 M/R cervical cancer patients. Patients were treated with 10 mg/kg every three weeks for a total of four cycles, followed by four additional cycles of maintenance therapy every 12 weeks for patients with radiologic response or stabilization. There was only one partial response and 10 patients had stable disease. The median progression-free survival (PFS) was only 2.5 months and the median overall survival was 8.5 months [1].

Pembrolizumab, an anti-PD-1 antibody, was evaluated in 98 M/R cervical cancer patients regardless of the PD-L1 status (KEYNOTE-158), at the dose of 200 mg intravenously every three weeks for up to 24 months or until confirmed disease progression, intolerable toxicity, or death. PD-L1-positivity, defined by PD-L1 combined positive score ≥1, was reported in 83% of patients. The overall response rate was only 12.2%, with complete responses seen in three patients and partial response in nine patients; 17 patients had stable disease and the disease control rate was 31%. All 12 responses were in patients with PD-L1-positive tumors. Of those who experienced response, nearly 70% (9/12) had a response lasting >9 months. A total of 12% of patients had grade 3/4 adverse events [2]. A second trial (KEYNOTE-028) evaluated pembrolizumab at the dose 10 mg/kg every two weeks for up to 24 months in 24 PD-L1-positive patients with advanced or recurrent disease. Overall response rate was 17%, all of them partial responses, with a median duration of only

5.4 months [3]. Based on results of both nonrandomized studies, FDA granted approval for the use of pembrolizumab in PD-L1-positive patients with metastatic or recurrent disease. However, it remains unclear if PD-L1 is a reliable biomarker in this setting to discriminate patients most likely to achieve a response. Also, the overall response rates in the enriched PD-L1 population reported with pembrolizumab does not seem to be different from those observed with second-line chemotherapy in the salvage setting such as irinotecan, topotecan, capecitabine, gemcitabine, vinorelbine, and pemetrexed [4].

Another anti-PD-1 agent, nivolumab at the dose of 240 mg intravenously every two weeks, was evaluated in a phase I/II study (CheckMate-358). CheckMate-358 is an ongoing phase I/II study that is investigating nivolumab-based therapies in virus-associated cancers, regardless of tumor cell PD-L1 expression. In a cohort with 19 advanced cervical patients with ≤2 prior systemic therapies, the overall response rate of nivolumab alone was 26.3%, with a disease control rate of 68% [5]. The CheckMate-358 study has also explored two different regimens combining nivolumab and ipilimumab. A total of 91 patients who had received up to two prior systemic therapies for M/R disease were randomized to either nivolumab at 3 mg/kg every two weeks plus ipilimumab at 1 mg/kg every six weeks (nivo3 + ipi1) or nivolumab at 1 mg/kg plus ipilimumab at 3 mg/kg, given every three weeks for four doses followed by nivolumab at 240 mg every two weeks (nivo1 + ipi3). In the nivo3 + ipi1 arm, median PFS was 13.8 months (95% CI: 2.1–not reached) in the patients not previously treated with systemic therapy for M/R disease and 3.6 months (95% CI: 1.9–5.1) in those with previous systemic therapy. In the nivo1 + ipi3 arm, the median PFS was 8.5. months (95% CI: 3.7–not reached) in the patients with no prior systemic therapy and 5.8 months (95% CI: 3.5–17.2) in those who had received prior systemic therapy. In the nivo3 + ipi1 arm, the objective response rate (ORR) was 31.6% in those patients who received no prior systemic therapy and 23.1% in those with prior systemic therapy. The ORR in the nivo1 + ipi3 arm were 45.8% and 36.4%, respectively. Although promising, this is a "pick a winner cohort," and CheckMate-358 continues to enroll patients with M/R cervical cancer for mature conclusions [6].

An international phase III study is evaluating the role of cisplatin, paclitaxel, and bevacizumab with or without atezolizumab (anti-PD-L1 antibody) in first-line therapy for advanced cervical cancer with overall survival as the primary endpoint. The role of immune checkpoint inhibitors has also been tested in locally advanced cervical cancer with durvalumab (anti-PD-L1 antibody), in a phase III study designed to compare durvalumab with and following chemoradiotherapy versus chemoradiotherapy alone with PFS as the primary endpoint. In the same scenario, pembrolizumab in addition to chemoradiotherapy has also been evaluated.

Conclusion

Therefore, based on the actual data, the role of immunotherapy in cervical cancer at this moment is uncertain. There are few phase I/II studies, no quality of life analysis, limited responses for the majority of patients at high cost, and no clear superiority over second-line chemotherapy (but obviously more expensive). Also, immunomediated toxicity is not negligible and there is no definitive biomarker to discriminate efficacy and toxicity. Lastly, the phase III trials either as first-line therapy for locally advanced or metastatic disease or as salvage therapy are still ongoing in order to support a possible role of immunotherapy in this setting with level 1 evidence.

References

1. Lheureux S, et al. Association of ipilimumab with safety and antitumor activity in women with metastatic or recurrent human papillomavirus–related cervical carcinoma. *JAMA Oncol* 2018;4(7):e173776.

2. Chung HC, et al. Efficacy and safety of pembrolizumab in previously treated advanced cervical cancer: results from the phase II KEYNOTE-158 study. *J Clin Oncol* 2019;37(17):1470–1478.

3. Frenel J-S, et al. Safety and efficacy of pembrolizumab in advanced, programmed death ligand 1–positive cervical cancer: results from the phase Ib KEYNOTE-028 Trial. *J Clin Oncol* 2017;35(36):4035–4041.

4. Boussios S, et al. Management of patients with recurrent/advanced cervical cancer beyond first line platinum regimens: where do we stand? A literature review. *Crit Rev Oncol/Hematol* 2016;108:164–174.

5. Naumann RW, et al. Safety and efficacy of nivolumab monotherapy in recurrent or metastatic cervical, vaginal, or vulvar carcinoma: results from the phase I/II CheckMate 358 Trial. *J Clin Oncol* 2019;37(31):2825–2834.

6. Naumann RW, et al. Efficacy and safety of nivolumab plus ipilimumab in patients with recurrent /metastatic cervical cancer: results from Checkmate 358. *Ann Oncol* 2019;30 (Suppl. 5):v851–v934.

Debate

48A

Should the Subsequent Management of Patients with Vulvar Cancer and a Positive Sentinel Lymph Node be Complete Groin Lymph Node Dissection or Radiation Therapy?

Dissection

Lilian T. Gien

Debate

Vulvar cancer is a rare disease, representing 4% of gynecologic malignancies, with 90% squamous cell histology. The most important prognostic factor for survival is lymph node metastasis. Patients with negative groin nodes have an excellent five-year overall survival (OS) rate (90%) versus those with groin metastasis (0–51%). The presence of groin metastasis increases risk of groin recurrence which is fatal in almost all patients. Therefore, the appropriate primary management of the groins at diagnosis of vulvar cancer is of utmost importance.

Surgery remains the primary treatment for early-stage vulvar cancer, but has shifted from radical to more limited surgery. Instead of complete inguinofemoral lymph node dissection (IFLD), associated with high rates of lymphedema (30–70%) and wound breakdown (20–40%), groin assessment is now done by sentinel lymph node (SLN) biopsy. The GROINSS-V study was an observational study of 403 women with early-stage (<4 cm) vulvar cancer, depth of >1 mm and clinically nonsuspicious groin nodes, of which 276 patients had a negative SLN [1]. Isolated groin recurrence was 2.5% with median follow-up of 105 months. Ten-year disease-specific survival was 91% in those SLN negative. There were significantly lower wound breakdown, cellulitis, or lymphedema among those with SLN biopsy compared to those with IFLD for positive nodes. Similarly, the Gynecologic Oncology Group (GOG) protocol 173 was an observational study of 452 patients with tumor size 2–6 cm who underwent a SLN biopsy and a complete IFLD [2]. SLN biopsy had a sensitivity of 91.7%, and a false negative predictive value of 2% for those with tumors <4 cm. Based on these two major studies, SLN biopsy is now the standard of care for vulvar cancer, which has led to a substantial reduction in surgical morbidity.

The importance of adjuvant radiation was demonstrated in GOG37, where 114 patients with positive groin nodes were randomized to adjuvant radiation therapy (RT) to the groin/pelvis versus pelvic node resection. Survival was superior in the adjuvant RT group with the most significant benefit in those with ≥2 positive groin nodes, demonstrating how RT is an integral part of managing positive groin nodes in vulvar cancer. Therefore, although patients with a negative SLN can avoid a full IFLD, for patients with a positive SLN, should the subsequent management be a complete IFLD which can potentially introduce surgical morbidity, or is it sufficient to offer adjuvant RT? Based on existing data, the standard of care remains complete surgical dissection of the groin nodes in order to maximize patient survival.

In GOG88, patients with clinically negative groin nodes were randomized to full IFLD or RT [3]. However, this trial was stopped early because the groin recurrence rate in the radiation only arm was unacceptably high at 18.5%. This trial emphasized that resection of clinically negative groins could not be substituted with radiation alone, and that surgical resection of microscopic positive nodes remains necessary. There are several criticisms of this trial, including the depth of treatment by RT resulting in insufficient dose of radiation to the groin. Despite the criticisms however, no other randomized controlled trial (RCT) has been done to re-evaluate this question, given the fatality associated with groin recurrence, reluctance to randomize, and the rarity of this disease. A Cochrane Review of this topic was completed in 2011, however GOG88 was the only RCT included. The conclusion of this systematic review was that there is not enough evidence to prove that primary RT is as effective to control tumors in the groin and surgery is the first-choice treatment for groin nodes in early invasive vulvar cancer.

In the era of SLN biopsy, there is little data regarding the prognostic significance of the size of the SLN metastasis. In an evaluation of the SLN positive patients in GROINSS-V, the proportion of patients with non-SLN metastasis increased with size of SLN metastasis [4]. Disease-specific survival for patients with SLN metastasis >2 mm was lower than those with metastasis ≤2 mm (69.5% vs. 94.4%, p=0.001). There was no size cut-off below which chances of non-SLN metastasis were close to zero, concluding that all patients with SLN metastasis necessitate additional groin treatment, regardless of the size of metastasis, and for those with metastasis >2 mm this includes a full IFLD.

GROINSS-V II was a second multicentered international observational study that evaluated whether adjuvant RT could be given for those with a positive SLN without IFLD [5]. At the start of the study all patients with a positive SLN were included. However, after interim analysis of 82 patients with metastatic SLN, there were nine groin recurrences. Those at risk for groin recurrence had metastases >2 mm and/or extranodal tumor growth. Therefore, the protocol was amended such that those with macrometastasis received IFLD and RT whereas only patients with micrometastasis (≤ 2 mm) could receive adjuvant RT without IFLD. There were 1544 eligible patients, 158 with micrometastatic SLNs. The isolated groin recurrence rate was 1.7% after two years in patients with micrometastasis treated with adjuvant RT. Based on the recurrence rate with RT for macrometastatic disease, radiotherapy with a total dose of 50 Gy was no safe alternative to IFLD.

Conclusion

A RCT is not possible in this patient population and decision guidelines will continue to be based on prospective observational studies. GROINSS-V III is the next planned observational study, which asks the question of whether patients with macrometastatic disease in the SLN can avoid a full IFLD. All patients enrolled in this study will have adjuvant RT at an increased dose of 56 Gy combined with concurrent chemotherapy, with the hypothesis that the addition of cisplatin and increased radiation dose could potentially overcome the need for IFLD in patients with a positive SLN >2 mm. However, the results of this study will not be available for several years, and safety monitoring with interim analysis will be crucial. In the meantime, the strongest data available in the literature support that the standard of care for patients with a positive SLN is IFLD, which should not be substituted by RT.

References

1. Van der Zee AGJ, et al. Sentinel node dissection is safe in the treatment of early-stage vulvar cancer. *J Clin Oncol* 2008;26:884–889.

2. Levenback CF, et al. Lymphatic mapping and sentinel lymph node biopsy in women with squamous cell carcinoma of the vulva: a Gynecologic Oncology Group study. *J Clin Oncol* 2012;30:3786–3791.

3. Stehman FB, et al. Groin dissection vs groin radiation in carcinoma of the vulva: a Gynecologic Oncology Group study. *Int J Rad Oncol Biol Phys* 1992;24:389–396.

4. Oonk MHM, et al. Size of sentinel-node metastasis and chances of non-sentinel-node involvement and survival in early-stage vulvar cancer: results from GROINSS-V, a multicentre observational study. *Lancet Oncol* 2010;11:646–652.

5. Oonk MHM, et al. Radiotherapy instead of inguinofemoral lymphadenectomy in vulvar cancer patients with a metastatic sentinel node: results of GROINSS-V II. *Int J Gynecol Cancer* 2019;29 (Suppl. 4):A14.

Debate

Should the Subsequent Management of Patients with Vulvar Cancer and a Positive Sentinel Lymph Node be Complete Groin Lymph Node Dissection or Radiation Therapy?

Radiation Therapy

Ryan M. Kahn and Wui-Jin Koh

Debate

Squamous cell carcinoma (SCC) of the vulva is a rare disease accounting for nearly 6% of all gynecologic malignancies, with an estimated 6300 newly diagnosed cases and 1500 deaths in the United States in 2022 [1]. The traditional primary treatment of early-stage disease with >1 mm of invasion consisted of radical excision of the tumor with elective inguinofemoral lymphadenectomy (IFL). However, only 25–35% of women with early-stage disease will be found to have lymph node metastases. Additionally, IFL has the potential to cause significant morbidity. with a 30–70% risk of long-term lymphedema as well as infection or wound breakdown in 20–40% of patients [2].

Recent evidence has shown that performing a sentinel lymph node (SLN) biopsy of the inguinofemoral lymph node basin – a less invasive approach resulting in decreased morbidity – is safe and feasible [2]. Long-term follow-up of the Groningen International Study on Sentinel nodes in Vulvar cancer (GROINSS-V-I) demonstrated that SLN biopsy with negative findings was associated with an isolated groin recurrence rate of 2.5% among 377 patients with unifocal disease over a median follow-up of 105 months, with a 10-year disease-specific survival (DSS) of 91% [3] The Gynecologic Oncology Group (GOG)-173 study – a prospective, multi-institutional validation trial – demonstrated similar findings. proving SLN biopsy is a reasonable alternative to IFL in select patients [4]. SLN biopsy has now currently become the standard of care over IFL in patients with early-stage SCC of the vulva – which includes patients with a unifocal tumor <4 cm as well as a negative clinical and or radiologic groin examination. However, a standardized treatment paradigm following the findings of a positive SLN remains lacking.

The known postoperative morbidity risks following IFL led to the follow-up study (GROINSS-V-II), investigating whether inguinofemoral radiation therapy (RT) is a saf alternative to IFL in patients with positive SLN findings. This study was a prospective, multicenter phase II single-arm study of patients with early-stage SCC of the vulva who underwent primary local excision and a SLN biopsy. If the SLN was positive with metastasis of any size, inguinofemoral RT was administered within six weeks after surgery. The RT regimen consisted of a total dose of 50 Gray (Gy) in 25–28 fractions of 1.8–2 Gy, five fractions per week, which was considered an effective dose for subclinical disease [5].

GROINSS-V-II study registered 1535 patients between the years of 2005–2016, with SLN metastasis identified in 322 cases. The stopping rule was temporarily activated in 2010 as the isolated groin recurrence rate in the RT group exceeded the study's predefined threshold – among 10 patients with an isolated groin recurrence, nine had SLN metastases of >2 mm and/or extracapsular spread. The protocol was then amended so patients with SLN macrometastases were assigned to IFL as the standard of care (with adjuvant RT for multiple LN involvement and/or extracapsular spread), whereas patients with SLN micrometastases (≤2 mm) continued to receive inguinofemoral RT alone [4]. At study conclusion, among 160 patients with SLN micrometastases, 126 received inguinofemoral RT alone per protocol, with a two-year ipsilateral isolated groin recurrence rate of 1.6%. While adjuvant RT added low-grade acute morbidity compared with SLN biopsy alone, chronic lymphedema was greatly decreased as compared to IFL with rates of 11% versus 23% respectively at 12 months. Ultimately, the authors of GROINSS-V-II concluded that inguinofemoral RT could spare patients with early SCC of the vulva with SLN micrometastases from the long-term morbidity of complete IFL [5].

The data is less clear for those with a macrometastasis (>2 mm) on SLN biopsy. GROINSS-V-II suggested inadequate control with postoperative RT alone, without further IFL. For the 162 patients with SLN macrometastases, the two-year groin recurrence rate was 22% in the RT cohort versus 6.9% in patients who underwent IFL with or without further RT (p=0.011) [5]. However, the RT approach used in GROINS-V-II has been challenged as possibly inadequate in coverage and dose for patients with a macrometastatic SLN [6]. It is informative to note that in the GOG-101 study, patients with initially unresectable grossly positive, fixed or ulcerated groin nodes underwent preoperative wide-field RT with concurrent 5FU and cisplatin, and demonstrated significant clinical response permitting resection in 95% of cases, and complete histologic clearance of all nodal disease in 15 of 37 patients [7]. The efficacy of appropriately designed adjuvant RT, with dose escalation and given with concurrent cisplatin, is being evaluated in GROINSS-VIII for patients with macrometastatic SLN.

Conclusion

Overall, the management of early-stage vulvar cancer has undergone major advances over the past decade. In patients with early-stage disease, clinicians must balance the proven benefits of adjuvant treatment options with the risks of toxicities and quality of life outcomes. Based on data from GROINSS-V-II, patients with SLN micrometastasis of ≤2 mm benefit from inguinofemoral RT over complete groin lymph node dissection. Further prospective trials are necessary to evaluate RT dose escalation in combination with chemotherapy in hopes to establish future standardized guidelines, especially in the adjuvant treatment of macroscopic SLN cases.

References

1. American Cancer Society. *Cancer Facts & Figures 2022*. Atlanta, GA: American Cancer Society, 2022.

2. Van der Zee AG, et al. Sentinel node dissection is safe in the treatment of early-stage vulvar cancer. *J Clin Oncol* 2008;26(6):884–889.

3. Te Grootenhuis NC, et al. Sentinel nodes in vulvar cancer: long-term follow-up of the GROningen INternational Study on Sentinel nodes in Vulvar cancer (GROINSS-V) I. *Gynecol Oncol* 2016;140 (1):8–14.

4. Levenback CF, et al. Lymphatic mapping and sentinel lymph node biopsy in women with squamous cell carcinoma of the vulva: a Gynecologic Oncology Group study. *J Clin Oncol* 2012;30(31):3786–3791.

5. Oonk MHM, et al. Radiotherapy versus inguinofemoral lymphadenectomy as treatment for vulvar cancer patients with micrometastases in the sentinel node: results of GROINSS-V II. *J Clin Oncol* 2021;39 (32):3623–3632.

6. Glaser S, et al. Inguinal nodal radiotherapy for vulvar cancer: are we missing the target again? *Gynecol Oncol* 2014;135(3):583–585.

7. Montana GS, et al. Preoperative chemo-radiation for carcinoma of the vulva with N2/N3 nodes: a Gynecologic Oncology Group study. *Int J Radiat Oncol Biol Phys* 2000;48(4):1007–1013.

What is the Best Treatment for Stage I Vulvar Squamous Cell Carcinoma with either a Close or Positive Surgical Margin?

49A

Re-excision

Sabrina M. Bedell and Britt K. Erickson

Debate

To date there are no prospective studies that directly evaluate outcomes for re-excision versus adjuvant radiation for close or positive margins in patients with stage I squamous cell carcinoma of the vulva. However, given available evidence as well as consideration of morbidities associated with radiotherapy, we suggest that re-excision is the preferred method of management for stage I vulvar cancer with close or positive margins. Observation may also be considered for patients with close margins.

Determining the true recurrence rates for patients with close or positive surgical margins is challenging. Importantly, unlike other tumor types, local recurrence in vulvar cancer is usually salvageable and distant recurrence is almost universally fatal. In the largest early-stage prospective Gynecologic Oncology Group (GOG) study, the salvage rate for local recurrence was 80% [1]. The majority of studies examining recurrence rates by margin status combine all stages of disease, which majorly confounds survival. Studies that report on only stage I tumors are limited by small sample size.

Additionally, the definition of "close margins" has changed over time. Historically, close margins have been defined as less than 8 mm [2]. However, recent data demonstrate that for patients with true stage I disease, 2–3 mm may better define those at increased risk of recurrence [3]. Additionally, these studies suggest that other factors such as age and presence of lichen sclerosis may be a more important predictor of recurrence compared to margin status. The most recent NCCN guidelines define a pathologic close margin as 1–3 mm [4].

In our series of 47 patients with stage I vulvar squamous cell carcinoma, which represents the largest series of stage I patients with sufficient treatment and survival outcome data, we found no difference in the rate of recurrence between patients who received any further treatment (vulvar radiation or re-excision) versus those who received no further treatment [5]. Notably, there were no distance recurrences and of the seven local recurrences, one was lost to follow-up and the remaining six were salvaged with excision, radiation, chemotherapy, or combination therapy. No patients died of disease.

Another multi-institutional cohort study evaluated outcomes following re-excision, stratified by pathology of the re-excision specimen margin, and found that for patients with stage I vulvar cancer, the mean time to recurrence was 58 months for those with VIN at re-excision margins, versus 9.4 months for those that had carcinoma at re-excision margins. Further, five of the six with local recurrences were salvaged with repeat excision and had no evidence of disease at time of follow-up – the sixth patient had no further follow-up [6]. Thus, successful re-excision resulted in improved outcomes, and those with stage I disease that did recur locally were often successfully salvaged with re-excision.

Adjuvant radiation has a host of morbid side effects including skin desquamation, pain, necrosis, and urinary, bowel, and sexual dysfunction. Of the few studies that report on complication rates for vulvar radiation, one indicates a conservative 42% rate of grade III Radiation Therapy Oncology Group (RTOG) acute skin reactions and 13% rate of grade III RTOG late skin reactions [7], while a second study indicates 100% rate of acute skin desquamation (the equivalent of RTOG grade IV acute skin reaction), and 5.5% rate of late skin reaction. It should be noted that in the latter study 22% of patients had died within one year of treatment, limiting the ability to draw conclusions regarding long-term side effects. The risk of long-term morbidity from adjuvant vulvar radiation is too high to be an acceptable adjuvant treatment for stage I vulvar cancer.

In addition, adjuvant radiation complicates treatment of future recurrences by (1) hampering healing following re-excision, and (2) eliminating radiation as a treatment option at that time. Radiation causes depletion of dermal stem cells, fibroblast dysfunction, defective collagen cross-linking, upregulation of pro-inflammatory cytokines, and microvascular changes that all contribute to chronic fibrosis and poor wound healing. Multiple strategies to improve wound healing of fibrotic tissue have been explored, but the only reliable strategy thus far is the use of vascularized flaps from tissue outside of the radiation field.

In contrast, re-excision likely reduces the risk of recurrence while minimizing morbidity. Although re-excision can be associated with temporary wound breakdown, published rates for wound breakdown and infection following modified vulvectomy are much lower than radiation side effect rates, at approximately 18% [8].

Conclusion

In conclusion, although there is a potential for adjuvant vulvar radiation to decrease recurrence, there is no data on the true risk reduction in stage I patients. The associated long-term morbidity far outweighs the potential benefits. Efforts should be made to re-excise close or positive margins for patients with stage I vulvar cancer and observation may also be considered, particularly in cases of close margins. Radiation therapy should be saved for the rare cases of positive margins or local recurrence that are not amendable to re-excision.

References

1. Stehman F, et al. Early stage I carcinoma of the vulva treated with ipsilateral superficial inguinal lymphadenectomy and modified radical hemivulvectomy: a prospective study of the Gynecologic Oncology Group. *Obstet Gynecol* 1992;79(4):490–497.

2. Heaps JM, et al. Surgical-pathologic variables predictive of local recurrence in squamous cell carcinoma of the vulva.

Gynecol Oncol 1990;38(3):309–314. https://doi.org/10.1016/0090-8258(90)90064-R

3. Arvas M, et al. The role of pathological margin distance and prognostic factors after primary surgery in squamous cell carcinoma of the vulva. *Int J Gynecol Cancer* 2018;28:623–631.

4. Bradley K, et al. (Squamous Cell Carcinoma) Vulvar Cancer. 2020.

5. Bedell SM, et al. Role of adjuvant radiation or re-excision for early stage vulvar squamous cell carcinoma with positive or close surgical margins. *Gynecol Oncol* 2019;154(2):276–279. https://doi.org/10.1016/j.ygyno.2019.05.028

6. Ioffe YJ, et al. Low yield of residual vulvar carcinoma and dysplasia upon re-excision for close or positive margins. *Gynecol Oncol* 2013;129(3):528–532. https://doi.org/10.1016/j.ygyno.2013.02.033

7. Faul CM, et al. Adjuvant radiation for vulvar carcinoma: improved local control. *Int J Radiat Oncol Biol Phys* 1997;38(2):381–389. https://doi.org/10.1016/S0360-3016(97)82500-X

8. Gaarenstroom KN, et al. Postoperative complications after vulvectomy and inguinofemoral lymphadenectomy using separate groin incisions. *Int J Gynecol Cancer* 2003;13(4):522–527. https://doi.org/10.1046/j.1525-1438.2003.13304.x

Debate

49B

What is the Best Treatment for Stage I Vulvar Squamous Cell Carcinoma with either a Close or Positive Surgical Margin?
Adjuvant Radiation

Rachel C. Sisodia

Debate

Of the 6120 women who are projected to develop vulvar malignancy in 2021, the majority of them will have disease which is confined to the vulva, of squamous cell etiology, and potentially curable [1]. The cornerstone of management for women with localized disease such as this is surgery. While surgery for vulva cancer was initially envisioned as an en-bloc radical resection with bilateral inguinofemoral lymphadenectomy (Basset-Way radical vulvectomy, 1912), over the decades, gynecologic oncologists have continued to improve the operation in the pursuit of lessening morbidity for our patients. Currently, management of a clinical stage I vulvar cancer is radical excision with a 1–2 cm negative margin on normal tissue and an 8 mm margin on fixed tissue; clinical stage IB tumors will also undergo nodal evaluation. Yet despite the desire for a less morbid, more conservative approach to surgery, multiple retrospective studies have shown that in regard to vulvar cancer, tumor-free margin matters. In a retrospective study of 135 patients with vulvar cancer, no patient with an 8 mm or greater tumor-free margin recurred. However, 48% of the women with a margin of less than 8 mm recurred, and local recurrence was associated with a 67% chance of death from metastatic disease [2]. In addition, close or positive margins are common. Given the frequency of close/positive margins, as well as the unacceptably high mortality rate due to local recurrence, it is incumbent upon gynecologic oncologists to actively manage close or positive margins in women with vulvar malignancy. Two choices are available for the woman with concerning margin status after vulvar resection: re-excision or radiation. Based on the increased morbidity with repeat excision, and the compromised quality of life associated with resection of critical perineal structures (anus, clitoris, urethra, vagina), radiotherapy is the most reasonable choice for management.

The role of adjuvant radiation in vulvar cancer has been studied for decades; since the 1990s, radiation oncologists and gynecologic oncologists have specifically studied its role in women with close or positive surgical margins [3]. Radiation fields consist of 45 Gy to 60 Gy to the area of the previous excision, and can be contoured to include the entire perineum, inguinal and pelvic nodes if indicated [4]. In regard to efficacy, while adjuvant radiation does not impact overall survival in women with negative margins, it is highly efficacious in the patient with close or positive surgical margins. In a study of 257 women with primary squamous cell carcinoma of the vulva, adjuvant radiation for women with close/positive surgical margins improved five-year overall survival dramatically (67.6% vs. 29%, p=0.038), bringing it equivalent to the overall survival rates seen in women with negative margins [3]. Furthermore, with the evolution of intensity modulated radiation therapy (IMRT), some of the previous concerns about radiation toxicity (skin desquamation, vaginal stenosis, pain, sexual dysfunction, and body image issues) can be ameliorated. In the largest study examining patient-reported outcomes in a routine clinical population of women with vulvar cancer, women who underwent radiation did not have statistically significantly different rates of pain, bleeding, discharge, bowel or bladder function, quality of life, or overall health than women who underwent a simple resection [4]. Furthermore, the single greatest predictor of impaired or diminished quality of life was local recurrence [4]. As such, it stands to reason that aggressively pursuing close or positive surgical margins with adjuvant radiation is an acceptable trade-off to the patient to guarantee long-term survival and high quality of life.

Conclusion

Finally, though radiation or re-excision has long been a mainstay of vulvar cancer treatment, more recent investigations have called this paradigm into question. In an intriguing manuscript by Grootenhuis et al. examining the specimens of 287 patients with primary vulvar squamous cell carcinoma and a close (but not positive) margin, tumor-free margin distance (≤8 mm, ≤ 5 mm, or ≤3 mm) did not impact the risk of local recurrence (HR=1.03, 95% CI: 0.99–1.06) [5]. However, local recurrence was seen more frequently in patients with differentiated vulvar intraepithelial neoplasia (dVIN) (HR=2.76, 95% CI: 1.62–4.71) and/or lichen sclerosis (HR=2.14, 95% CI: 1.11–4.12) in the margin, suggesting that local recurrence is more about tumor biology than a close margin. These findings are that of a single retrospective study and do not yet change the standard of care, but they do highlight the need for continued research into the pathogenesis and management of vulvar cancer. In the interim, gynecologic oncologists will need to continue to use available therapies to help cure women with vulvar cancer, and based on its high efficacy and manageable side-effect profile, radiation continues to be the therapy of choice for close/positive margins after resection.

References

1. SEER Database: Vulvar Cancer. Available from: https://seer.cancer.gov/statfacts/html/vulva.html [last accessed November 9, 2022].

2. Heaps JM, et al. Surgical pathologic variables predictive of local recurrence in squamous cell carcinoma of the vulva. *Gynecol Oncol* 1990;38 (3):309.

3. Ignatov T, et al. Adjuvant radiotherapy for vulvar cancer with close or positive surgical margins. *J Cancer Res Clin Oncol* 2016;142:489–495.

4. Alimena S, et al. Patient reported outcome measures among patients with vulvar cancer at various stages of treatment, recurrence and survivorship. *Gynecol Oncol* 2021;160:252–259.

5. Grootenhuis NC, et al. Margin status revisited in vulvar squamous cell carcinoma. *Gynecol Oncol* 2019;154(2):266–275.

Should Adjuvant Radiation be Given to Women with Single Node Positive Vulvar Cancer?

Yes

Rachel C. Sisodia

Debate

Vulvar cancer is a rare and poorly studied disease. While the majority of women will present with disease localized to the vulva, a significant percentage will present with more advanced disease involving at least one inguinal lymph node. In addition, lymph node involvement often occurs quite early in disease course. In a sentinel study examining 177 cases of clinical stage I vulvar squamous cell carcinomas examining depth of invasion as a predictor for lymph node metastases, occult metastases were found in 10.5% of women with a depth of invasion between 1.1 mm and 2 mm, and with risk increasing up to 42.9% when the depth of invasion was more than 5 mm [1]. The presence of positive lymph nodes is considered the single most important prognostic indicator for women with vulvar carcinoma, and is associated with markedly reduced survival. As such, assessment of the inguinofemoral nodes is part of all staging surgery for lesions that are clinically larger than 2 cm or have more than 1 mm of invasion [2].

While there is ubiquitous agreement that macro-metastases or multiple involved nodes must be treated for a patient to have a chance at survival, controversy exists over how to manage women with a single positive node. Historically, it was believed that after undergoing full lymphadenectomy, node-positive women should undergo radiation therapy or chemoradiation. A sentinel report in the field, the AGO-CaRE-1 study, examined 447 women with node-positive vulvar cancer and demonstrated a statistically significant survival benefit with radiation as opposed to inguinal dissection alone (HR=0.63, 95% CI: 0.43–0.91) [3]. While there was a trend for improved survival in women with one positive node who were radiated, only women with two or more positive nodes met statistical significance for a difference in survival rate. Further confounding the results of this study is the fact that women had a drop in their overall survival even with one positive node. This finding supports the idea that even a single positive node is a harbinger of worsened prognosis. Both findings had also been reported in older studies [3]. Conversely, a large SEER database study examining women with stage III, single-node positive vulvar cancer showed that adjuvant radiation had a clear survival benefit over women receiving no further therapy with a five-year overall survival (OS) of 77% versus 61.2% (p =0.02). This effect was particularly pronounced when the patient had <12 lymph nodes removed [4]. Of note, given the uncertainty around radiation in the setting of one macro-metastases, we are currently unable to opine on the management of a patient found to have a micro-metastases or isolated tumor cells on sentinel node biopsy. The GROningen International Study on Sentinel nodes in Vulvar Cancer (GROINS-V-II)/Gynecologic Oncology Group 270 protocol, which is ongoing, seeks to provide insight to management of micro-metastases found after sentinel node removal.

With such conflicting literature, what is the gynecologic oncologist to do in the patient with a single positive groin node? While the literature allows for an argument to be made for either adjuvant radiation or full lymphadenectomy alone, based on the above data the most prudent course of action would be to perform radiation. While Mahner et al. was unable to prove a statistically significant benefit in radiating patients with a single positive groin node, there was a clear trend towards improved progression-free survival and OS with administration of radiation after surgery [3]. Furthermore, even having one positive node correlates with a lower OS (three-year OS, 7.8%) when compared to stage I or stage II disease. In addition, a SEER review of 490 patients showed a benefit in disease-specific survival in women with a single groin node that were radiated. Though this effect was greatest when there were only a limited number of nodes removed (study comments on <12 cut-off), one must understand that this cut-off was a statistical outcome of the study and difficult to extrapolate to any one individual woman (who may have more or less lymphatic tissue).

Conclusion

For women with vulvar cancer, groin recurrence is a serious event which almost invariably is fatal. As such, in an area where there is conflicting data, it is incumbent on the patient's physician to err on the side of being conservative. Until clearer data is available, patients with a single positive groin node should be administered radiation therapy at curative attempt.

References

1. Hacker NF, et al. Individualization of treatment for stage I squamous cell vulvar carcinoma. *Obstet Gynecol* 1984;63 (2):155.

2. National Comprehensive Cancer Network. NCCN guidelines. Available from: www .nccn.org/professionals/physician_gls/pdf/v ulvar.pdf

3. Mahner S, et al. Adjuvant therapy in lymph node positive vulvar cancer: the AGO-CaRE-1 study. *J Natl Cancer Inst* 2015;107(3):dju426.

4. Parthasarathy A, et al. The benefit of adjuvant radiation therapy in single node positive squamous cell vulvar carcinoma. *Gynecol Oncol* 2006;103:1095–1099.

Debate

50B Should Adjuvant Radiation Therapy be Given to Patients with Single Node Positive Vulvar Cancer?

No

Aaron M. Praiss and Kaled M. Alektiar

Debate

Vulvar cancer is rare, accounting for <1% of all cancers in women and 6% of cancers of the female reproductive tract. A total of 6330 new diagnoses of vulvar cancer and 1560 deaths from vulvar cancer are estimated in 2022. Squamous cell carcinoma (SCC) is the most common histology of vulvar cancer (>90%). Vulvar cancer metastasizes through three main methods: local extension, lymphatic embolization to regional inguino-femoral lymph nodes (IFLN), and hematogenous spread to distant sites. From an anatomic perspective, vulvar lymphatics drain first into the superficial inguinal lymph nodes located within the femoral triangle, and then beyond that into the pelvic nodal basins.

The most important prognostic factor for vulvar cancer is IFLN metastasis. Survival is reduced to 50% in patients with positive IFLNs, and recurrences often occur within two years of primary treatment. Five-year disease-specific survival ranges from 25–40% in patients with positive IFLNs versus 70–93% in patients with negative IFLNs [1]. Risk of IFLN metastases rises with increasing depth of invasion (DOI) of the primary tumor: <1% risk for IFLN metastasis with DOI <1 mm, 6–12% risk for IFLN metastasis with DOI 1.1–3 mm, and 15–20% risk for IFLN metastasis with DOI 3.1–5 mm.

The controversy regarding adjuvant radiotherapy for single IFLN positive vulvar cancer started with Gynecologic Oncology Group (GOG) protocol 37 [2]. This prospective randomized trial from the 1980s investigated the value of pelvic lymphadenectomy compared with pelvic and groin radiation therapy after vulvectomy and IFLN dissection. Overall, this study demonstrated an improved two-year overall survival (OS) (68% vs. 54%, p=0.03) in favor of the radiotherapy group. More importantly, however, the number of positive nodes impacted survival based on this data. Within the radiotherapy arm patients with one positive IFLN had a two-year survival of 80% versus 66% for those with two or more positive IFLNs. Multiple trials since have further demonstrated improved oncologic outcomes for patients with two or more positive IFLNs receiving adjuvant radiotherapy.

Fast forward 30 years, and Mahner et al. further studied this controversy in the AGO-CaRE-1 study [3]. This retrospective exploratory multicenter cohort study utilized data from 29 gynecologic centers in Germany from 1998 to 2008. A total of 802 patients with surgically proven negative IFLNs and 447 patients with positive IFLNs wer

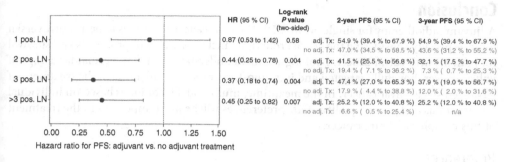

	HR (95 % CI)	Log-rank P value (two-sided)	2-year PFS (95 % CI)	3-year PFS (95 % CI)
1 pos. LN	0.87 (0.53 to 1.42)	0.58	adj. Tx: 54.9 % (39.4 % to 67.9 %) no adj. Tx: 47.0 % (34.5 % to 58.5 %)	54.9 % (39.4 % to 67.9 %) 43.6 % (31.2 % to 55.2 %)
2 pos. LN	0.44 (0.25 to 0.78)	0.004	adj. Tx: 41.5 % (25.5 % to 56.8 %) no adj. Tx: 19.4 % (7.1 % to 36.2 %)	32.1 % (17.5 % to 47.7 %) 7.3 % (0.7 % to 25.3 %)
3 pos. LN	0.37 (0.18 to 0.74)	0.004	adj. Tx: 47.4 % (27.0 % to 65.3 %) no adj. Tx: 17.9 % (4.4 % to 38.8 %)	37.9 % (19.0 % to 56.7 %) 12.0 % (2.0 % to 31.6 %)
>3 pos. LN	0.45 (0.25 to 0.82)	0.007	adj. Tx: 25.2 % (12.0 % to 40.8 %) no adj. Tx: 6.6 % (0.5 % to 25.4 %)	25.2 % (12.0 % to 40.8 %) n/a

Hazard ratio for PFS: adjuvant vs. no adjuvant treatment

Figure 50B.1 Forest plot of progression-free survival in nodal subgroups with regards to adjuvant radiotherapy [3].

included in the final analysis, of which 38.5% had one positive IFLN and 22.8% had two positive IFLNs. Progression-free survival (PFS) and OS decreased significantly with increasing number of positive nodes. Three-year PFS ranged from 47.6% for one positive IFLN to 21.2% for more than three positive IFLNS (p<0.001). OS followed a similar trend with three-year OS ranging from 72.8% for one positive IFLN to 33.0% for more than three positive IFLNs (p<0.001). More importantly, in multivariable analysis, the OS hazard ratio for adjuvant radiotherapy in two positive IFLNs versus single IFLN positive vulvar cancer was 2.52 (1.69, 5.24) p<0.001, indicating a significant impact of adjuvant radiotherapy in patients with two or more positive IFLN vulvar cancer. A forest plot of PFS by nodal subgroup also clearly demonstrates a lack of benefit of adjuvant radiotherapy for the single IFLN positive group (Figure 50B.1) [3]. Even though this study is retrospective, this is the largest study in this debate, demonstrating no improved survival benefit for patients with one positive IFLN receiving adjuvant radiotherapy or surveillance.

Two other recent studies have tried to address this question. Fons et al. were unable to demonstrate a significant benefit of adjuvant radiotherapy in patients with single IFLN positive disease, both with regards to PFS and OS [4]. Furthermore, recurrence rates were comparable between the adjuvant radiotherapy and observation arms (39% vs. 32%). Using the Surveillance Epidemiology and End Result database (SEER), Parthasarathy et al. demonstrated improved outcomes for patients with single IFLN positive vulvar cancer receiving adjuvant radiotherapy as compared to observation [5]. However, the SEER database study lacked key information regarding size and location of the IFLNs.

It is important to note the poor survival for any node-positive cases (three-year OS, 33–72%) and high recurrence rates (30–40%) in all these studies. Beyond the question of survival benefit from adjuvant radiotherapy in single IFLN positive vulvar cancer, there are postoperative and postradiotherapy complications and quality of life concerns that need to be considered in this patient population. Wound breakdown and infection are reported to occur in up to 40% of patients after IFLN dissection, and lymphocyst formation and lymphedema are reported from 20% to 40%. The addition of adjuvant radiotherapy can lead to further complications including gastrointestinal toxicity, desquamation, fistula formation, and bone fractures. As such, weighing the risks and benefits of adjuvant radiotherapy in single-node positive disease, one must consider quality of life altering complications and long-term radiotherapy sequelae for what remains an unclear survival benefit.

Conclusion

Adjuvant radiotherapy for single positive IFLN vulvar cancer continues to be a controversial topic, especially considering the crucial role IFLN metastases play in prognosis and survival for patients with vulvar cancer. Looking ahead, in understanding the molecular landscape of vulvar cancer, hopefully targeted and immuno-therapies will find a role in the treatment of advanced stage vulvar cancer. In the meantime, multimodal techniques based on individual disease status and patient quality of life preferences will be most important in the treatment of this complex and rare cancer.

References

1. Woelber L, et al. Prognostic role of lymph node metastases in vulvar cancer and implications for adjuvant treatment. *Int J Gynecol Cancer* 2012;22 (3):503–508.

2. Homesley HD, et al. Radiation therapy versus pelvic node resection for carcinoma of the vulva with positive groin nodes. *Obstet Gynecol* 1986;68(6):733–740.

3. Mahner S, et al. Adjuvant therapy in lymph node-positive vulvar cancer: the AGO-CaRE-1 study. *J Natl Cancer Inst* 2015;107(3):dju426.

4. Fons G, et al. Adjuvant radiotherapy in patients with vulvar cancer and one intra capsular lymph node metastasis is not beneficial. *Gynecol Oncol* 2009;114 (2):343–345.

5. Parthasarathy A, et al. The benefit of adjuvant radiation therapy in single-node-positive squamous cell vulvar carcinoma. *Gynecol Oncol* 2006;103(3):1095–1099.

51A

Is Pelvic Exenteration an Option for a Pelvic Recurrence of a Vulvar/ Vaginal Melanoma after Previous Radiation Therapy?
Yes

John P. Geisler and Kelly J. Manahan

Debate

Many controversies exist in all aspects of gynecologic oncology. Some of these can be answered by clinical trials because of higher incidence and prevalence of specific cancers. However, some gynecologic cancers are infrequent, requiring observational studies and logic to determine appropriate treatment plans. Vulvo-vaginal melanomas fall into this category.

Although melanoma is the second most common histology of vulvar cancer, it is still very uncommon [1]. Melanomas are malignant tumors which originate in melanocytes. Vulvo-vaginal melanomas are classified into three categories: nodular, mucosal, and superficial spreading [2]. While nodular melanomas are more common in the vagina, superficial spreading and mucosal are more common in the vulva [2]. As a general rule, for patients who are operative candidates, surgical excision is the initial treatment of choice. The overall prognosis for vulvo-vaginal melanomas is significantly lower than for cutaneous melanoma [3]. A Surveillance Epidemiology and End Results database review demonstrates that this may occur because of the advanced depth of invasion and stage at initial presentation for vulvo-vaginal melanomas. The extent of initial excision is guided by many factors: anatomic location of the lesion, presence of locally advanced (or unresectable) disease, presence of metastatic disease and depth of stromal invasion [4,5]. For example, an anterior pelvic exenteration may be needed initially even for a small lesion of the anterior middle vagina overlying the proximal urethra. Look and colleagues established that lymph node dissection was more prognostic than therapeutic in vulvar melanomas [6].

Although melanomas are relatively radiation resistant, radiation is used on a case-by-case basis, especially for lymph node metastatic disease [7]. Frumovitz and colleagues noted that the use of radiation after wide local excision of vaginal melanomas decreased local recurrence and increased mean overall survival from 16 to 29 months [5]. Unfortunately, local recurrences were far less common than distant recurrence in this same study.

How does the gynecologic oncologist approach a patient with a vulvar or vaginal melanoma that has recurred in the vulva or vagina after radiation? A repeat biopsy (not cytology) to prove recurrence and to check for treatable mutations (i.e., *BRAF*v600 or *KIT*) is the first step. The next step is to assess for the presence of metastatic disease. Multiple studies have demonstrated that positron emission tomography/computed tomography (PET/CT) has the best sensitivity for detection of metastases [8]. Once these steps are completed and the results are known, an informed discussion can be undertaken with the patient and their caregivers. If metastatic disease exists, undertaking an exenteration is not advisable, just as undertaking an exenteration is not advisable if adequate resection margins cannot be achieved in the previously radiated field. If treatable mutations exist in the tumor, especially a previously untreated *BRAF*v600 or *KIT* mutation is present, systemic treatment is recommended over ultra-radical surgery. Although a pelvic exenteration can be curative for patients with small central recurrences without metastases, exenterations can affect quality of life and be challenging to recover from both physically and psychologically [9]. Changes in techniques from the use of robotic systems, for the supra-levator portion of the surgery, vascularized muscle-flaps to fill the pelvis, J-pouches rather than end-to-end colo-coloanastamosis, and enhanced recovery strategies all make an exenteration more tolerable in the well-chosen patient [10].

Conclusion

There are some clinical controversies in gynecologic oncology that even with large multinational cooperative groups will not be able to be answered with randomized trials. The use of pelvic exenterations after radiation for recurrent vulvo-vaginal melanoma is one of these clinical questions. Primary exenteration has been shown to be effective in well-chosen patients [4,5]. In the absence of randomized trials, the gynecologic oncologist has to look at other available data including other treatment options (immunotherapy, chemotherapy), the experience of the anesthesia, surgical, and postoperative teams, as well as the patient's ability to cope with the physical and psychological stressors of ultra-radical surgery. Until a randomized trial shows no benefit, or better nonsurgical treatments evolve, pelvic exenteration for resectable, central, recurrent vulvo-vaginal melanoma in a radiated pelvis should remain an option.

References

1. Boer FL, et al. Vulvar malignant melanoma: pathogenesis, clinical behaviour and management: review of the literature. *Cancer Treat Rev* 2019;73:91–103.

2. Saito T, et al. Japan Society of Gynecologic Oncology guidelines 2015 for the treatment of vulvar cancer and vaginal cancer. *Int J Clin Oncol* 2018;23:201–234.

3. Mert I, et al. Vulvar/vaginal melanoma: an updated surveillance epidemiology and end results database review, comparison with cutaneous melanoma and significance of racial disparities. *Int J Gynecol Cancer* 2013;23:1118–1125.

4. Geisler JP, et al. Pelvic exenteration for malignant melanomas of the vagina or urethra with over 3 mm of invasion. *Gyneco. Oncol* 1995;59:338–341.

5. Frumovitz M, et al. Primary malignant melanoma of the vagina. *Obstet Gynecol* 2010;116:1358–1365.

6. Look KY, et al. Vulvar melanoma reconsidered. *Cancer* 1993;72:143–146.

7. Agrawal S, et al. The benefits of adjuvant radiation therapy after therapeutic lymphadenectomy for clinically advanced, high-risk, lymph node-metastatic melanoma. *Cancer* 2009;115:5836–5844.

8. Xing Y, et al. Contemporary diagnostic imaging modalities for the staging and surveillance of melanoma patients: a meta-analysis. *J Natl Cancer Inst* 2011;103:129–142.

9. Rezk YA, et al. A prospective study of quality of life in patients undergoing pelvic exenteration: interim results. *Gynecol Oncol* 2013;128:191–197.

10. Schneider A, et al. Current developments for pelvic exenteration in gynecologic oncology. *Curr Opin Obstet Gynecol* 2009;21:4–9.

Is Pelvic Exenteration an Option for a Pelvic Recurrence of a Vulvar/ Vaginal Melanoma after Previous Radiation Therapy?

No

Mario M. Leitao, Jr.

Debate

Until recently, therapy for any type of melanoma was limited, and outcomes were dismal in those with advanced or recurrent disease. At a time when there were no viable options for vulvovaginal melanomas, pelvic exenteration may have seemed like a good treatment approach. Today, however, pelvic exenteration should not be considered in patients with vulvovaginal melanomas, either newly diagnosed or recurrent . . . except possibly as a last resort in rare, highly select cases. Due to the rarity of these tumors, data to direct treatment are limited to case series, and although they are often treated as one entity, vulvar and vaginal melanomas are different, with varying incidence and mortality rates.

Vulvovaginal melanomas are associated with worse overall survival (OS) compared to vulvar carcinomas, as well as cutaneous melanomas [1]. The five-year OS rate for newly diagnosed, locally advanced, American Joint Committee on Cancer (AJCC) stage II vulvar melanoma is approximately 50%, and decreases with increasing stage. Vaginal melanomas are associated with even worse outcomes, and many of the recurrences are distant. In the primary setting, therefore, a highly morbid procedure with risk of postoperative mortality, permanent stomas, and body disfigurement does not seem like a good approach. Overall survival is even worse in patients with recurrence that requires exenteration, especially after prior radiation, in whom the risk/benefit ratio is unfavorable. Surgical resection can be considered in patients with recurrence in the vulva or vagina, and even the groins, if a nonexenterative resection is possible.

Patients who present with newly diagnosed, locally advanced, or recurrent vulvovaginal melanoma may be best treated with hypofractionated radiation therapy combined with immunotherapy. This approach has been our standard of care since we treated a young woman with vaginal melanoma using 3000 cGy external-beam radiation therapy in five fractions, along with ipilimumab [2]. The patient experienced a pathologic complete response and remains disease free, without recurrence, 100 months (8+ years) since her initial diagnosis. The combination of radiation therapy and ipilimumab was prospectively assessed in a single-arm study of 10 patients with locally advanced melanoma, of which only one had mucosal melanoma [3]. A radiographic complete response was achieved in four out of 10 patients. Three patients achieved a partial response. These three patients all underwent a surgical resection for what was considered residual disease. Two of these three patients achieved a pathologic complete response. The use of hypofractionated radiation therapy is controversial and debatable. Some may prefer to use combination immunotherapy or dabrafenib/trametinib (for *BRAF V600E/K*-mutated cases) without radiation.

The National Comprehensive Cancer Network (NCCN) does not recommend routine molecular profiling for stage I and II resected melanomas but does recommend it for stage III/IV, unresectable, and/or recurrent melanomas to help guide treatment [4]. This principle would generally apply to vulvovaginal melanomas, but considering the rarity of these tumors, it is reasonable to at least perform molecular analysis for *KIT, BRAF,* and *NRAS* in all cases. Broader genomic analysis when obtaining molecular testing, if possible, may provide a better understanding of this disease and also identify other potentially targetable mutations and/or triage cases for select clinical trials. The value of routine testing for programmed death-ligand 1 (PD-L1) expression in melanoma is unclear and not recommended by the NCCN [4].

Nivolumab and pembrolizumab, anti-PD-1 (programmed cell death protein 1) monoclonal antibodies, as well as other more recently developed anti-PD1 and PD-L1 agents, are preferred over ipilimumab. The anti-tumor activity of these agents is not affected by the presence of *BRAF* mutations. Combination cytotoxic T-lymphocyte-associated protein 4 (CTLA-4) and PD-1 therapies have higher responses but are more toxic. Single-agent anti-PD-1 therapy is preferred with hypofractionated therapy, but combinations are acceptable if radiation is not given. Patients with *BRAF V600E* or *V600 K* mutations will benefit from targeted therapy using dual MAPK pathway inhibition with a BRAF and a MEK inhibitor. This combination has an overall response rate of 65%, with a median OS of 33.6 months in patients with metastatic and/or recurrent cutaneous melanoma [5].

Conclusion

Resection of locally (vulva, vagina, pelvis, and/or groins) and metastatic recurrent melanoma may be an option in those in whom a negative-margin, limited-morbidity procedure is possible [4,6]. There is an extensive body of literature on treatment options for recurrent and metastatic melanoma that includes chemotherapeutics, radiation therapy, and other available and novel agents. We recommend following published guidelines, such as those provided by the NCCN [4]. Pelvic exenteration, even after prior pelvic radiation and isolated to the pelvis, should not be considered outside a "last resort" option in very rare, select cases. Such cases may include patients in whom disease remains truly confined to the pelvis and has stabilized without further response to other therapies or in those who require palliation of symptoms without other alternatives.

References

1. Mert I, et al. Vulvar/vaginal melanoma: an updated Surveillance Epidemiology and End Results Database review, comparison with cutaneous melanoma and significance of racial disparities. *Int J Gynecol Cancer* 2013;23:1118–1125.

2. Schiavone MB, et al. Combined immunotherapy and radiation for treatment

of mucosal melanomas of the lower genital tract. *Gynecol Oncol Rep* 2016;16:42–46.

3. Salama AKS, et al. Ipilimumab and radiation in patients with high risk resected or regionally advanced melanoma. *Clin Cancer Res* 2021;27(5):1287–1295.

4. National Comprehensive Cancer Network. Melanoma: cutaneous (Version 1.2021). Available from: www.nccn.org/profes sionals/physician_gls/pdf/cutaneous_mela noma.pdf

5. Dummer R, et al. Overall survival in patients with BRAF-mutant melanoma receiving encorafenib plus binimetinib versus vemurafenib or encorafenib (COLUMBUS): a multicenter, open-label, randomized, phase 3 trial. *Lancet Oncol* 2018;19:1315–1327.

6. Wasif N, et al. Does metastatectomy improve survival in patients with stage IV melanoma? A cancer registry analysis of outcomes. *J Surg Oncol* 2011;104:111–115.

Index

Printed in the United States
by Baker & Taylor Publisher Services